T0227152

Non-Hodgkin Lymphoma

Editor

CARON A. JACOBSON

HEMATOLOGY/ONCOLOGY CLINICS OF NORTH AMERICA

www.hemonc.theclinics.com

Consulting Editors
GEORGE P. CANELLOS
H. FRANKLIN BUNN

August 2019 • Volume 33 • Number 4

ELSEVIER

1600 John F. Kennedy Boulevard ● Suite 1800 ● Philadelphia, Pennsylvania, 19103-2899

http://www.theclinics.com

HEMATOLOGY/ONCOLOGY CLINICS OF NORTH AMERICA Volume 33, Number 4
August 2019 ISSN 0889-8588, ISBN 13: 978-0-323-68225-1

Editor: Stacy Eastman
Developmental Editor: Kristen Helm

Hematology/Oncology Clinics (ISSN 0889-8588) is published bimonthly by Elsevier Inc., 360 Park Avenue South, New York, NY 10010-1710. Months of issue are February, April, June, August, October, and December. Business and Editorial Offices: 1600 John F. Kennedy Blvd., Ste. 1800, Philadelphia, PA 19103–2899. Customer Service Office: 3251 Riverport Lane, Maryland Heights, MO 63043. Periodicals postage paid at New York, NY and at additional mailing offices. Subscription prices are $430.00 per year (domestic individuals), $830.00 per year (domestic institutions), $100.00 per year (domestic students/residents), $480.00 per year (Canadian individuals), $1028.00 per year (Canadian institutions) $547.00 per year (international individuals), $1028.00 per year (international institutions), and $255.00 per year (international and Canadian students/residents). International air speed delivery is included in all *Clinics* subscription prices. All prices are subject to change without notice. **POSTMASTER:** Send address changes to *Hematology/Oncology Clinics of North America*, Elsevier Health Sciences Division, Subscription Customer Service, 3251 Riverport Lane, Maryland Heights, MO 63043. Customer Service (orders, claims, online, change of address): Elsevier Health Sciences Division, Subscription **Customer Service, 3251 Riverport Lane, Maryland Heights, MO 63043. Tel: 1-800-654-2452 (U.S. and Canada); 314-447-8871 (outside U.S. and Canada). Fax: 314-447-8029. E-mail: journalscustomerservice-usa@elsevier.com (for print support); journalsonlinesupport-usa@elsevier.com (for online support)**.

Reprints. For copies of 100 or more, of articles in this publication, please contact the Commercial Reprints Department, Elsevier Inc., 360 Park Avenue South, New York, New York 10010-1710; Tel.: 212-633-3874, Fax: 212-633-3820, E-mail: reprints@elsevier.com.

Hematology/Oncology Clinics of North America is covered in *MEDLINE/PubMed (Index Medicus)*, *EMBASE/ Excerpta Medica, and BIOSIS*.

Contributors

CONSULTING EDITORS

GEORGE P. CANELLOS, MD
William Rosenberg Professor of Medicine, Department of Medical Oncology, Dana-Farber Cancer Institute, Boston, Massachusetts, USA

H. FRANKLIN BUNN, MD
Professor of Medicine, Division of Hematology, Brigham and Women's Hospital, Harvard Medical School, Boston, Massachusetts, USA

EDITOR

CARON A. JACOBSON, MD, MMSc
Assistant Professor of Medicine, Harvard Medical School, Medical Director, Immune Effector Cell Therapy Program, Dana-Farber Cancer Institute, Boston, Massachusetts, USA

AUTHORS

RAMI ALSHARIF, MD
Hematology/Oncology Fellow, George Washington University Cancer Center, George Washington University, Washington, DC, USA

PHILIPPE ARMAND, MD, PhD
Medical Oncology, Associate Professor of Medicine, Harvard Medical School, Dana-Farber Cancer Institute, Boston, Massachusetts, USA

JORGE J. CASTILLO, MD
Bing Center for Waldenstrom Macroglobulinemia, Dana-Farber Cancer Institute, Harvard Medical School, Boston, Massachusetts, USA

CARLA CASULO, MD
James P. Wilmot Cancer Institute, University of Rochester Medical Center, University of Rochester, Rochester, New York, USA

YI-BIN CHEN, MD
Massachusetts General Hospital, Boston, Massachusetts, USA

BRUCE D. CHESON, MD, FACP, FAAAS, FASCO
Professor of Medicine, Lombardi Comprehensive Cancer Center, MedStar Georgetown University Hospital, Washington, DC, USA

UGONMA N. CHUKWUEKE, MD
Department of Medical Oncology, Center for Neuro-Oncology, Dana-Farber Cancer Institute, Department of Neurology, Brigham and Women's Hospital, Harvard Medical School, Boston, Massachusetts, USA

JENNIFER L. CROMBIE, MD
Medical Oncology, Instructor of Medicine, Harvard Medical School, Dana-Farber Cancer Institute, Boston, Massachusetts, USA

BENJAMIN DIAMOND, MD
Fellow, Department of Medicine, Medical Oncology, Lymphoma Department, Memorial Sloan Kettering Cancer Center, New York, New York, USA

KIERON DUNLEAVY, MD
Professor of Medicine, Director of Lymphoma, George Washington University Cancer Center, George Washington University, Washington, DC, USA

ALEX F. HERRERA, MD
Assistant Professor, Department of Hematology and Hematopoietic Cell Transplantation, City of Hope National Medical Center, Duarte, California, USA

BRADLEY D. HUNTER, MD, MPH
Dana-Farber Cancer Institute, Massachusetts General Hospital, Boston, Massachusetts, USA

ERIC D. JACOBSEN, MD
Assistant Professor of Medicine, Department of Medical Oncology, Dana-Farber Cancer Institute, Boston, Massachusetts, USA

CARON A. JACOBSON, MD, MMSc
Assistant Professor of Medicine, Harvard Medical School, Medical Director, Immune Effector Cell Therapy Program, Dana-Farber Cancer Institute, Boston, Massachusetts, USA

LUIS M. JUÁREZ-SALCEDO, MD
Department of Hematology, Gregorio Marañon University Hospital, Madrid, Spain

ANITA KUMAR, MD
Lymphoma Department, Memorial Sloan Kettering Cancer Center, Attending, Department of Medicine, Lymphoma Service, New York, New York, USA

CECILIA A. LAROCCA, MD
Instructor, Department of Dermatology, Center for Cutaneous Oncology, Brigham and Women's Hospital, Dana-Farber Cancer Institute, Harvard Medical School, Boston, Massachusetts, USA

NICOLE R. LeBOEUF, MD, MPH
Assistant Professor, Department of Dermatology, Center for Cutaneous Oncology, Brigham and Women's Hospital, Dana-Farber Cancer Institute, Harvard Medical School, Boston, Massachusetts, USA

MAYUR NARKHEDE, MD
Clinical Fellow, Lombardi Comprehensive Cancer Center, MedStar Georgetown University Hospital, Washington, DC, USA

LAKSHMI NAYAK, MD
Department of Medical Oncology, Center for Neuro-Oncology, Dana-Farber Cancer Institute, Department of Neurology, Brigham and Women's Hospital, Harvard Medical School, Boston, Massachusetts, USA

SAMUEL Y. NG, MD, PhD
Instructor of Medicine, Department of Medical Oncology, Dana-Farber Cancer Institute, Boston, Massachusetts, USA

RUSSELL JAMES HUBBARD RYAN, MD
Assistant Professor, Department of Pathology, University of Michigan Medical School, Ann Arbor, Michigan, USA

KARIM WELAYA, MBBCh
James P. Wilmot Cancer Institute, University of Rochester Medical Center, University of Rochester, Rochester, New York, USA

RYAN ALAN WILCOX, MD, PhD
Assistant Professor, Division of Hematology and Oncology, Department of Internal Medicine, University of Michigan Medical School, Ann Arbor, Michigan, USA

MARYAM SARRAF YAZDY, MD
Assistant Professor of Medicine, Lombardi Comprehensive Cancer Center, MedStar Georgetown University Hospital, Washington, DC, USA

Contents

Mature B- and T-cell lymphomas are diverse in their biology, etiology, genetics, clinical behavior, and response to specific therapies. Here, the authors review the principles of diagnostic classification for non-Hodgkin lymphomas, summarize the characteristic features of major entities, and place recent biological and molecular findings in the context of principles that are applicable across the spectrum of mature lymphoid cancers.

Diffuse large B-cell lymphoma (DLBCL), the most common subtype of non-Hodgkin lymphoma, is characterized by both clinical and molecular heterogeneity. Despite efforts to tailor therapy for individual patients, treatment remains uniform and a subset of patients have poor outcomes. The past decade has witnessed a dramatic expansion of our understanding of the genomic underpinnings of this disease, especially with the application of next-generation sequencing. In this review, the authors highlight the current genomic landscape of DLBCL and how this information provides a potential molecular framework for precision medicine-based strategies in this disease.

Burkitt lymphoma (BL) is highly aggressive and requires very intensive chemotherapy approaches for successful treatment. Although "standard" approaches are tolerated in young patients, this is not the case in older adults, and new approaches that lower toxicity but maintain high curability are needed and are currently in development. Recently, high-grade B-cell lymphomas with MYC and BCL2 and/or BCL6 rearrangements have been categorized separately from diffuse large B-cell lymphoma or BL. These have poor outcomes and many exciting novel approaches are being tested in an attempt to augment curability. These diseases harbor many interesting targets for rational small molecule inhibition in future trials.

> Primary central nervous system lymphoma (PCNSL) is an uncommon sub-
> type of extranodal non-Hodgkin lymphoma (NHL) with less than 1500
> cases annually. Incidence of PCNSL has remained stable in the post–
> highly active antiretroviral therapy era, owing to increasing incidence in
> elderly, immunocompetent patients. Most PCNSL is diffuse large B cell
> in origin, with less frequent involvement of T-cell and Burkitt lymphoma.
> Secondary central nervous system lymphoma is more likely to occur in
> the relapsed setting of a systemic NHL. Methotrexate forms the backbone
> of management for prophylaxis and treatment of disease. Treatments are
> currently under investigation for both disease entities.

> Mantle cell lymphoma (MCL) is biologically and clinically heterogeneous
> with no clear standard of care. Overexpression of cyclin D1 is a hallmark
> of MCL. Evolving characterization of other molecular drivers explain a va-
> riety of disease phenotypes. These molecular profiles challenge risk strat-
> ification techniques. TP53-deleted disease is associated with adverse
> outcomes. Frontline treatment programs include intensive chemoimmuno-
> therapy and autologous stem cell transplantation. Minimal residual
> disease may change management of MCL and guide therapy. As
> commonly dysregulated pathways become enumerated, novel biologically
> targeted agents and their combinations have been developed that will
> increasingly replace older, more toxic, and less efficacious regimens.

> Follicular lymphoma is the most common indolent lymphoma in the United
> States. In this review article, the authors discuss the different prognostic
> biomarkers available for follicular lymphoma. Treatment options, including
> observation, immunotherapy versus chemoimmunotherapy, in both the
> frontline and the relapse setting are also discussed in detail. Patients
> with follicular lymphoma with unmet needs include those with early
> relapse, with multiple relapses, and with histologic transformation. The
> treatment options for these patients are not well defined, and the authors
> discuss the available data for treating these patients.

> Lymphoplasmacytic lymphoma (LPL) and marginal zone lymphoma (MZL)
> are indolent subtypes of non-Hodgkin lymphoma. Both are typically CD5
> and CD10 negative. In recent years, there have been several scientific ad-
> vances that have helped improve the diagnosis of these conditions. These
> conditions have been managed similarly in previous years with observation
> in asymptomatic patients and systemic therapy in advanced stages.

However, there are specific differences. Differential responses are also seen with novel agents such as the BTK inhibitor ibrutinib. It is encouraging to see that there several clinical trials specific for patients with LPL and MZL ongoing.

ranging in behavior from indolent to highly aggressive. For many years, the traditional treatment of NHL centered on chemotherapy. However, the introduction of rituximab ushered in the era of immunotherapy for NHLs. This article reviews novel immune therapies that have been used for the treatment of NHL. The data supporting the use of rituximab have been reviewed extensively; this article focuses on novel immunotherapies other than rituximab that remain in use or are actively being studied in clinical trials.

Mayur Narkhede, Maryam Sarraf Yazdy, and Bruce D. Cheson

Chemotherapy nonspecifically affects all cells undergoing DNA replication and has severe side effects. Understanding of the biology of non-Hodgkin lymphomas has led to development of drugs that target specific lymphoma cell functions and tumor microenvironment. Targeted agents used in combination with chemotherapy pave the way to a chemotherapy-free world. These drugs target multiple oncogenic pathways and modulate the immune system, with better outcomes. Such combinations should be administered only in clinical trials. Incorporating studies of the biology and genetics of these tumors into therapeutic studies may lead to a chemotherapy-free world with improved outcomes and reduced toxicities.

HEMATOLOGY/ONCOLOGY
CLINICS OF NORTH AMERICA

SERIES OF RELATED INTEREST

Surgical Oncology Clinics of North America

THE CLINICS ARE AVAILABLE ONLINE!
Access your subscription at:
www.theclinics.com

Preface

Redefining Non-Hodgkin Lymphoma: Using Genomic Subtypes to Improve Treatment Options

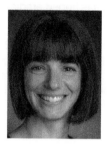

Caron A. Jacobson, MD, MMSc
Editor

The evolution of genomic analyses of the tumor and its microenvironment has led to a shift in the way in which we think about lymphoma, its classification, and its therapy. Genomic annotation of disease subgroups previously defined on the basis of morphology and immunohistochemistry has identified tremendous heterogeneity within the field that has both predictive and prognostic importance when considering responsiveness to standard chemoimmunotherapies. This advancement comes in parallel with the rapid development and availability of new drugs that target genetic and immunologic vulnerabilities of these tumors, and, as such, we stand on the precipice of significant progress within the field.

Take, for example, the most common subtype of B-cell non-Hodgkin lymphoma (NHL), diffuse large B-cell lymphoma (DLBCL). This disease, once thought of as a single entity, is now recognized as potentially 5 genetically distinct subtypes, all of which carry different sensitivities to chemotherapy and may each benefit from specific novel agents and treatment strategies. In addition, the efficacy of chimeric antigen receptor T cells in these diseases marks the largest breakthrough in DLBCL since the advent of rituximab. Recent randomized studies combining traditional chemotherapy with targeted agents have failed to show an overall benefit, but perhaps inclusion onto these trials was too broad and results will be more promising if we instead use the more refined genomic classifications. Similarly, the importance of perturbations in PD-L1 and PD-L2 in primary mediastinal large B-cell lymphoma, T-cell/histiocyte-rich large B-cell lymphoma, and Epstein-Barr virus–positive large B-cell lymphoma has paved the way for the use of immunotherapy in these lymphomas. Such strategies

Hematol Oncol Clin N Am 33 (2019) xiii–xiv
https://doi.org/10.1016/j.hoc.2019.04.005
0889-8588/19/© 2019 Published by Elsevier Inc.

hemonc.theclinics.com

are also effective in primary testicular lymphoma and primary central nervous system lymphoma, which are also defined, but recurrent alterations in genes of the toll-like receptor pathway are thus susceptible to Bruton tyrosine kinase inhibition, thereby offering progress for diseases in relapse that had limited options to date. Finally, a genomic understanding of T-cell lymphomas, a previously poorly characterized and understood collection of diseases, has identified new pathways to target, and new and effective drugs to treat, these historically very high-risk malignancies.

In this issue of *Hematology/Oncology Clinics of North America*, the refinement in our classification of NHL, away from a purely histologic and toward a genetically annotated classification, is discussed in general and for each of the NHL subtypes. This lays the groundwork for exploration of therapeutic advances, taking advantage of new oncogenic and immunologic targets for the treatment and it is hoped eradication of these lymphomas.

Caron A. Jacobson, MD, MMSc
Dana-Farber Cancer Institute
450 Brookline Avenue
Boston, MA 02215, USA

E-mail address:
caron_jacobson@dfci.harvard.edu

Ontogeny, Genetics, Molecular Biology, and Classification of B- and T-Cell Non-Hodgkin Lymphoma

Russell James Hubbard Ryan, MD[a],*, Ryan Alan Wilcox, MD, PhD[b]

KEYWORDS

- B-cell lymphoma • T-cell lymphoma • Lymphoma classification • Lymphomagenesis

KEY POINTS

- Clinical classification of lymphomas requires integrated assessment of histology, phenotype, genetics, other laboratory findings, and clinical presentation/history.
- Lymphomas alter their local microenvironment and may rely on other cell types for contact signals and soluble growth factors required for lymphoma cell homeostasis.
- Lymphomas recapitulate gene expression programs that are characteristic of stages in normal lymphoid development.
- Driver genetic alterations in lymphoma include rearrangement of cis-regulatory elements, gene fusions, amplifications, gain-of-function mutations, and inactivating events.
- Mutated pathways include immune receptor signaling, metabolic regulation, transcription and chromatin state, trafficking, DNA damage response, cell-cycle regulation, apoptosis, and immunosurveillance.

INTRODUCTION

The advent of genome-scale profiling technologies has dramatically improved our understanding of the biological basis of mature B- and T-cell lymphomas. The purpose of this review is to place newer biological and molecular findings in the context of principles that are applicable across the spectrum of mature lymphoid malignancies.

PRINCIPLES OF DIAGNOSIS AND CLASSIFICATION

Lymphoid cancers are diverse in their clinical behavior and response to therapies; therefore, accurate subclassification of lymphomas is indispensable for clinical care.

[a] Department of Pathology, University of Michigan Medical School, 4306 Rogel Cancer Center, 1500 East Medical Center Drive, Ann Arbor, MI 48109-5936, USA; [b] Division of Hematology and Oncology, Department of Internal Medicine, University of Michigan Medical School, 4310 Rogel Cancer Center, 1500 East Medical Center Drive, Ann Arbor, MI 48109-5936, USA
* Corresponding author.
E-mail address: rjhryan@med.umich.edu

Hematol Oncol Clin N Am 33 (2019) 553–574
https://doi.org/10.1016/j.hoc.2019.04.003
0889-8588/19/© 2019 Elsevier Inc. All rights reserved.

Under the broadly accepted World Health Organization (WHO) classification system,[1] each lymphoma subtype is defined by a unique combination of characteristic findings that may include cytologic appearance, immunophenotype, microscopic growth pattern, anatomic sites of involvement as assessed by physical examination and radiological studies, genetic mutations, chromosomal rearrangements/copy number abnormalities, and other specific laboratory findings. Clinical history may also be central to the definition of certain lymphoid neoplasms, as in the case of posttransplant lymphoproliferative disorders. Evaluation of lymphoid architecture and heterogeneity is essential for lymphoma classification, and therefore, an excisional lymph node biopsy should be procured whenever feasible for initial diagnosis.[2] Accurate classification of lymphoid malignancies remains challenging, and reclassification may be anticipated in ≈20% of cases following expert hematopathology review.[3]

RELATIONSHIP OF LYMPHOMA TO NORMAL LYMPHOID DEVELOPMENT

Most lymphomas recapitulate characteristic morphologic, phenotypic, epigenetic, and gene expression features of specific stages in normal lymphoid cell development, although altered to varying degrees by genetic or epigenetic aberrations (**Fig. 1** and **Table 1**). For example, follicular lymphoma (FL) recapitulates the morphology and immunophenotype of B-cell populations in the germinal center (GC) light zone, whereas marginal zone lymphomas (MZL) can show a spectrum of differentiation that resembles specific non-GC B-cell and plasma cell subpopulations, and

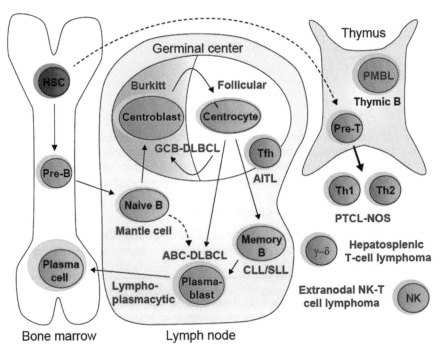

Fig. 1. Relationship of lymphomas to normal lymphocyte development. Stages of lymphoid development, with corresponding mature B-, T-, and natural killer–cell lymphoma subtypes indicated in red text. Proliferative stages of B-cell development are colored violet. HSC, hematopoietic stem cell. Lymphomas are abbreviated as indicated in **Table 1**.

Table 1
Subtypes and features of selected non-Hodgkin mature lymphoid cancers

Lymphoma Subtype	Abbreviation	Key Diagnostic Features	Genomic Aberrations (Selected)	Suggested Precursor	Clinical Aggressiveness	Notes
B cell						
Follicular lymphoma	FL	Small & large cells in follicles. CD10+, BCL6+, BCL2+(most)	IGH-BCL2, KMT2D, CREBBP, TNFRSF14, EZH2, mTOR pathway	In situ follicular neoplasia	Low (grade 1–2) to moderate (grade 3)	Low-grade FL can be partially or (rarely) entirely diffuse
Nodal marginal zone lymphoma	NMZL	Expanded marginal zones, small/ colonized follicle centers	KMT2D, NOTCH2, PTPRD, KLF2, BCR pathway	Unknown	Low to moderate	Rare and challenging to diagnose due to lack of distinctive markers
Extranodal marginal zone lymphoma of mucosa-associated lymphoid tissue	MALT lymphoma	Clonal small B cells and plasma cells. Lymphoepithelial lesions and follicular colonization	BIRC3-MALT1, IGH-MALT1, BCL10-IGH, FOXP1-IGH, TNFAIP3, other BCR pathway, TP53, MYD88, NOTCH2, BCL6-R	Clonal B cells in setting of localized chronic inflammation (eg, lymphoepithelial sialadenitis)	Low	Common sites of origin include stomach, intestine, ocular adnexa, salivary glands, lung, thyroid, skin, and soft tissues
Splenic marginal zone lymphoma	SMZL	Marrow sinusoidal infiltrate and aggregates, splenomegaly w/ expanded white pulp	KLF2, NOTCH2, TRAF3, TNFAIP3, MYD88, TP53, BCR pathway	Monoclonal B-cell lymphocytosis, non-CLL type	Low	Cells in peripheral blood may show characteristic "polar villi"

(continued on next page)

Table 1
(continued)

Lymphoma Subtype	Abbreviation	Key Diagnostic Features	Genomic Aberrations (Selected)	Suggested Precursor	Clinical Aggressiveness	Notes
Lympho-plasmacytic lymphoma	LPL	Plasmacytoid lymphocytes, Dutcher bodies, IgM paraprotein	MYD88 L265P (>90%), CXCR4, CD79B, KMT2D, TP53, ARID1A	IgM monoclonal gammopathy of undetermined significance	Low	Also known as Waldenstrom macroglob-ulinemia
Chronic lymphocytic leukemia/small lymphocytic lymphoma	CLL/SLL	Small cells in blood with proliferation centers in nodes. CD5+, CD23+, LEF1+, FMC7−	del(13q14), +12, NOTCH1, SF3B1, ATM, TP53, CHD2, BIRC3, Toll-like receptor pathway	Monoclonal B-cell lymphocytosis, CLL type	Low (IGHV-mut) to moderate (TP53 or ATM mutated)	Early genetic events may occur in an abnormal hematopoietic stem cell clone
Mantle cell lymphoma	MCL	Uniform small cells or blastoid. CD5+, CyclinD1+, Sox11+(most).	IGH-CCND1, UBR5, ATM, TP53, NOTCH1/2, BIRC3, TRAF2	In situ mantle cell neoplasia	Moderate, low (Sox11-neg), or high (blastoid)	Rare cyclin D1-neg cases identifiable with Sox11
Hairy cell leukemia	HCL	Cytoplasmic projections. CyclinD1+, Annexin A1+	BRAF V600E (~100%)	Abnormal hematopoietic stem cell > clonal B cell	Moderate	Hairy cell variant has mutations in other MAP kinase genes
Diffuse large B-cell lymphoma, germinal center B-cell subtype	GCB-DLBCL	Large cells growing in sheets. CD20+, CD10+, BCL6+, GCET1+, LMO2+.	BCL2-R, CREBBP, EZH2, KMT2D, TNFRSF14, GNA13, MEF2B, PTEN, SGK1, NFKBIA/E, REL-Amp, MYC-R	Evidence for 2 genetic subgroups; BCL2-R group may share origin with FL	High	High-grade lymphomas with concurrent MYC and BCL2 rearrangements are more aggressive & separately classified. Mixed evidence for significance of MYC-R + BCL6-R.
Diffuse large B-cell lymphoma, activated B-cell subtype	ABC-DLBCL	Large cells growing in sheets. CD20+, IRF4+, FOXP1+, BCL6−/+. EBER + classified separately	CD79B MYD88, CDKN2A, ETV6, PIM1, TBL1XR1, BCL6-R, BCL2-Amp, PRDM1, TNFAIP3, NOTCH2, MYC-R	Multiple subgroups. NOTCH2/BCL6-R subgroup may be related to marginal zone	High	

Primary mediastinal large B-cell lymphoma	PMBL	Large cells in sheets. CD20+, CD30+, CD23+, MAL+, c-Rel nuc+	CIITA-R, CD274/PDCD1LG2-R/Amp, REL-Amp, SOCS1, STAT6, PTPN1	Unknown	High	"Gray zone": features of both PMBL and Hodgkin lymphoma
Burkitt lymphoma	BL	Blastoid, CD10+, BCL6+, BCL2–neg, simple karyotype with MYC-R	MYC-R, ID3/TCF3, DDX3X, FOXO1, ARID1A, SMARCA4, CCND3, FBXO11	Endemic: EBV-infected B cell w/concurrent malaria (?)	Very high	Most African endemic and HIV-associated cases are EBER+
T/NK cell						
Adult T-cell leukemia/lymphoma	ATLL	Flower-like nuclei, CD25+, HTLV-1 serology positive, hypercalcemia	PLCG1, PRKCB, CCR4/7, STAT3, TP53, VAV1, NOTCH1, RHOA, CD274-R	HTLV-1-infected T cells, usually since infancy	Low to high	HTLV-1-endemic regions (Japan, Caribbean, Africa, South America)
T-cell prolymphocytic leukemia	T-PLL	Circulating medium-sized T cells, CD4+/CD8– or double-positive	TRA-TCL1A/B, TRA-MTCP1, JAK3, JAK1, STAT5B	Unknown	High	Increased occurrence in patients with ataxia–telangiectasia
Angio-immunoblastic T-cell lymphoma	AITL	Follicular dendritic proliferation. BCL6+, CD10+, PD1+ T cells. EBV+ B cells	TET2, DNMT3A, IDH2, RHOA, CD28, PLCG1	Abnormal hematopoietic stem cell > T follicular helper cell	High	T follicular helper phenotype seen in subset of non-ATIL lymphomas
Peripheral T-cell lymphoma, NOS	PTCL-NOS	Polymorphous, often with eosinophils and histiocytes. Clonal T cells with antigen loss.	TET2/3, DNMT3A, GNA13, RHOA, CD58, FYN, CD28	Unknown	High	Expression of GATA2 vs T-Bet may denote biologically distinct subtypes

(continued on next page)

Table 1
(continued)

Lymphoma Subtype	Abbreviation	Key Diagnostic Features	Genomic Aberrations (Selected)	Suggested Precursor	Clinical Aggressiveness	Notes
Hepatosplenic T-cell lymphoma	HSTL	Usually TCR gamma-delta+, often CD4– and CD8–	+7q, STAT5B, STAT3, SETD2, INO80, ARID1B, SMARCA2, TET2/3, DNMT3A	Unknown	High	Predisposed by immunosupression due to solid organ transplant
Anaplastic large cell lymphoma, ALK+	ALK + ALCL	Large cells with sinusoidal growth. ALK+, CD30+, cytotoxic granule+	NPM1-ALK or other ALK-R	Unknown	High	Variants with atypical morphology (small cell, etc) are ALK+
Anaplastic large cell lymphoma, ALK–	ALK-negative ALCL	Classic ALCL features, CD30+, ALK–, cytotoxic granule protein+	DUSP22/IRF4-R, TP63-R, ROS1-R, TYK2-R, FRK-R. JAK1, STAT3, PRDM1	Unknown	High	Significantly better prognosis in DUSP22/IRF4-R vs TP63-R
Extranodal NK-/T-cell lymphoma, nasal type	ENKTL	Angiocentric & angiodestructive. cytoplasmic CD3+, CD56+, EBER+	DDX3X, TP53, KMT2D, STAT3	EBV-infected NK or T cell	High	Most common in Asian populations

Note: "Genomic aberrations" lists symbols of genes involved in gene fusion or regulatory element rearrangements ("-R" or partner loci linked by hyphen), amplifications ("-Amp") or mutation/inactivation (no suffix).
Abbreviation: IgM, immunoglobulin M.

angioimmunoblastic T-cell lymphoma (AITL) recapitulates the appearance and gene expression program of T-follicular helper cells (Tfh). In diffuse large B-cell lymphoma (DLBCL), major subgroups show gene expression programs characteristic of normal GC B cells (GCB-DLBCL) or in vitro activated peripheral blood B cells (ABC-DLBCL).[4] Distinguishing these subgroups is of ongoing interest in clinical trials for targeted agents, but remains challenging in routine practice due to the imprecision of immuno-histochemical classification algorithms, limited availability of more precise RNA-based classifier technologies,[5] and likelihood that additional subgroups exist.[6,7]

Like DLBCL, peripheral T-cell lymphoma not otherwise specified (PTCL-NOS) is a heterogeneous category of biologically diverse aggressive lymphomas. The T-cell transcription factors GATA-3 and T-bet define normal T helper cell subsets (Th2 and Th1) and distinguish 2 clinically, molecularly, and genetically distinct subtypes of PTCL-NOS.[8–10] As in DLBCL, distinguishing these subtypes reliably in a clinical context remains challenging, but could hold significant diagnostic, prognostic, and therapeutic implications.[11,12]

The concept of a normal developmental lymphoid stage that is biologically most similar to a given lymphoma subtype has come to be known as "cell of origin" in the lymphoma field. This does not necessarily refer to the cell type in which the neoplastic process began, as lymphomagenesis is a multistep process. For example, chromosomal rearrangements that lead to activation of the oncogenes BCL2 or CCND1 in B-cell lymphomas result from aberrant VDJ recombination in the immature B-cell stage.[13] Early oncogenic driver events in chronic lymphocytic leukemia/small lymphocytic lymphoma (CLL/SLL)[14] and hairy cell leukemia[15] can occur in multipotent hematopoietic progenitors, although the fully evolved cancers are most similar to mature memory B cells. Likewise, mutations associated with T-cell lymphomas, including DNMT3A and TET2, commonly occur in the hematopoietic stem cell compartment and may represent a T-cell lymphoma precursor event.[16]

Lymphoma grade, corresponding roughly to growth rate, is a critical determinant of lymphoma clinical behavior and therapeutic approach. Transformation of low-grade lymphomas to higher-grade lymphomas (typically DLBCL-like) is an ominous clinical event that is often associated with acquisition of additional genetic events, such as inactivation of TP53 or activating MYC rearrangements.[17,18]

THE LYMPHOMA MICROENVIRONMENT

Relationships between neoplastic lymphoid cells and their microenvironment define the biology of many lymphomas. Early clonal precursors of some lymphomas can be recognized by their immunophenotype in an otherwise architecturally normal lymph node; examples include in situ follicular neoplasia (a precursor of FL)[19] and in situ mantle cell neoplasia (a likely precursor of mantle cell lymphoma [MCL]).[20] These clones bear the same oncogene-activating rearrangements as fully evolved lymphomas but lack the ability to expand beyond the normal microanatomical compartment.

In contrast, fully evolved lymphomas have gained additional genetic hits and are characterized by their ability to alter the normal architecture of the lymph node or other organ in which they arise.[21] Nonetheless, many well-differentiated lymphomas remain dependent on altered lymphoid structures, such as the expanded follicular dendritic cell meshworks that are essential to the biology of FL and AITL. Recognition of dependency on the follicular microenvironment is critical to the distinction between grade 3 FL and DLBCL, which can be cytologically and immunophenotypically identical. Altered chemokine and chemokine receptor expression or mutations in genes that regulate lymphocyte trafficking may mediate relationships between neoplastic cells and the follicular stroma in germinal center-derived B- and T-cell lymphomas.[22,23] Some lymphomas occurring in distinct anatomic sites, such as duodenal-type primary gastrointestinal follicular lymphoma, show dramatically different clinical behavior from genetically and histologically similar systemic lymphomas, potentially due to unique aspects of tumor cell-microenvironment interactions.[24,25]

Lymphomas that grow diffusely, such as DLBCL and many PTCL-NOS, are also greatly influenced by microenvironmental factors such as lymphoma-associated macrophages (LAM), blood vessels, fibroblasts, and other stromal elements. LAM provide ligands for pathogenic antigen and costimulatory receptors that are expressed by malignant lymphocytes.[21,26] Some lymphomas seem to shape a growth-promoting stromal microenvironment via gene mutations that result in altered cytokine secretion and stromal cell activation/recruitment.[27,28] Gene expression signatures derived from stromal populations are associated with outcomes in several lymphoma types.[29,30]

In T-cell lymphomas, gain-of-function mutations in costimulatory receptors[31–33] may potentiate responsiveness of lymphoma cells to ligand presented by LAM and other nonneoplastic cell populations, whereas deletions of the checkpoint receptor PD-1 may allow evasion of inhibitory microenvironmental signals.[34] LAM and regulatory T cells may also promote the evasion of host antitumor immunity by providing checkpoint ligands and immunoregulatory cytokines.[35–38] Recurrent mutations in genes such as *TET2* that are associated with clonal hematopoiesis may be present in both T-cell lymphoma cells and in constituents of the microenvironment,[39] potentially contributing to lymphomagenesis.

PREDISPOSING FACTORS

Genetic predisposition for some mature B-lymphoid cancers, including CLL/SLL and DLBCL, is relatively high compared with common epithelial cancers, based on family registry–based data.[40] Genome-wide association studies (GWAS) have identified genetic polymorphisms linked to increased risk for CLL/SLL, DLBCL, FL, and others, but the specific loci identified to date account for only a fraction of the overall apparent familial risk for these cancers.[40] Genetic variants mapping to the human leukocyte antigen (HLA) loci seem to strongly contribute to risk for several lymphoma subtypes.[41] Many lymphoma risk polymorphisms identified in GWAS studies affect noncoding regions with possible roles in gene regulation. For example, a GWAS-identified single-nucleotide polymorphism (SNP) linked to altered risk for CLL/SLL[42] lies near *MYC* regulatory elements that have been implicated in CLL/SLL and MCL,[43–45] whereas SNPs linked to DLBCL risk[46] are located on the opposite side of the *MYC* gene, in a region containing candidate DLBCL *MYC* enhancers.[44] Ubiquitous (eg, Epstein–Barr virus [EBV]) and endemic (eg, HTLV-1) viruses play direct roles in the development of some lymphomas, whereas chronic antigenic stimulation due to infection is central to the development of others, such as *Helicobacter pylori*–associated gastric mucosa-associated lymphoid tissue (MALT) lymphoma.[47] Some lymphomas may be predisposed by complex interactions between genetic, infectious, and/or environmental factors. For example, EBV-associated T- and natural killer (NK)-cell lymphomas are more common in populations of Asian and Indigenous American versus European genetic background, despite similar rates of EBV infection.[48] Concurrent EBV and malaria infection have been implicated in the high endemic rate of Burkitt lymphoma (BL) in equatorial Africa.[49]

IMMUNE RECEPTORS AS DRIVERS OF LYMPHOMAGENESIS

Surface immunoglobulin (IG) mediates signaling that is critical for the survival of normal B cells and lymphomas. Utilization of particular immunoglobulin heavy chain

(IGH) gene segments in lymphoma out of proportion to their usage in normal B-cell populations, such as *IGHV1-2* or *IGHV4* in splenic marginal zone lymphoma[50] or *IGHV3-7* and *IGHV3-23*[51] in lymphoplasmacytic lymphomas, suggests that recognition of specific antigens (autoantigens or exposure to specific pathogens) may drive prooncogenic signaling in many cases. A phenomenon of cell-autonomous B-cell receptor signaling observed in many cases of CLL/SLL is thought to be mediated by surface IG molecules that are capable of homophilic interactions in the absence of antigen.[52] Similarly, many cases of ABC-DLBCL depend on chronic active B-cell receptor signaling[53] mediated by B-cell receptors with strong autonomous or autoantigen-dependent signaling activity.[54] The somatic hypermutation status of immunoglobulin genes seems to segregate with high- and low-risk forms of both CLL/SLL[55] and MCL,[56] likely reflecting different natural histories with regard to transit through the germinal center, as well as different co-occurring oncogenic mechanisms.[57,58]

Similarly, the T-cell receptor (TCR) mediates signaling that is critical for the survival of normal and malignant T cells. Expression of TCR and downstream scaffold proteins and kinases is maintained in most nodal T-cell lymphomas, with the notable exception of ALK+ ALCL.[26] For example, the interleukin 2 (IL-2)-inducible T-cell kinase regulates the spatiotemporal localization of the TCR signalosome and is a critically important mediator of TCR signaling[59] and is frequently overexpressed in T-cell lymphomas.[60,61] Biased TCR Vβ usage and recurrent gain-of-function alterations in signaling intermediates immediately downstream from the TCR, further implicate the TCR in T-cell lymphomagenesis,[26] and have significant therapeutic implications for these lymphomas.[12]

MECHANISMS OF ONCOGENE DYSREGULATION IN LYMPHOMA

B and T lymphocytes use unique machinery to alter the structure and sequence of antigen receptor genes during normal development, and aberrations in these processes are important contributors to lymphomagenesis. Many recurrent genomic rearrangements seen in mature B- and T-cell cancers are caused by errors in V(D)J recombination in immature B cells, whereas other recurrent rearrangements and point mutations are due to off-target activity of activation-induced cytosine deaminase,[62,63] which normally catalyzes *IGH* class switch recombination and somatic hypermutation in the germinal center. Many rearrangements activate oncogene expression by an "enhancer hijacking" mechanism that involves 3-dimensional looping of distal enhancers present on the partner loci to activate promoters of the involved oncogenes,[44,64–67] whereas a minority of rearrangements encode fusion oncoproteins. Given the variability of genomic breakpoints, particularly for enhancer-hijacking rearrangements, fluorescence in-situ hybridization is the most definitive method for their identification in clinical settings, although some rearrangements (*IGH-BCL2, IGH-CCND1, ALK*) can be inferred based on immunohistochemisty.

Genome-wide evaluation of gene mutations and copy number aberrations has identified fundamental genetic drivers of B-cell lymphomagenesis and supported the existence of genetically determined subtypes of CLL/SLL,[58] MCL,[57] and DLBCL.[6,7] More recently, genome-wide CRISPR-Cas9 knockout studies in cell lines have highlighted genes and pathways that are essential for specific lymphoma subtypes,[68–70] often corresponding to the same pathways that are altered by recurrent mutations.

DRIVER MUTATIONS: SIGNALING, MOTILITY, AND METABOLISM

Discovery of recurrent mutations in genes encoding cytoplasmic signaling pathways have provided important clues regarding potentially targetable pathways in specific lymphoma subtypes. For example, discovery of the MYD88 L265P mutations in greater than 90% of lymphoplasmacytic lymphoma revealed the central importance of toll-like receptor signaling in that disease.[71] Gain-of-function MYD88 mutations are also seen in ABC-DLBCL[72] and frequently co-occur with mutations of the proximal B-cell receptor signaling complex gene CD79B in large cell lymphomas arising in extranodal sites.[73–75] Recent work uncovered a novel mechanism of oncogenic signaling via direct physical interactions between the mutant MYD88-containing TLR signaling complex, the BCR/CD79 signaling complex, and the metabolism-regulating mechanistic complex of rapamycin (mTOR) complex within endolysosomal membranes in both DLBCL and LPL.[68] This complex therefore seems to directly regulate both metabolic signaling to mTOR, as well as signaling to nuclear factor (NF)-κB via the CARD11-BCL10-MALT1 (CBM) axis. The CBM pathway seems to be a unique dependency of ABC-DLBCL as opposed to GCB-DLBCL based on CRISPR screen data[68] and is the direct target of oncogene-activating rearrangements and tumor suppressor gene deletions in MALT lymphoma.[47] Bruton's tyrosine kinase (BTK) which mediates signaling from the BCR to the CBM complex can be effectively targeted by small molecule inhibitors such as ibrutinib for the therapy of CLL/SLL and MCL, although a subset of lymphomas may develop resistance due to mutations in BTK or PLCG2, which encodes a direct target of the BTK kinase.[76–78]

Genetic alteration of mTOR regulation seems to be central to the biology of FL, which shows recurrent mutations in RRAGC, ATP6V1B2, and ATP6AP1,[79,80] genes encoding the amino acid sensing machinery that controls mTOR activation in response to nutrient availability. ATP6V1B2 mutations seem to decouple mTOR activation from autophagy, potentially sustaining lymphoma cell survival in specific low-nutrient conditions.[81] In GCB-DLBCL, the PI3K-AKT-mTOR signaling axis is dysregulated by inactivating mutations of PTEN, amplification of the negative PTEN-regulating MIR17 locus, and change-of-function mutations affecting the downstream transcription factor FOXO1.[82] The PI3-kinase delta inhibitor idelalisib is effective in the treatment of CLL/SLL,[83] possibly due to the requirement for tonic/autonomous BCR signaling via PI3K in that disease.

Genetic alteration of Janus kinase (JAK) signaling is a prominent feature of primary mediastinal large B-cell lymphoma (PMBL) in which activity of the pathway is increased by JAK2 gene amplification[84] and inactivation of the negative regulators SOCS1 and PTPN1.[85] Increased JAK2 signaling is thought to contribute to phosphorylation of STAT6 protein and the STAT target gene activation that is characteristic of the PMBL gene expression program. STAT6 mutations occur in PMBL,[86] classic Hodgkin lymphoma (cHL),[87] and follicular lymphoma.[88] The function of mutant STAT6 proteins remains unclear, as they show reduced activation-associated phosphorylation,[86] but other evidence points to increased or altered transactivation function.[87,88] STAT3 mutations are infrequent but recurrent in GCB-DLBCL.[6,89] Apparent loss-of-function mutations affecting the STAT3 phosphatase-encoding gene PTPRD seem to be a specific finding in nodal MZL.[90] Mutations in STAT3 and STAT5B are common driver events in mature T-cell neoplasms, including T-cell large granulocytic leukemia[91,92] and hepatosplenic gamma-delta T-cell lymphoma.[93] STAT signaling is also activated by ALK fusions and other mutationally activated tyrosine kinases in ALK+ and ALK-negative ALCL.[94]

Gene mutations affecting the MAP kinase pathway are common in several mature B-cell cancers. The BRAF V600E mutation is ubiquitous in hairy cell leukemia,[95] which responds clinically to the BRAF V600E-specific inhibitor vemurafenib,[96] whereas MAP2K1 (MEK1) mutations are common in hairy cell leukemia-variant[97] and pediatric-type follicular lymphoma.[98] BRAF mutations also occur in a subset of DLBCL.[6]

Mutations also affect signaling pathways related to lymphocyte chemokine response and trafficking, such as *CXCR4* in LPL/WM.[99] Genes encoding a set of regulators (*S1PR2, P2RY8, GNA13, ARGEF1*) that converge on RhoA signaling are recurrently mutated in germinal center B-cell lymphomas,[22] affecting both trafficking and PI3K-AKT signaling. Mutations of the *RHOA* gene itself are common in AITL,[100,101] further highlighting the importance of this pathway in germinal center–derived lymphomas. A gain-of-function mutation in the chemokine receptor gene *CCR4* in adult T-cell leukemia/lymphoma impairs receptor internalization and promotes PI3K/AKT signaling on ligand binding.[102]

The diversity of signaling pathway mutations in lymphoma may reflect the degree to which these pathways are "rewired" in different stages of B- and T-cell development. Understanding lymphoma subtype–specific signaling dependencies will be critical for prioritizing the growing list of signaling pathway–targeted therapies and for anticipating and overcoming mechanisms of resistance.

DRIVER MUTATIONS: EPIGENETIC AND TRANSCRIPTIONAL REGULATORS

Another large category of recurrently mutated genes in lymphoma comprises genes encoding chromatin and epigenetic regulatory proteins. *EZH2*, which encodes a repressive histone methyltransferase, is targeted by recurrent gain-of-function mutations in GCB-DLBCL and FL.[103–105] EZH2 methyltransferase activity is essential for GCB-DLBCL and normal germinal center B cells,[106] and specific EZH2 inhibitors have shown promising activity in early phase clinical trials for B-cell lymphoma.[107] The histone methyltransferase gene *KMT2D* and acetyltransferase gene *CREBBP* undergo recurrent inactivating mutations in several B-cell lymphoma types,[89,108] suggesting that the encoded proteins play a tumor suppressor role in lymphoma, possibly by promoting activation of differentiation genes. Recurrent mutations that alter linker histone genes may also affect chromatin regulation in DLBCL.[109]

Genetic alteration of DNA methylation pathways have been strongly implicated in AITL, which bears mutations in the DNA methyltransferase *DNMT3A* and the demethylation pathway gene *TET2*,[110] as well as change-of-function mutations in the metabolic enzyme *IDH2*[111] that result in oncometabolite-dependent inhibition of DNA and histone demethylation. T-cell lymphomas harboring concurrent *TET2* and *IDH2* mutations have distinct gene expression and epigenetic profiles, most notably upregulation of Tfh-associated genes.[112] Mouse models of concurrent *TET2* and *RHOA* mutations result in highly penetrant AITL-like lymphomas with strong activation of PI3K and mTOR signaling.[113,114]

Other mutations alter transcriptional regulators that act more selectively at DNA sequence–specific targets. In the setting of genomic rearrangements, overexpressed c-Myc (or in rare cases of MCL, N-Myc[115]) directly binds genes that sustain anabolic cellular metabolism and cell cycle progression.[116] The transcriptional repressor BCL6 blocks expression of several classes of tumor suppressor genes, including cell-cycle inhibitors, DNA damage response genes, and regulators of differentiation.[117] BCL6 expression is activated in lymphomas by several distinct mechanisms. Activating rearrangements such as *IGH-BCL6* occur most commonly in non–germinal center phenotype lymphomas.[6,89,118] In contrast, GCB-DLBCL and normal centroblasts show activation of distal BCL6 super-enhancers,[119,120] which in turn are bound and activated by the transcription factor MEF2B.[44,121] High-level BCL6 expression is also facilitated by noncoding mutations that alter repressive BCL6 protein–binding sites in the BCL6 promoter.[122] MEF2B itself is a target of recurrent mutations in B-cell lymphoma that alter DNA-binding properties and interactions with corepressors,[121,123,124] although the effect of these mutations on the MEF2B regulome remains poorly understood. Inactivating mutations of *PRDM1* (BLIMP1) are common in ABC-DLBCL,[6,125] where they likely function to prevent terminal differentiation. Many other developmental transcription factors are recurrently mutated in DLBCL, including *EBF1*, *POU2AF1*, *POU2F2*, *IKZF3*, *IRF4*, and *IRF8*.[6,126] Gain-of-function mutations in *TCF3* or inactivating mutations of its negative regulator *ID3* are genetic hallmarks of BL.[127] Other developmental TF gene aberrations with apparent lymphoma subtype–specific roles include *KLF2*, which is recurrently inactivated in splenic and nodal MZL,[50,90] and *FOXP1*-activating rearrangements in MALT lymphoma and extranodal DLBCL.[128,129]

NOTCH1 and *NOTCH2*, which encode proteins that serve as both cell-surface receptors and transcription factors, undergo truncating PEST domain mutations in several small B-cell lymphoma types (CLL,[130] MCL,[131] MZL,[90,132,133] and FL[134]) that increase the stability of the active intracellular form of the protein. Similar gain-of-function Notch gene mutations are enriched in recently described genetic subtypes of DLBCL,[6,7] often in concert with BCL6 rearrangements. Since PEST mutations alone do not seem to initiate Notch signaling, interactions with Notch ligand–expressing stromal cells might be critical for Notch-dependent lymphomas, a concept supported by immunohistochemical detection of active Notch in most CLL lymph node biopsies,[135] although active Notch can also be seen in some circulating CLL cells.[45] Intracellular Notch sustains the growth of some MCL cell lines by binding and activating B-cell–specific *MYC* enhancers, and several lines of evidence point to a similar role for Notch in CLL.[43,45,136] Whether inhibitors of Notch signaling might play a role in B-cell lymphoma therapy remains to be determined.

The NF-κB family of transcriptional regulators are known to play a critical role in ABC-DLBCL as major downstream effectors of BCR signaling via BTK and the CBM complex[53,137] This canonical pathway of BCR signaling to NF-κB seems to be essential for a subset of MCL but is dispensable for MCL with mutations in the alternative NF-κB pathway, which may confer resistance to BCR signaling inhibitors.[78] Focal amplification of the NF-κB gene *REL* is thought to contribute to NF-κB activation in PMBL and cHL.[138,139] Although the canonical pathway of BCR signaling to NF-κB is inactive in GCB-DLBCL, this disease also shows recurrent focal *REL* amplifications[139] and inactivating mutations of the NF-κB inhibitor genes *NFKBIA* and *NFKBIE*,[6] suggesting that NF-κB activation by alternate mechanisms may play a role in a subset of GCB-DLBCL.

DRIVER MUTATIONS: DNA DAMAGE RESPONSE, CELL-CYCLE REGULATION, AND SURVIVAL

Mutations or genomic deletions affecting genes that regulate DNA damage response are critical in several lymphoma subtypes. Inactivation of *ATM* on 11q (often involving concurrent deletion of *BIRC3)* is common in MCL,[57] while *ATM* and *TP53*-inactivating lesions are associated with more aggressive behavior in CLL.[140] In DLBCL, *TP53* mutation is a genetic hallmark of a distinct subgroup characterized by frequent copy number aberrations.[6]

Genetic alteration of cell-cycle regulatory genes in lymphoma includes the *CCND1* rearrangements seen in most MCL, as well as rarer activating rearrangements of *CCND2* or *CCND3*.[115] Unlike *CCND1*, *CCND3* is often expressed in B cells in the absence of rearrangement, and gain-of-function point mutations can lead to increased CCND3 protein stability in BL and other high-grade B-cell lymphomas.[127] Deletion of the cell-cycle inhibitory genes *CDKN2A* and *RB1* is also recurrent in DLBCL.[6]

Low levels of antiapoptotic proteins leave normal germinal center B cells highly prone to apoptosis, but this vulnerability is overcome in many FL and GCB-DLBCL by *BCL2*-activating rearrangements. The small-molecule BCL2 inhibitor Venetoclax is effective in CLL/SLL,[141] which expresses *BCL2* in the absence of an activating genetic event, whereas early clinical evidence suggests efficacy in at least a subset of patients with other lymphoma subtypes, including DLBCL, MCL, and FL.[142]

IMMUNOSURVEILLANCE AND IMMUNE EVASION IN LYMPHOMAGENESIS

The normal immune system plays an important role in fighting emerging lymphoma clones. Patients treated with immunosuppressive therapy following organ or bone marrow transplantation, or in the setting of an autoimmune disorder, are therefore at increased risk for development of lymphoproliferative disorders. Some lymphoid malignancies arising in these settings may show a therapeutic response to a decrease or cessation of immunosuppressive therapy alone. Escape from immunosurveillance also likely plays a role in the development of lymphoproliferative disorders arising in sites that are physiologically immune privileged (central nervous system, testes) or pathologically sequestered from the immune system.

Immune evasion may be particularly important in the development of virally driven lymphoid malignancies, such as B- and T-/NK-cell lymphomas driven by EBV, or in adult T-cell leukemia/lymphoma driven by human T-lymphotropic virus 1, because certain antigens produced by these viruses can be highly immunogenic. However, it is now clear that even nonvirally driven lymphomas occurring in immune-competent persons frequently select for genetic mutations that promote escape from immune surveillance. Genomic deletion of HLA loci is common in DLBCLs occurring in immune-privileged sites.[143] Other DLBCLs show recurrent mutations in immune-interaction genes such as *CD83*, *CD58*, and *CD70*,[89] and these mutations may be particularly enriched in specific genetic subgroups.[6] Mutations in *B2M*,[144] a gene required for self-antigen presentation to T cells via HLA-class 1, and *CIITA*, a gene required for HLA class 2 expression and antigen presentation, are also recurrent in large B-cell lymphomas. Mutations that alter chromatin and transcriptional regulation may also contribute to immune evasion, as gain-of-function mutant EZH2 was recently implicated in suppression of major histocompatibility complex gene expression in DLBCL,[145] suggesting a mechanism by which EZH2 inhibitor therapy might restore immune-mediated lymphoma cell eradication. Rearrangements and amplifications that increase expression of *PDCD1LG2* and/or *CD274*, the genes encoding the T-cell checkpoint ligands PD-L2 and PD-L1, are particularly common in PMBL.[84,146–148]

Monoclonal antibodies such as rituximab that direct immune responses to neoplastic cells are already a mainstay of lymphoma therapy,[149] and as checkpoint inhibitors and cellular immunotherapies continue to emerge as appealing therapeutic options for patients with advanced lymphoma,[150–152] mechanisms of immune escape are likely to be of even greater therapeutic significance in the future.

SUMMARY

Basic research continues to provide novel insights regarding the cause, genetics, and biological diversity of mature lymphoid cancers. As therapeutic options continue to expand, integration of traditional diagnostic approaches and molecular analyses will likely be essential for optimal lymphoma patient care.

ACKNOWLEDGEMENTS

The authors gratefully acknowledge support from the U.S. National Institutes of Health, grants K08CA208013 (RR) and R01CA217994 (RW). We regret that many important works could not be cited due to length constraints.

REFERENCES

1. Swerdlow SH, Campo E, Harris NL, et al. WHO classification of tumors of haematopoietic and lymphoid tissues. Revised 4th edition. Lyon (France): World Health Organization; 2017.
2. Zelenetz AD, Gordon LI, Abramson JS, et al. B-cell lymphomas. NCCN guidelines version 1. 2019. Available at: https://www.nccn.org/professionals/physician_gls/pdf/b-cell.pdf. Accessed February 12, 2019.
3. Laurent C, Baron M, Amara N, et al. Impact of expert pathologic review of lymphoma diagnosis: Study of patients from the French Lymphopath network. J Clin Oncol 2017;35(18):2008–17.
4. Alizadeh AA, Elsen MB, Davis RE, et al. Distinct types of diffuse large B-cell lymphoma identified by gene expression profiling. Nature 2000;403(6769):503–11.
5. Scott DW, Wright GW, Williams PM, et al. Determining cell-of-origin subtypes of diffuse large B-cell lymphoma using gene expression in formalin-fixed paraffin embedded tissue. Blood 2014;123(8):1214–7.
6. Chapuy B, Stewart C, Dunford AJ, et al. Molecular subtypes of diffuse large B cell lymphoma are associated with distinct pathogenic mechanisms and outcomes. Nat Med 2018;24(5):679–90.
7. Schmitz R, Wright GW, Huang DW, et al. Genetics and pathogenesis of diffuse large B-cell lymphoma. N Engl J Med 2018;378(15):1396–407.
8. Wang T, Feldman AL, Wada DA, et al. GATA-3 expression identifies a high-risk subset of PTCL, NOS with distinct molecular and clinical features. Blood 2014; 123(19):3007–15.
9. Iqbal J, Wilcox R, Naushad H, et al. Genomic signatures in T-cell lymphoma: how can these improve precision in diagnosis and inform prognosis? Blood Rev 2016;30(2):89–100.
10. Iqbal J, Wright G, Wang C, et al. Gene expression signatures delineate biological and prognostic subgroups in peripheral T-cell lymphoma. Blood 2014; 123(19):2915–23.
11. de Leval L, Gaulard P. Cellular origin of T-cell lymphomas. Blood 2014;123(19): 2909–10.
12. Wang T, Lu Y, Polk A, et al. T-cell receptor signaling activates an ITK/NF-κB/GATA-3 axis in T-cell lymphomas facilitating resistance to chemotherapy. Clin Cancer Res 2017;23(10):2506–15.
13. Tsujimoto Y, Louie E, Bashir MM, et al. The reciprocal partners of both the t(14; 18) and the t(11; 14) translocations involved in B-cell neoplasms are rearranged by the same mechanism. Oncogene 1988;2(4):347–51.
14. Damm F, Mylonas E, Cosson A, et al. Acquired initiating mutations in early hematopoietic cells of CLL patients. Cancer Discov 2014;4(9):1088–101.
15. Chung SS, Kim E, Park JH, et al. Hematopoietic stem cell origin of BRAFV600E mutations in hairy cell leukemia. Sci Transl Med 2014;6(238):238ra71.
16. Quivoron C, Couronné L, Della Valle V, et al. TET2 inactivation results in pleiotropic hematopoietic abnormalities in mouse and is a recurrent event during human lymphomagenesis. Cancer Cell 2011;20:25–38.

17. Rossi D, Spina V, Deambrogi C, et al. The genetics of Richter syndrome reveals disease heterogeneity and predicts survival after transformation. Blood 2011; 117(12):3391–401.

18. Pasqualucci L, Khiabanian H, Fangazio M, et al. Genetics of follicular lymphoma transformation. Cell Rep 2014;6(1):130–40.

19. Jegalian AG, Eberle FC, Pack SD, et al. Follicular lymphoma in situ: clinical implications and comparisons with partial involvement by follicular lymphoma. Blood 2011;118(11):2976–84.

20. Carvajal-Cuenca A, Sua LF, Silva NM, et al. In situ mantle cell lymphoma: clinical implications of an incidental finding with indolent clinical behavior. Haematologica 2012;97(2):270–8.

21. Scott DW, Gascoyne RD. The tumour microenvironment in B cell lymphomas. Nat Rev Cancer 2014;14(8):517–34.

22. Muppidi JR, Schmitz R, Green J a, et al. Loss of signalling via Gα13 in germinal centre B-cell-derived lymphoma. Nature 2014;516(7530):254–8.

23. Wilcox RA. Myeloid-derived suppressor cells: therapeutic modulation in cancer. Front Biosci (Elite Ed) 2012;4:838–55.

24. Hellmuth JC, Louissaint A, Szczepanowski M, et al. Duodenal-type and nodal follicular lymphomas differ by their immune microenvironment rather than their mutation profiles. Blood 2018;132(16):1695–702.

25. Bende RJ, Smit LA, Bossenbroek JG, et al. Primary follicular lymphoma of the small intestine: α4β7 expression and immunoglobulin configuration suggest an origin from local antigen-experienced B cells. Am J Pathol 2003;162(1): 105–13.

26. Wilcox RA. A three-signal model of T-cell lymphoma pathogenesis. Am J Hematol 2016;91(1):113–22.

27. Boice M, Salloum D, Mourcin F, et al. Loss of the HVEM tumor suppressor in lymphoma and restoration by modified CAR-T cells. Cell 2016;167(2):405–18.e13.

28. Gayden T, Sepulveda FE, Khuong-Quang D-A, et al. Germline HAVCR2 mutations altering TIM-3 characterize subcutaneous panniculitis-like T cell lymphomas with hemophagocytic lymphohistiocytic syndrome. Nat Genet 2018; 50(12):1650–7.

29. Dave SS, Wright G, Tan B, et al. Prediction of survival in follicular lymphoma based on molecular features of tumor-infiltrating immune cells. N Engl J Med 2004;351(21):2159–69.

30. Lenz G, Wright G, Dave SS, et al. Stromal gene signatures in large-B-cell lymphomas. N Engl J Med 2008;359(22):2313–23.

31. Ungewickell A, Bhaduri A, Rios E, et al. Genomic analysis of mycosis fungoides and Sézary syndrome identifies recurrent alterations in TNFR2. Nat Genet 2015; 47(9):1056–60.

32. Sekulic A, Liang WS, Tembe W, et al. Personalized treatment of Sézary syndrome by targeting a novel CTLA4 : CD28 fusion. Mol Genet Genomic Med 2015;3(2):130–6.

33. Rohr J, Guo S, Huo J, et al. Recurrent activating mutations of CD28 in peripheral T-cell lymphomas. Leukemia 2016;30(5):1062–70.

34. Wartewig T, Kurgyis Z, Keppler S, et al. PD-1 is a haploinsufficient suppressor of T cell lymphomagenesis. Nature 2017;552(7683):121–5.

35. Wilcox RA, Feldman AL, Wada DA, et al. B7-H1 (PD-L1, CD274) suppresses host immunity in T-cell lymphoproliferative disorders. Blood 2009;114(10): 2149–58.

36. Wilcox RA, Wada DA, Ziesmer SC, et al. Monocytes promote tumor cell survival in T-cell lymphoproliferative disorders and are impaired in their ability to differentiate into mature dendritic cells. Blood 2009;114(14):2936–44.

37. Keane C, Vari F, Hertzberg M, et al. Ratios of T-cell immune effectors and checkpoint molecules as prognostic biomarkers in diffuse large B-cell lymphoma: a population-based study. Lancet Haematol 2015;2(10):e445–55.

38. Yang Z-Z, Novak AJ, Stenson MJ, et al. Intratumoral CD4+CD25+ regulatory T-cell-mediated suppression of infiltrating CD4+ T cells in B-cell non-Hodgkin lymphoma. Blood 2006;107(9):3639–46.

39. Schwartz FH, Cai Q, Fellmann E, et al. TET2 mutations in B cells of patients affected by angioimmunoblastic T-cell lymphoma. J Pathol 2017;242(2):129–33.

40. Sampson JN, Wheeler WA, Yeager M, et al. Analysis of heritability and shared heritability based on genome-wide association studies for thirteen cancer types. J Natl Cancer Inst 2016;107(12):1–11.

41. Vijai J, Kirchhoff T, Schrader KA, et al. Susceptibility loci associated with specific and shared subtypes of lymphoid malignancies. PLoS Genet 2013;9(1): e1003220.

42. Crowther-Swanepoel D, Broderick P, Di Bernardo MC, et al. Common variants at 2q37.3, 8q24.21, 15q21.3 and 16q24.1 influence chronic lymphocytic leukemia risk. Nat Genet 2010;42(2):132–6.

43. Ryan RJH, Petrovic J, Rausch DM, et al. A B cell regulome links notch to downstream oncogenic pathways in small B cell lymphomas. Cell Rep 2017;21(3): 784–97.

44. Ryan RJH, Drier Y, Whitton H, et al. Detection of enhancer-associated rearrangements reveals mechanisms of oncogene dysregulation in B-cell lymphoma. Cancer Discov 2015;5(10):1058–71.

45. Fabbri G, Holmes AB, Viganotti M, et al. Common nonmutational NOTCH1 activation in chronic lymphocytic leukemia. Proc Natl Acad Sci U S A 2017;114(14): E2911–9.

46. Cerhan JR, Berndt SI, Vijai J, et al. Genome-wide association study identifies multiple susceptibility loci for diffuse large B cell lymphoma. Nat Genet 2014; 46(11):1233–8.

47. Sagaert X, Van Cutsem E, De Hertogh G, et al. Gastric MALT lymphoma: a model of chronic inflammation-induced tumor development. Nat Rev Gastroenterol Hepatol 2010;7(6):336–46.

48. Cohen JI, Kimura H, Nakamura S, et al. Epstein-Barr virus-associated lymphoproliferative disease in non-immunocompromised hosts: a status report and summary of an international meeting, 8-9 September 2008. Ann Oncol 2009; 20(9):1472–82.

49. Moormann AM, Snider CJ, Chelimo K. The company malaria keeps: How co-infection with Epstein-Barr virus leads to endemic Burkitt lymphoma. Curr Opin Infect Dis 2011;24(5):435–41.

50. Clipson A, Wang M, de Leval L, et al. KLF2 mutation is the most frequent somatic change in splenic marginal zone lymphoma and identifies a subset with distinct genotype. Leukemia 2015;29(5):1177–85.

51. Gachard N, Parrens M, Soubeyran I, et al. IGHV gene features and MYD88 L265P mutation separate the three marginal zone lymphoma entities and Waldenström macroglobulinemia/lymphoplasmacytic lymphomas. Leukemia 2013; 27(1):183–9.

52. Minden MD, Übelhart R, Schneider D, et al. Chronic lymphocytic leukaemia is driven by antigen-independent cell-autonomous signalling. Nature 2012; 489(7415):309–12.
53. Davis RE, Ngo VN, Lenz G, et al. Chronic active B-cell-receptor signalling in diffuse large B-cell lymphoma. Nature 2010;463(7277):88–92.
54. Young RM, Wu T, Schmitz R, et al. Survival of human lymphoma cells requires B-cell receptor engagement by self-antigens. Proc Natl Acad Sci U S A 2015; 112(44):13447–54.
55. Hamblin TJ, Davis Z, Gardiner A, et al. Unmutated Ig V(H) genes are associated with a more aggressive form of chronic lymphocytic leukemia. Blood 1999;94(6): 1848–54.
56. Fernàndez V, Salamero O, Espinet B, et al. Genomic and gene expression profiling defines indolent forms of mantle cell lymphoma. Cancer Res 2010; 70(4):1408–18.
57. Beà S, Valdés-Mas R, Navarro A, et al. Landscape of somatic mutations and clonal evolution in mantle cell lymphoma. Proc Natl Acad Sci U S A 2013; 110(45):18250–5.
58. Puente XS, Beà S, Valdés-Mas R, et al. Non-coding recurrent mutations in chronic lymphocytic leukaemia. Nature 2015;526(7574):519–24.
59. Singleton KL, Gosh M, Dandekar RD, et al. Itk controls the spatiotemporal organization of T cell activation. Sci Signal 2011;4(193):1–12.
60. Agostinelli C, Rizvi H, Paterson J, et al. Intracellular TCR-signaling pathway: novel markers for lymphoma diagnosis and potential therapeutic targets. Am J Surg Pathol 2014;38(10):1349–59.
61. Liang PI, Chang ST, Lin MY, et al. Angioimmunoblastic T-cell lymphoma in Taiwan shows a frequent gain of ITK gene. Int J Clin Exp Pathol 2014;7(9): 6097–107.
62. Qian J, Wang Q, Dose M, et al. B cell super-enhancers and regulatory clusters recruit AID tumorigenic activity. Cell 2014;159(7):1524–37.
63. Meng F, Du Z, Federation A, et al. Convergent transcription at intragenic super-enhancers targets AID-initiated genomic instability. Cell 2014;159(7):1538–48.
64. Banerji J, Olson L, Schaffner W. A lymphocyte-specific cellular enhancer is located downstream of the joining region in immunoglobulin heavy chain genes. Cell 1983;33(3):729–40.
65. Pettersson S, Cook GP, Brüggemann M, et al. A second B cell-specific enhancer 3' of the immunoglobulin heavy-chain locus. Nature 1990;344(6262):165–8.
66. Gostissa M, Yan CT, Bianco JM, et al. Long-range oncogenic activation of Igh-c-myc translocations by the Igh 3' regulatory region. Nature 2009;462:803–7.
67. Chong LC, Ben-Neriah S, Slack GW, et al. High-resolution architecture and partner genes of MYC rearrangements in lymphoma with DLBCL morphology. Blood Adv 2018;2(20):2755–65.
68. Phelan JD, Young RM, Webster DE, et al. A multiprotein supercomplex controlling oncogenic signalling in lymphoma. Nature 2018;560(7718):387–91.
69. Reddy A, Zhang J, Davis NS, et al. Genetic and functional drivers of diffuse large B cell lymphoma. Cell 2017;171(2):481–94.e15.
70. Ng SY, Yoshida N, Christie AL, et al. Targetable vulnerabilities in T- and NK-cell lymphomas identified through preclinical models. Nat Commun 2018;9(1):2024.
71. Treon SP, Xu L, Yang G, et al. MYD88 L265P somatic mutation in Waldenström's macroglobulinemia. N Engl J Med 2012;367(9):826–33.
72. Ngo VN, Young RM, Schmitz R, et al. Oncogenically active MYD88 mutations in human lymphoma. Nature 2011;470(7332):115–9.

73. Chapuy B, Roemer MGM, Stewart C, et al. Targetable genetic features of primary testicular and primary central nervous system lymphomas. Blood 2016; 127(7):869–81.

74. Schrader AMR, Jansen PM, Willemze R, et al. High prevalence of MYD88 and CD79B mutations in intravascular large B-cell lymphoma. Blood 2018;131(18): 2086–9.

75. Mareschal S, Pham-Ledard A, Viailly PJ, et al. Identification of somatic mutations in primary cutaneous diffuse large B-cell lymphoma, leg type by massive parallel sequencing. J Invest Dermatol 2017;137(9):1984–94.

76. Woyach JA, Furman RR, Liu T-M, et al. Resistance mechanisms for the Bruton's tyrosine kinase inhibitor ibrutinib. N Engl J Med 2014;370(24):2286–94.

77. Martin P, Maddocks K, Leonard JP, et al. Postibrutinib outcomes in patients with mantle cell lymphoma. Blood 2016;127(12):1559–63.

78. Rahal R, Frick M, Romero R, et al. Pharmacological and genomic profiling identifies NF-κB-targeted treatment strategies for mantle cell lymphoma. Nat Med 2014;20(1):87–92.

79. Ying ZX, Jin M, Peterson LF, et al. Recurrent mutations in the MTOR regulator RRAGC in follicular lymphoma. Clin Cancer Res 2016;22(21):5383–93.

80. Okosun J, Wolfson RL, Wang J, et al. Recurrent mTORC1-activating RRAGC mutations in follicular lymphoma. Nat Genet 2016;48(2):183–8.

81. Wang F, Gatica D, Ying ZX, et al. Follicular lymphoma-associated mutations in vacuolar ATPase ATP6V1B2 activate autophagic flux and mTOR. J Clin Invest 2019;130:1626–40.

82. Trinh DL, Scott DW, Morin RD, et al. Analysis of FOXO1 mutations in diffuse large B-cell lymphoma. Blood 2013;121(18):3666–74.

83. Furman RR, Sharman JP, Coutre SE, et al. Idelalisib and rituximab in relapsed chronic lymphocytic leukemia. N Engl J Med 2014;370(11):997–1007.

84. Rosenwald A, Wright G, Leroy K, et al. Molecular diagnosis of primary mediastinal B cell lymphoma identifies a clinically favorable subgroup of diffuse large B cell lymphoma related to Hodgkin lymphoma. J Exp Med 2003;198(6):851–62.

85. Gunawardana J, Chan FC, Telenius A, et al. Recurrent somatic mutations of PTPN1 in primary mediastinal B cell lymphoma and Hodgkin lymphoma. Nat Genet 2014;46(4):329–35.

86. Ritz O, Guiter C, Castellano F, et al. Recurrent mutations of the STAT6 DNA binding domain in primary mediastinal B-cell lymphoma. Blood 2009;114(6): 1236–42.

87. Tiacci E, Ladewig E, Schiavoni G, et al. Pervasive mutations of JAK-STAT pathway genes in classical Hodgkin lymphoma. Blood 2018;131(22):2454–65.

88. Yildiz M, Li H, Bernard D, et al. Activating STAT6 mutations in follicular lymphoma. Blood 2014;125(4):668–80.

89. Morin RD, Mendez-Lago M, Mungall AJ, et al. Frequent mutation of histone-modifying genes in non-Hodgkin lymphoma. Nature 2011;476(7360):298–303.

90. Spina V, Khiabanian H, Messina M, et al. The genetics of nodal marginal zone lymphoma. Blood 2016;128(10):1362–74.

91. Koskela HLM, Eldfors S, Ellonen P, et al. Somatic STAT3 mutations in large granular lymphocytic leukemia. N Engl J Med 2012;366(20):1905–13.

92. Rajala HLM, Eldfors S, Kuusanmäki H, et al. Discovery of somatic STAT5b mutations in large granular lymphocytic leukemia. Blood 2013;121(22):4541–50.

93. Nicolae a, Xi L, Pittaluga S, et al. Frequent STAT5B mutations in γδ hepatosplenic T-cell lymphomas. Leukemia 2014;28(11):2244–8.

94. Crescenzo R, Abate F, Lasorsa E, et al. Convergent mutations and kinase fusions lead to oncogenic STAT3 activation in anaplastic large cell lymphoma. Cancer Cell 2015;27(4):516–32.

95. Tiacci E, Trifonov V, Schiavoni G, et al. BRAF mutations in hairy-cell leukemia. N Engl J Med 2011;364:2305–15.

96. Tiacci E, Park JH, De Carolis L, et al. Targeting mutant BRAF in relapsed or refractory hairy-cell leukemia. N Engl J Med 2015;373(18):1733–47.

97. Waterfall JJ, Arons E, Walker RL, et al. High prevalence of MAP2K1 mutations in variant and IGHV4-34-expressing hairy-cell leukemias. Nat Genet 2014;46(1): 8–10.

98. Louissaint A, Schafernak KT, Geyer JT, et al. Pediatric-type nodal follicular lymphoma: a biologically distinct lymphoma with frequent MAPK pathway mutations. Blood 2016;128(8):1093–100.

99. Roccaro AM, Sacco A, Jimenez C, et al. C1013G/CXCR4 acts as a driver mutation of tumor progression and modulator of drug resistance in lymphoplasmacytic lymphoma. Blood 2014;123(26):4120–31.

100. Palomero T, Couronné L, Khiabanian H, et al. Recurrent mutations in epigenetic regulators, RHOA and FYN kinase in peripheral T cell lymphomas. Nat Genet 2014;46(2):166–70.

101. Sakata-Yanagimoto M, Enami T, Yoshida K, et al. Somatic RHOA mutation in angioimmunoblastic T cell lymphoma. Nat Genet 2014;46(2):171–5.

102. Nakagawa M, Schmitz R, Xiao W, et al. Gain-of-function CCR4 mutations in adult T cell leukemia/lymphoma. J Exp Med 2014;211(13):2497–505.

103. Morin RD, Johnson NA, Severson TM, et al. Somatic mutations altering EZH2 (Tyr641) in follicular and diffuse large B-cell lymphomas of germinal-center origin. Nat Genet 2010;42(2):181–5.

104. Ryan RJH, Nitta M, Borger D, et al. EZH2 codon 641 mutations are common in BCL2-rearranged germinal center B cell lymphomas. PLoS One 2011;6(12): e28585.

105. Sneeringer CJ, Scott MP, Kuntz KW, et al. Coordinated activities of wild-type plus mutant EZH2 drive tumor-associated hypertrimethylation of lysine 27 on histone H3 (H3K27) in human B-cell lymphomas. Proc Natl Acad Sci U S A 2010;107(49):20980.

106. Béguelin W, Popovic R, Teater M, et al. EZH2 is required for germinal center formation and somatic EZH2 mutations promote lymphoid transformation. Cancer Cell 2013;23(5):677–92.

107. Italiano A, Soria JC, Toulmonde M, et al. Tazemetostat, an EZH2 inhibitor, in relapsed or refractory B-cell non-Hodgkin lymphoma and advanced solid tumours: a first-in-human, open-label, phase 1 study. Lancet Oncol 2018;19(5): 649–59.

108. Pasqualucci L, Dominguez-Sola D, Chiarenza A, et al. Inactivating mutations of acetyltransferase genes in B-cell lymphoma. Nature 2011;471(7337):189–95.

109. Lohr JG, Stojanov P, Lawrence MS, et al. Discovery and prioritization of somatic mutations in diffuse large B-cell lymphoma (DLBCL) by whole-exome sequencing. Proc Natl Acad Sci U S A 2012;109(10):3879–84.

110. Couronné L, Bastard C, Bernard OA. TET2 and DNMT3A mutations in human T-cell lymphoma. N Engl J Med 2012;366(1):95–6.

111. Odejide O, Weigert O, Lane AA, et al. A targeted mutational landscape of angioimmunoblastic T-cell lymphoma. Blood 2014;123(9):1293–6.

112. Wang C, McKeithan TW, Gong Q, et al. IDH2R172 mutations define a unique subgroup of patients with angioimmunoblastic T-cell lymphoma. Blood 2015; 126(15):1741–52.

113. Cortes JR, Ambesi-Impiombato A, Couronné L, et al. RHOA G17V Induces T Follicular Helper Cell Specification and Promotes Lymphomagenesis. Cancer Cell 2018;33(2):259–73.e7.

114. Ng SY, Brown L, Stevenson K, et al. RhoA G17V is sufficient to induce autoimmunity and promotes T-cell lymphomagenesis in mice. Blood 2018;132(9): 935–47.

115. Wlodarska I, Dierickx D, Vanhentenrijk V, et al. Translocations targeting CCND2, CCND3, and MYCN do occur in t(11;14)-negative mantle cell lymphomas. Blood 2008;111(12):5683–90.

116. Kress TR, Sabò A, Amati B. MYC: connecting selective transcriptional control to global RNA production. Nat Rev Cancer 2015;15(10):593–607.

117. Hatzi K, Melnick A. Breaking bad in the germinal center: how deregulation of BCL6 contributes to lymphomagenesis. Trends Mol Med 2014;2:1–10.

118. Iqbal J, Greiner TC, Patel K, et al. Distinctive patterns of BCL6 molecular alterations and their functional consequences in different subgroups of diffuse large B-cell lymphoma. Leukemia 2007;21(11):2332–43.

119. Ramachandrareddy H, Bouska A, Shen Y, et al. BCL6 promoter interacts with far upstream sequences with greatly enhanced activating histone modifications in germinal center B cells. Proc Natl Acad Sci U S A 2010;107(26):11930–5.

120. Bunting KL, Soong TD, Singh R, et al. Multi-tiered reorganization of the genome during B cell affinity maturation anchored by a germinal center-specific locus control region. Immunity 2016;45(3):497–512.

121. Brescia P, Schneider C, Holmes AB, et al. MEF2B instructs germinal center development and acts as an oncogene in B cell lymphomagenesis. Cancer Cell 2018;34(3):453–65.e9.

122. Pasqualucci L, Migliazza A, Basso K, et al. Mutations of the BCL6 proto-oncogene disrupt its negative autoregulation in diffuse large B-cell lymphoma. Blood 2003;101(8):2914–23.

123. Ying CY, Dominguez-Sola D, Fabi M, et al. MEF2B mutations lead to deregulated expression of the oncogene BCL6 in diffuse large B cell lymphoma. Nat Immunol 2013;14(10):1084–92.

124. Pon JR, Wong J, Saberi S, et al. MEF2B mutations in non-Hodgkin lymphoma dysregulate cell migration by decreasing MEF2B target gene activation. Nat Commun 2015;6(1):7953.

125. Mandelbaum J, Bhagat G, Tang H, et al. BLIMP1 is a tumor suppressor gene frequently disrupted in activated B cell-like diffuse large B cell lymphoma. Cancer Cell 2010;18(6):568–79.

126. Morin RD, Mungall K, Pleasance E, et al. Mutational and structural analysis of diffuse large B-cell lymphoma using whole-genome sequencing. Blood 2013; 122(7):1256–65.

127. Schmitz R, Young RM, Ceribelli M, et al. Burkitt lymphoma pathogenesis and therapeutic targets from structural and functional genomics. Nature 2012; 490(7418):116–20.

128. Haralambieva E, Adam P, Ventura R, et al. Genetic rearrangement of FOXP1 is predominantly detected in a subset of diffuse large B-cell lymphomas with extranodal presentation. Leukemia 2006;20(7):1300–3.

129. Streubel B, Vinatzer U, Lamprecht A, et al. T(3;14)(p14.1;q32) involving IGH and FOXP1 is a novel recurrent chromosomal aberration in MALT lymphoma. Leukemia 2005;19(4):652–8.

130. Puente XS, Pinyol M, Quesada V, et al. Whole-genome sequencing identifies recurrent mutations in chronic lymphocytic leukaemia. Nature 2011;475(7354): 101–5.

131. Kridel R, Meissner B, Rogic S, et al. Whole transcriptome sequencing reveals recurrent NOTCH1 mutations in mantle cell lymphoma. Blood 2012;119(9): 1963–71.

132. Kiel MJ, Velusamy T, Betz BL, et al. Whole-genome sequencing identifies recurrent somatic NOTCH2 mutations in splenic marginal zone lymphoma. J Exp Med 2012;209(9):1553–65.

133. Rossi D, Trifonov V, Fangazio M, et al. The coding genome of splenic marginal zone lymphoma: activation of NOTCH2 and other pathways regulating marginal zone development. J Exp Med 2012;209(9):1537–51.

134. Karube K, Martínez D, Royo C, et al. Recurrent mutations of NOTCH genes in follicular lymphoma identify a distinctive subset of tumours. J Pathol 2014; 234(3):423–30.

135. Kluk MJ, Ashworth T, Wang H, et al. Gauging NOTCH1 activation in cancer using immunohistochemistry. PLoS One 2013;8(6):e67306.

136. Jitschin R, Braun M, Qorraj M, et al. Stromal cell – mediated glycolytic switch in CLL cells involves Notch-c-Myc signaling. Blood 2015;125(22):3432–7.

137. Davis RE, Brown KD, Siebenlist U, et al. Constitutive nuclear factor kappaB activity is required for survival of activated B cell-like diffuse large B cell lymphoma cells. J Exp Med 2001;194(12):1861–74.

138. Joos S, Menz CK, Wrobel G, et al. Classical Hodgkin lymphoma is characterized by recurrent copy number gains of the short arm of chromosome 2. Blood 2002; 99(4):1381–7.

139. Lenz G, Wright GW, Emre NCT, et al. Molecular subtypes of diffuse large B-cell lymphoma arise by distinct genetic pathways. Proc Natl Acad Sci U S A 2008; 105(36):13520–5.

140. Döhner H, Stilgenbauer S, Benner A, et al. Genomic aberrations and survival in chronic lymphocytic leukemia. N Engl J Med 2000;343(26):1910–6.

141. Roberts AW, Davids MS, Pagel JM, et al. Targeting BCL2 with venetoclax in relapsed chronic lymphocytic leukemia. N Engl J Med 2016;374(4):311–22.

142. Davids MS, Roberts AW, Seymour JF, et al. Phase I first-in-human study of venetoclax in patients with relapsed or refractory non-hodgkin lymphoma. J Clin Oncol 2017;35(8):826–33.

143. Riemersma SA, Jordanova ES, Schop RF, et al. Extensive genetic alterations of the HLA region, including homozygous deletions of HLA class II genes in B-cell lymphomas arising in immune-privileged sites. Blood 2000;96(10):3569–77.

144. Challa-Malladi M, Lieu YK, Califano O, et al. Combined genetic inactivation of β2-microglobulin and CD58 reveals frequent escape from immune recognition in diffuse large B cell lymphoma. Cancer Cell 2011;20(6):728–40.

145. Ennishi D, Takata K, Beguelin W, et al. Molecular and genetic characterization of MHC deficiency identifies EZH2 as therapeutic target for enhancing immune recognition. Cancer Discov 2019;9(4):546–63.

146. Steidl C, Shah SP, Woolcock BW, et al. MHC class II transactivator CIITA is a recurrent gene fusion partner in lymphoid cancers. Nature 2011;471(7338): 377–81.

147. Twa DDW, Chan FC, Ben-Neriah S, et al. Genomic rearrangements involving programmed death ligands are recurrent in primary mediastinal large B-cell lymphoma. Blood 2014;123(13):2062–5.

148. Green MR, Monti S, Rodig SJ, et al. Integrative analysis reveals selective 9p24.1 amplification, increased PD-1 ligand expression, and further induction via JAK2 in nodular sclerosing Hodgkin lymphoma and primary mediastinal large B-cell lymphoma. Blood 2010;116(17):3268–77.

149. Freeman CL, Sehn LH. A tale of two antibodies: obinutuzumab versus rituximab. Br J Haematol 2018;182(1):29–45.

150. Wang Y, Wu L, Tian C, et al. PD-1-PD-L1 immune-checkpoint blockade in malignant lymphomas. Ann Hematol 2018;97(2):229–37.

151. Zhang J, Medeiros LJ, Young KH. Cancer immunotherapy in diffuse large B-cell lymphoma. Front Oncol 2018;8:351.

152. Brown CE, Mackall CL. CAR T cell therapy: inroads to response and resistance. Nat Rev Immunol 2019;19(2):73–4.

Diffuse Large B-Cell Lymphoma and High-Grade B-Cell Lymphoma

Genetic Classification and Its Implications for Prognosis and Treatment

Jennifer L. Crombie, MD*, Philippe Armand, MD, PhD

KEYWORDS

- Diffuse large B-cell lymphoma • DLBCL • Cell of origin • Genomic classifications
- Targeted therapy • Precision medicine

KEY POINTS

- Diffuse large B-cell lymphoma (DLBCL) is a clinically and molecularly heterogeneous disease.
- Despite numerous robust prognostic biomarkers, predictive biomarkers are lacking.
- Attempts to use cell-of-origin classification for personalized therapy have thus far been unsuccessful.
- Recent advances in next-generation sequencing have advanced our understanding of the genomic heterogeneity of DLBCL.
- Prospective clinical trials are required to determine whether genomic-based classification of DLBCL can be used to guide treatment strategies.

INTRODUCTION

Diffuse large B-cell lymphoma (DLBCL) is the most common subtype of non-Hodgkin lymphoma, with approximately 27,000 new diagnoses in the United States each year.[1] DLBCL can occur de novo or as a result of transformation from a more indolent lymphoma. Although treatment with rituximab and multiagent chemotherapy results in cure for many patients, up to 40% of patients will have relapsed or refractory disease.[2]

Disclosure Statement: J. Crombie has no conflicts of interest to disclose. P. Armand: Consultancy: Merck, BMS, Pfizer, Affimed, Adaptive, Infinity. Research funding (inst): Merck, BMS, Affimed, Adaptive, Roche, Tensha, Otsuka, Sigma-Tau
Medical Oncology, Harvard Medical School, Dana-Farber Cancer Institute, 450 Brookline Avenue, Boston, MA 02215, USA
* Corresponding author.
E-mail address: jennifer_crombie@dfci.harvard.edu

hemonc.theclinics.com

Salvage chemotherapy followed by autologous stem cell transplantation remains the standard approach in this setting, yet fewer than half of patients will achieve long-term disease control.[3] Furthermore, patients who have refractory disease or relapse after transplant have limited therapeutic options with a poor overall survival.[4] Although chimeric antigen receptor T-cell therapy is a revolutionary treatment for patients with relapsed/refractory disease, still more than half of patients do not have a sustained response to treatment and are in urgent need of therapeutic options.[5]

Recently, comprehensive genomic analyses have allowed a better molecular characterization of DLBCL tumors, moving us closer toward the use of precision medicine in DLBCL. In this review, we highlight validated prognostic biomarkers as well as attempts made thus far to use them to personalize therapy in this heterogeneous disease. We also review the findings of more recent genomic analyses that could lead to a potential paradigm shift in management, possibly allowing for effective personalized therapy.

HETEROGENEITY OF DIFFUSE LARGE B-CELL LYMPHOMA

DLBCL has a clinically heterogeneous course, with approximately one-third of patients failing to respond durably to standard chemoimmunotherapy. This heterogeneity is thought to arise from the diverse origins of malignant lymphocytes, owing to antigen-exposed B cells transiting through the germinal center (**Fig. 1**). The germinal center is the site within a lymph node where B-lymphocytes, which have been exposed to antigens, undergo affinity maturation, developing the ability to produce high-affinity antibodies. Although this process is fundamental to immunologic function, it also involves mechanisms that predispose to malignant transformation. For

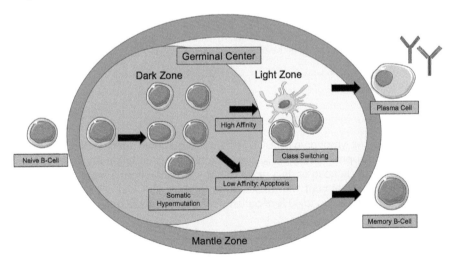

Fig. 1. B-cell development. This image represents the process of B-cell development within the germinal center of a lymph node. A naive B cell is exposed to an antigen before entering the germinal center. The B cell undergoes clonal expansion and somatic hypermutation in the process of affinity maturation. B cells that are able to make high-affinity antibodies will further undergo class switching before differentiating into a plasma cell or memory B cells. This process inherently leads to genomic instability that can promote lymphomagenesis. GCB-like DLBCL are thought to develop from B cells lacking markers of early postgerminal center cells, whereas ABC-like DLBCL display a transcriptional signature similar to cells before plasma cell differentiation.

example, high cellular proliferation rate, activation-induced cytidine deaminase-mediated immunoglobulin editing, and somatic hypermutation result in genomic instability, which can promote lymphomagenesis.[6,7] Genomic changes subsequently include multiple low-frequency genetic alterations including chromosomal translocations, somatic mutations, and copy-number alterations, which contribute to the high degree of molecular diversity seen in this disease and presumably lead to variable chemoresistance.[6,8]

VALIDATED PROGNOSTIC BIOMARKERS
International Prognostic Index

Currently a variety of prognostic factors are used to predict outcomes in DLBCL. The International Prognostic Index (IPI), which is based on 5 clinical characteristics, remains a mainstay of clinical risk stratification, highlighting disparities in outcomes in response to frontline therapy.[9,10] Clinical features comprising the IPI include age, lactate dehydrogenase, performance status, number of extranodal sites, and Ann Arbor stage. Whereas the IPI is a robust and accessible tool to effectively predict survival, it is unable to identify targetable vulnerabilities or guide the use of individualized therapy.

Cell-of-Origin Classification

Using gene expression profiling, molecularly distinct subtypes of DLBCL were identified in 2000, whose different genetic profile reflected different stages of B-cell development (see **Fig. 1**).[11,12] Germinal center B-cell (GCB)-like DLBCL expresses genes that define the germinal center B-cell signature and lack expression of early postgerminal center markers.[11,13] For example, recurrent t(14;18) translocations and amplification of the c-rel gene on chromosome 2p are found exclusively in this subtype of DLBCL.[12] The other main subtype of DLBCL is the activated B-cell (ABC)-like DLBCL, whose transcriptional signature resembles that of postgerminal center B cells blocked at plasmablastic differentiation. Recurrent trisomy 3, deletion of the inhibitor of kinase 4A-alternative reading frame (INK4A/ARF) locus and constitutive activation of the anti-apoptotic nuclear factor κB (NF-κB) signaling pathway are defining features of this subtype.[12,14,15] A smaller subset of tumors falls into a third group that does not express either set of genes at high levels. The cell-of-origin (COO) classification separates DLBCL tumors into the above 3 subtypes and has been repeatedly found to predict overall survival. Indeed, even with modern chemoimmunotherapy, patients with GCB subtype DLBCL often have superior outcomes following multiagent chemotherapy compared with patients with ABC-like DLBCL.[12] In 1 study, patients with GCB DLBCL had a 5-year survival of 60%, compared with 35% for those with ABC-like DLBCL following anthracycline-based chemotherapy.[12] Although the use of COO classification has become standard in clinical practice for prognostication, its prognostic validity has not been uniformly reproduced,[16] suggesting that potential residual heterogeneity within these subgroups may exist and carry important prognostic information. Furthermore, the difficulty of using standard immunohistochemistry markers to assign COO classification, which would facilitate the routine characterization of patients, has hampered the use of the COO classification for personalized therapy assignment.[17,18]

Comprehensive Clustering

An alternative transcriptional profiling classification, termed comprehensive consensus clustering (CCC), has also been used to subset distinct variants of

DLBCL.[19] This analysis identified 3 distinct groups: B-cell receptor, oxidative phosphorylation, and host response, highlighting the role of the tumor microenvironment and host inflammatory response as defining features in DLBCL. Although this study offered a nonoverlapping categorization from COO, and suggested potential rational therapeutic targets for each group, it has had a more limited role in clinical practice to date.

Double-Hit and Double-Expressor Status

Independently of the COO and CCC classifications, DLBCL molecular features involving the *MYC* oncogene have allowed the identification of a group of patients with aggressive clinical course. Specifically, within the GCB subtype, lymphomas with concurrent translocations involving *MYC* and *BCL-2* or *BCL-6*, termed double-hit lymphoma (DHL) or triple-hit lymphoma, have repeatedly been shown to have a particularly aggressive and refractory clinical course.[20,21] In the 2016 revision of the World Health Organization classification for lymphoma, a new entity, high-grade B-cell lymphoma with translocations involving *MYC* and *BCL-2* or *BCL-6*, was included, emphasizing the prognostic significance of these genomic aberrations. Even more recently, RNA sequencing data have also been used to define a gene expression signature that identifies GCB subtype DLBCL with a double-hit signature, even in the absence of *MYC* or *BCL-2* translocations, again identifying patients with a poorer prognosis.[22,23]

Efforts to use immunohistochemistry of MYC and BCL-2 to recapitulate the biology of DHL showed that combined increase in MYC and BCL-2 protein expression on the tumor cell surface, termed double-expressor lymphoma (DEL), is also an unfavorable subgroup with inferior outcomes after standard frontline therapy.[16,20] However, DEL and DHL are not identical or even strongly overlapping categorizations, and DEL status is not a surrogate of DHL status (or vice versa). Both DHL and DEL have also been associated with poor prognosis after autologous stem cell transplantation, with DHL and DEL associated with a reduction in progression-free survival (PFS) and DHL associated with a reduction in overall survival (OS).[24] Specifically, the 4-year PFS in patients with DEL compared with those with non-DEL was 48% versus 59% ($P = .049$) and the 4-year PFS in patients with DHL compared with those with non-DHL was 28% versus 57% ($P = .013$), and 4-year OS was 25% versus 61% ($P = .002$).[24] These data highlight that, although autologous stem cell transplantation remains a potentially curable option for patients with DLBCL, those with high-risk disease, such as those with DHL, are in need of novel treatment strategies both for frontline and for salvage treatment.

TRIALS TARGETING CELL-OF-ORIGIN SUBTYPES

Currently R-CHOP (rituximab, cyclophosphamide, doxorubicin, vincristine, and prednisone) remains the standard of care across most DLBCL subtypes in the frontline setting, although retrospective data suggest the value of more aggressive combination chemotherapy strategies in high-grade B-cell lymphoma with translocations involving *MYC* and *BCL-2* or *BCL-6*.[25–27] Despite the availability of numerous prognostic tools to predict therapy response, efforts to tailor therapeutic interventions for specific subtypes have so far been met with little success.

There have been numerous attempts to personalize therapy, especially across COO subtypes. Given the constitutive activation of NF-κB in ABC subtype DLBCL, which represents a high-risk subgroup of DLBCL, it has been hypothesized that inhibitors of NF-κB might sensitize cells to chemotherapy, thus improving outcomes.

Bortezomib is a proteasome inhibitor that blocks degradation of IkBα, consequently inhibiting NF-κB activity. Although there has been limited activity of bortezomib as a single agent in relapsed/refractory DLBCL, when combined with chemotherapy, a small study demonstrated that there were increased responses (83% vs 13%) and median OS (10.8 vs 3.4 months) in ABC compared with GCB DLBCL, respectively.[28] Although these data were encouraging, it should be noted that this study consisted of only 12 patients with ABC and 15 patients with GCB subtype DLBCL, and that the classification of COO used both gene expression profiling and the less-reliable method of immunohistochemistry.[28] Bortezomib was also tested in combination with R-CHOP for initial therapy for DLBCL, in which, unlike previous studies of R-CHOP alone, patients with GCB and ABC subtype DLBCL were found to have similar outcomes, suggesting potential selective improvement of outcome in ABC patients.[29] Based on these encouraging preliminary studies, a randomized phase 2 trial was developed comparing R-CHOP with R-CHOP plus bortezomib in patients with non-GCB subtype DLBCL as determined by immunohistochemistry.[30] Overall response rates with R-CHOP and R-CHOP plus bortezomib were 98% and 96%, respectively, and there was no significant OS with the addition of bortezomib.

Similar findings were seen with ibrutinib, an inhibitor of Bruton's tyrosine kinase (BTK). As ABC subtype DLBCL carry mutations that result in chronic active B-cell receptor signaling, ibrutinib was also theorized to have increased activity in this subtype. Although the phase 1/2 trial of ibrutinib monotherapy in relapsed/refractory DLBCL resulted in partial responses in 37% (14/38) of patients with ABC DLBCL, but in only 5% (1/20) of subjects with GCB DLBCL ($P = .0106$), confirmatory studies in the frontline setting have failed to demonstrate a benefit of adding ibrutinib to chemotherapy.[31] For example, a global, randomized, phase 3 trial of R-CHOP versus R-CHOP plus ibrutinib in patients with non-GCB DLBCL demonstrated no improvement in event-free survival with the addition of ibrutinib.[32] Similar studies with the addition of lenalidomide to frontline chemotherapy have also been performed, although phase 3 confirmatory studies are ongoing.[33–36]

GENOMIC UNDERPINNINGS OF DIFFUSE LARGE B-CELL LYMPHOMA

Growing evidence suggests that the failure of biomarkers such as COO to guide therapy stems from heterogeneity within traditional classification structures. More recently, techniques incorporating next-generation sequencing have exposed a more complex genomic variability in DLBCL. Such analyses have also identified a broad range of genomic aberrations that are potentially driving or contributing to lymphomagenesis.

Initial genomic analyses identified the genetic diversity of DLBCL, although they were limited by small sample size and limited scope.[37–39] One study, for example, identified frequent mutations in histone-modifying genes such as *MLL2*, which encodes a methyltransferase enzyme, and MEF2B, a calcium-regulated gene that cooperates with CREBBP and EP300 in acetylating histones.[37] In a subsequent study, whole-exome sequencing revealed recurrent mutations in genes known to be functionally relevant in DLBCL, including *MYD88*, *CARD11*, *EZH2*, and *CREBBP*, as well as in a variety of genes with unknown significance.[39] In addition to mutations, copy-number alterations are also common in DLBCL. In 1 small analysis of DLBCL samples, 90 copy-number alterations were identified across 6 individuals studied, with significant variability across samples.[38] Another analysis of a larger cohort of patients identified 47 recurrent copy-number alterations, including 21 copy gains and 26 copy losses, with frequencies of 4% to 27%, many of which resulted in decreased p53 activity and perturbed cell-cycle regulation.[8] Although these studies were fundamental to the recognition of the genomic complexity of DLBCL, given the small numbers of patients studied, they failed to identify a framework to categorize patients or guide the use of therapy.

More recently, larger-scale whole-exome sequencing and transcriptome analyses from a cohort of more than 1000 patients with DLBCL has comprehensively identified single-nucleotide variants, insertions/deletions (indels), and copy-number alterations in DLBCL, resulting in the discovery of approximately 150 recurrently mutated driver genes, including some that occur at low frequency and would be missed in smaller studies.[40] Although most identified mutations occurred in GCB and ABC subtypes, a small number of alterations were specific to each COO classification. For example, *EZH2*, *SGK1*, *GNA13*, *SOCS1*, *STAT6*, and *TNFRSF14* mutations were more frequently mutated in GCB DLBCLs, whereas *ETV6*, *MYD88*, *PIM1*, and *TBL1XR1* were more frequently mutated in ABC DLBCLs.[40] The functional roles of these mutations were also analyzed by unbiased CRISPR screens, identifying a much smaller subset of genes with functional relevance.

Additional studies have since been performed, incorporating analyses of a broad range of genomic aberrations in large cohorts of patients with DLBCL. In 1 study of 151 patients, a total of 761 potential driver mutations were identified and all tumors were found to have copy-number alterations, including frequent losses, gains, and amplifications.[41] The authors also analyzed the clinical influence of genetic alterations in predefined functional pathways. For example, mutations in the NOTCH signaling pathway and in *TP53/CDKN2A* were associated with poorer outcomes, whereas JAK/STAT pathway mutations were associated with improved outcomes.[41] They also found that 46% of patients had at least 1 genomic alteration that could be a predictive biomarker of drug response in DLBCL or other lymphomas and could potentially be exploited to guide targeted therapy.[41]

A similar study incorporated whole-exome and transcriptome sequencing, array-based copy-number analysis, and targeted amplicon resequencing in 574 DLBCL samples.[42] This study specifically investigated how such genetic aberrations could refine the categories of ABC or GCB subtypes. *CD79B* and *MYD88*^{L265P} mutations were enriched in ABC subtype DLBCLs, and *EZH2* mutations and *BCL-2* translocations were frequently found in the same tumor and were much more frequent in GCB tumors. Mutations such as *NOTCH2* and *BCL-6* fusions were less likely to be classifiable by COO. The authors used these finding to classify DLBCL tumors into 4 genomic subtypes, characterized by (1) *CD79B/MYD88*^{L265P} double mutations, (2) *NOTCH2* mutations or *BCL6* fusions in ABC or unclassified DLBCL, (3) *NOTCH1* mutations, and (4) *EZH2* mutations or *BCL2* translocations.[42] These subtypes had prognostic relevance even after accounting for COO assignment, with inferior responses found in patients with *CD79BMYD88*^{L265P} double mutations and *NOTCH1* mutations.[42] Of note, these genomic subtypes comprised just under half of the cases studied, suggesting that a distinct pattern of genomic heterogeneity might be identified in the remaining group of patients.

An additional analysis of a large of cohort of previously untreated patients with DLBCL identified distinct genomic subtypes of DLBCL using comprehensive genomic analyses.[6] Recurrent mutations, somatic copy-number alterations, and structural variants were used to characterize patient samples into distinct genomic clusters using nonnegative matrix factorization classification (**Table 1**), and genomic signatures subsequently correlated with outcome data. Interestingly, this genomic-based classification suggested heterogeneity even within the COO subgroups, with a newly identified poor-risk GCB subtype and a favorable-risk ABC subtype. Specific subsets of tumors

Table 1
Newly identified genomic clusters of DLBCL

	Cluster 1	Cluster 2	Cluster 3	Cluster 4	Cluster 5
Characteristic mutations	*BCL-6* structural variants with mutations in NOTCH2 signaling pathway components	Biallelic inactivation of *TP53*, 17p copy loss, 9p21.3/*CDKN2A* copy loss and associated genomic instability	*BCL2* structural variants, inactivating mutations and/or copy loss of *PTEN* and alterations of epigenetic enzymes	Alterations in JAK/STAT and BRAF pathway components and multiple histones	Near-uniform *BCL2* copy gain, frequent activating *MYD88*$^{L-265P}$, *CD79B* mutations
Cell of origin	ABC	COO independent	GCB	GCB	ABC
Risk	Low-risk		High-risk	Low-risk	High-risk
Other features	Features of extrafollicular, possibly marginal zone, lymphoma				Extranodal tropism

Data from Chapuy B, Stewart C, Dunford AJ, et al. Molecular subtypes of diffuse large B cell lymphoma are associated with distinct pathogenic mechanisms and outcomes. Nat Med 2018;24(5):679–90.

(clusters) with discrete genetic signatures included: (1) high-risk ABC DLBCLs with near-uniform *BCL2* copy gain, frequent activating *MYD88*[L265P], *CD79B* mutations, and extranodal tropism (cluster 5); (2) low-risk ABC DLBCLs with genetic features of an extrafollicular, possibly marginal zone, origin (cluster 1); (3) high-risk GCB DLBCLs with *BCL2* structural variants, inactivating mutations and/or copy loss of *PTEN* and alterations of epigenetic enzymes (cluster 3); (4) a newly defined group of low-risk GCB DLBCLs with distinct alterations in JAK/STAT and BRAF pathway components and multiple histones (cluster 4); and (5) an ABC/GCB-independent group of tumors with biallelic inactivation of *TP53*, 9p21.3/*CDKN2A* copy loss and associated genomic instability (cluster 2). The genetically distinct subtypes were found to have significant differences in PFS, with a significantly higher risk of relapse in cluster 5 ABC DLBCL and cluster 3 GCB DLBCL.

These recent comprehensive genomic analyses have shed light on the previously unappreciated genomic complexity of DLBCL, the limitations of gene expression-based classification systems, and the challenge of adopting a uniform treatment approach in this disease. They also suggest specific therapeutic approaches to genomically characterized subsets. For example, although ibrutinib did not improve outcomes when added to chemotherapy for patients with non-GCB DLBCL, there may be a role for BTK inhibition in distinct genomic subtypes of DLBCL, such as in patients with *CD79B/MYD88*[L265P] double mutations[42] or those within the high-risk ABC DLBCLs, with near-uniform *BCL2* copy gain, and frequently activating *MYD88*[L265P] and *CD79B* mutations, as recently described (cluster 5).[6,42] Similarly, there may be a role for other targeted therapies, including EZH2, PI3K, and BCL-2 inhibitors in distinct genomic subtypes of DLBCL. In fact, preclinical work has already identified preferential activity of targeted therapies in individual genomic subtypes of DLBCL that may have clinical implications.[43] Prospective clinical trials are required to validate the use of genomic classifications and to determine whether they can be used to guide the use of targeted therapy.

USE OF GENOMIC INFORMATION IN PATIENTS

Although major progress has been made in understanding the genomic landscape of DLBCL, this understanding has not yet translated into clinical success. Some of the limitations of using comprehensive genomic analyses for therapy selection include the high cost, long turn-around times, and necessary access to sophisticated sequencing platforms that are typically restricted to research centers. Further distillation of genomic data into more limited and more broadly useable sequencing panels will likely be necessary for the short-term deployment of genomically driven treatment strategies. In addition, continued investigation of the role of liquid biopsies, in which tumor DNA from the peripheral blood serves as a surrogate for tumor biopsies, may improve the availability of genomic information and provide a means to track genomic changes with time.[44] Overall, the expansion of genomic data and more sophisticated classification methods currently under development hold great promise to transform the treatment approach to this disease and to improve the outcomes for those with high-risk disease.

REFERENCES

1. Teras LR, DeSantis CE, Cerhan JR, et al. 2016 US lymphoid malignancy statistics by World Health Organization subtypes. CA Cancer J Clin 2016;66(6):443–59.
2. Sehn LH, Donaldson J, Chhanabhai M, et al. Introduction of combined CHOP plus rituximab therapy dramatically improved outcome of diffuse large B-cell lymphoma in British Columbia. J Clin Oncol 2005;23(22):5027–33.

3. Philip T, Guglielmi C, Hagenbeek A, et al. Autologous bone marrow transplantation as compared with salvage chemotherapy in relapses of chemotherapy-sensitive non-Hodgkin's lymphoma. N Engl J Med 1995;333(23):1540–5.
4. Crump M, Neelapu SS, Farooq U, et al. Outcomes in refractory diffuse large B-cell lymphoma: results from the international SCHOLAR-1 study. Blood 2017; 130(16):1800–8.
5. Neelapu SS, Locke FL, Bartlett NL, et al. Axicabtagene ciloleucel CAR T-cell therapy in refractory large B-cell lymphoma. N Engl J Med 2017;377(26):2531–44.
6. Chapuy B, Stewart C, Dunford AJ, et al. Molecular subtypes of diffuse large B cell lymphoma are associated with distinct pathogenic mechanisms and outcomes. Nat Med 2018;24(5):679–90.
7. Basso K, Dalla-Favera R. Germinal centres and B cell lymphomagenesis. Nat Rev Immunol 2015;15(3):172–84.
8. Monti S, Chapuy B, Takeyama K, et al. Integrative analysis reveals an outcome-associated and targetable pattern of p53 and cell cycle deregulation in diffuse large B cell lymphoma. Cancer Cell 2012;22(3):359–72.
9. International Non-Hodgkin's Lymphoma Prognostic Factors Project. A predictive model for aggressive non-Hodgkin's lymphoma. N Engl J Med 1993;329(14): 987–94.
10. Ziepert M, Hasenclever D, Kuhnt E, et al. Standard International prognostic index remains a valid predictor of outcome for patients with aggressive CD20+ B-cell lymphoma in the rituximab era. J Clin Oncol 2010;28(14):2373–80.
11. Alizadeh AA, Eisen MB, Davis RE, et al. Distinct types of diffuse large B-cell lymphoma identified by gene expression profiling. Nature 2000;403(6769):503–11.
12. Rosenwald A, Wright G, Chan WC, et al. The use of molecular profiling to predict survival after chemotherapy for diffuse large-B-cell lymphoma. N Engl J Med 2002;346(25):1937–47.
13. Pasqualucci L, Dalla-Favera R. Genetics of diffuse large B-cell lymphoma. Blood 2018;131(21):2307–19.
14. Bea S, Zettl A, Wright G, et al. Diffuse large B-cell lymphoma subgroups have distinct genetic profiles that influence tumor biology and improve gene-expression-based survival prediction. Blood 2005;106(9):3183–90.
15. Lenz G, Wright G, Dave SS, et al. Stromal gene signatures in large-B-cell lymphomas. N Engl J Med 2008;359(22):2313–23.
16. Staiger AM, Ziepert M, Horn H, et al. Clinical impact of the cell-of-origin classification and the MYC/BCL2 dual expresser status in diffuse large B-cell lymphoma treated within prospective clinical trials of the German High-Grade Non-Hodgkin's Lymphoma Study Group. J Clin Oncol 2017;35(22):2515–26.
17. Hans CP, Weisenburger DD, Greiner TC, et al. Confirmation of the molecular classification of diffuse large B-cell lymphoma by immunohistochemistry using a tissue microarray. Blood 2004;103(1):275–82.
18. Meyer PN, Fu K, Greiner TC, et al. Immunohistochemical methods for predicting cell of origin and survival in patients with diffuse large B-cell lymphoma treated with rituximab. J Clin Oncol 2011;29(2):200–7.
19. Monti S, Savage KJ, Kutok JL, et al. Molecular profiling of diffuse large B-cell lymphoma identifies robust subtypes including one characterized by host inflammatory response. Blood 2005;105(5):1851–61.
20. Green TM, Young KH, Visco C, et al. Immunohistochemical double-hit score is a strong predictor of outcome in patients with diffuse large B-cell lymphoma treated with rituximab plus cyclophosphamide, doxorubicin, vincristine, and prednisone. J Clin Oncol 2012;30(28):3460–7.

21. Johnson NA, Savage KJ, Ludkovski O, et al. Lymphomas with concurrent BCL2 and MYC translocations: the critical factors associated with survival. Blood 2009;114(11):2273–9.

22. Ennishi D, Jiang A, Boyle M, et al. Double-hit gene expression signature defines a distinct subgroup of germinal center B-cell-like diffuse large B-cell lymphoma. J Clin Oncol 2019;37(3):190–201.

23. Sha C, Barrans S, Cucco F, et al. Molecular high-grade B-cell lymphoma: defining a poor-risk group that requires different approaches to therapy. J Clin Oncol 2019;37(3):202–12.

24. Herrera AF, Mei M, Low L, et al. Relapsed or refractory double-expressor and double-hit lymphomas have inferior progression-free survival after autologous stem-cell transplantation. J Clin Oncol 2017;35(1):24–31.

25. Wilson W, sin-Ho J, Pitcher B, et al. Phase III randomized study of R-CHOP versus DA-EPOCH-R and molecular analysis of untreated diffuse large B-cell lymphoma: CALGB/alliance 50303. Blood 2016;128:469.

26. Oki Y, Noorani M, Lin P, et al. Double hit lymphoma: the MD Anderson Cancer Center clinical experience. Br J Haematol 2014;166(6):891–901.

27. Petrich AM, Gandhi M, Jovanovic B, et al. Impact of induction regimen and stem cell transplantation on outcomes in double-hit lymphoma: a multicenter retrospective analysis. Blood 2014;124(15):2354–61.

28. Dunleavy K, Pittaluga S, Czuczman MS, et al. Differential efficacy of bortezomib plus chemotherapy within molecular subtypes of diffuse large B-cell lymphoma. Blood 2009;113(24):6069–76.

29. Ruan J, Martin P, Furman RR, et al. Bortezomib plus CHOP-rituximab for previously untreated diffuse large B-cell lymphoma and mantle cell lymphoma. J Clin Oncol 2011;29(6):690–7.

30. Leonard JP, Kolibaba KS, Reeves JA, et al. Randomized phase II study of R-CHOP with or without bortezomib in previously untreated patients with non-germinal center B-cell-like diffuse large B-cell lymphoma. J Clin Oncol 2017;35(31):3538–46.

31. Wilson WH, Young RM, Schmitz R, et al. Targeting B cell receptor signaling with ibrutinib in diffuse large B cell lymphoma. Nat Med 2015;21(8):922–6.

32. Younes A, Sehn LH, Johnson P, et al. Randomized Phase III Trial of Ibrutinib and Rituximab Plus Cyclophosphamide, Doxorubicin, Vincristine, and Prednisone in Non-Germinal Center B-Cell Diffuse Large B-Cell Lymphoma. J Clin Oncol 2019. [Epub ahead of print].

33. Castellino A, Chiappella A, LaPlant BR, et al. Lenalidomide plus R-CHOP21 in newly diagnosed diffuse large B-cell lymphoma (DLBCL): long-term follow-up results from a combined analysis from two phase 2 trials. Blood Cancer J 2018;8(11):108.

34. Nowakowski GS, LaPlant B, Macon WR, et al. Lenalidomide combined with R-CHOP overcomes negative prognostic impact of non-germinal center B-cell phenotype in newly diagnosed diffuse large B-cell lymphoma: a phase II study. J Clin Oncol 2015;33(3):251–7.

35. Nowakowski GS, Chiappella A, Witzig TE, et al. ROBUST: lenalidomide-R-CHOP versus placebo-R-CHOP in previously untreated ABC-type diffuse large B-cell lymphoma. Future Oncol 2016;12(13):1553–63.

36. King RL, Nowakowski GS, Witzig TE, et al. Rapid, real time pathology review for ECOG/ACRIN 1412: a novel and successful paradigm for future lymphoma clinical trials in the precision medicine era. Blood Cancer J 2018;8(3):27.

37. Morin RD, Mendez-Lago M, Mungall AJ, et al. Frequent mutation of histone-modifying genes in non-Hodgkin lymphoma. Nature 2011;476(7360):298–303.
38. Pasqualucci L, Trifonov V, Fabbri G, et al. Analysis of the coding genome of diffuse large B-cell lymphoma. Nat Genet 2011;43(9):830–7.
39. Lohr JG, Stojanov P, Lawrence MS, et al. Discovery and prioritization of somatic mutations in diffuse large B-cell lymphoma (DLBCL) by whole-exome sequencing. Proc Natl Acad Sci U S A 2012;109(10):3879–84.
40. Reddy A, Zhang J, Davis NS, et al. Genetic and functional drivers of diffuse large B cell lymphoma. Cell 2017;171(2):481–94.e15.
41. Karube K, Enjuanes A, Dlouhy I, et al. Integrating genomic alterations in diffuse large B-cell lymphoma identifies new relevant pathways and potential therapeutic targets. Leukemia 2018;32(3):675–84.
42. Schmitz R, Wright GW, Huang DW, et al. Genetics and pathogenesis of diffuse large B-cell lymphoma. N Engl J Med 2018;378(15):1396–407.
43. Bojarczuk K, Wienand K, Ryan JA, et al. Targeted inhibition of PI3Kalpha/delta is synergistic with BCL-2 blockade in genetically defined subtypes of DLBCL. Blood 2019;133(1):70–80.
44. Scherer F, Kurtz DM, Newman AM, et al. Distinct biological subtypes and patterns of genome evolution in lymphoma revealed by circulating tumor DNA. Sci Transl Med 2016;8(364):364ra155.

Burkitt Lymphoma and Other High-Grade B-Cell Lymphomas with or without MYC, BCL2, and/or BCL6 Rearrangements

Rami Alsharif, MD, Kieron Dunleavy, MD*

KEYWORDS

- Burkitt lymphoma • Risk-adapted • High-grade B-cell lymphoma
- MYC with BCL2 and/or BCL6

KEY POINTS

- Burkitt lymphoma (BL) is a highly curable aggressive lymphoma, and although young patients have excellent outcomes, toxicity with standard approaches is a challenge to delivering optimal therapy in older patients.
- Currently "intermediate" intensity approaches are being developed with the goal of maintaining high cure rates but with much less toxicity.
- There are aggressive B-cell lymphomas that have features in between BL and diffuse large B-cell lymphoma (DLBCL), and in a recent revision to the WHO Classification these have been categorized separately from BL or DLBCL and are called high-grade B-cell lymphoma (HGBCL) with or without *MYC*, *BCL2*, and *BCL6* translocations.
- Recent progress in elucidating and understanding the molecular biology of BL and HGBL has identified many novel and critical targets for rational drug development in the future.

INTRODUCTION

Since the publication of the fourth edition of the World Health Organization (WHO) Classification of Hematopoietic and Lymphoid Tumors in 2008, the authors have made significant strides in better understanding the pathobiology and clinical characteristics of highly aggressive B-cell lymphomas. This led to a major revision in 2016, which serves as an update to the fourth edition.[1] Although Burkitt lymphoma

Dr R. Alsharif has no disclosures. Dr K. Dunleavy has had consultant/advisory roles for Abbvie, Adaptive, Amgen, Celgene, Janssen, Seattle Genetics, Pharmacyclics, Kite.
George Washington University Cancer Center, Department of Hematology and Oncology, 2150 Pennsylvania Avenue, Washington, DC 20037, USA
* Corresponding author.
E-mail address: kdunleavy@mfa.gwu.edu

Hematol Oncol Clin N Am 33 (2019) 587–596
https://doi.org/10.1016/j.hoc.2019.04.001
0889-8588/19/© 2019 Elsevier Inc. All rights reserved.

hemonc.theclinics.com

(BL), characterized by the translocation and deregulation of the *MYC* gene is a well-defined entity, there exists a subset of aggressive B-cell lymphomas (previously categorized as diffuse large B-cell lymphoma [DLBCL]) that are not. These frequently have Burkitt-like features, distinct morphology, and often harbor genetic aberrations such as rearrangements of *MYC* and *BCL2*. They are also associated with an inferior outcome compared with DLBCLs without these features. This group of high-grade B-cell lymphomas (HGBLs) have been recognized for years and were captured in previous classification systems under various labels such as "B-cell lymphoma un-classifiable (BCLU) with features intermediate between DLBCL and BL" (2008 WHO classification). Such labels are now obsolete. The current revision proposes a distinct category called "HGBL with or without *MYC*, *BCL2*, and/or *BCL6* translo-cations"—the nontranslocated cases are called HGBL, not otherwise specified (NOS). In the revision, BL cases that lack a *MYC* translocation are included in a pro-visional entity called "Burkitt-like Lymphoma with 11q aberration."[1] This new revision is helpful in developing new and hopefully more effective approaches for these diseases.

BURKITT LYMPHOMA

BL is a rare and highly aggressive B-cell lymphoma. It was first described over 50 years ago by Denis Burkitt in Ugandan children with unusual jaw tumors in association with other specific anatomic sites.[2] This "endemic" variant occurs in equatorial Africa and other specific geographic regions and typically affects men between the ages of 4 and 7 years (**Table 1**).[3] Sporadic BL affects children and young adults in all world regions and also has a male predominance.[4] Immunodeficiency-associated BL is associated with the human immunodeficiency virus (HIV) virus and typically affects men with rela-tively preserved immune function.[5]

Pathobiology of Burkitt Lymphoma

BL has a very high proliferative/apoptotic rate, and this accounts for its classic "starry sky pattern" observed on low magnification under the microscope. At higher power, BL tumor cells are classically monomorphic; intermediate in size; and contain round nuclei, multiple dark nucleoli, and basophilic cytoplasm.[6] BL is derived from a germinal center B-cell, with tumor cells expressing B-cell–associated antigens (CD19, CD20, CD22, CD79a) and germinal center–associated markers (CD10 and BCL6). BL lacks expression of CD5, B-cell leukemia/lymphoma 2 (BCL2), terminal deoxynucleotidyl transferase (TdT), and typically CD23. BCL6 staining is independent of the presence of a BCL6 gene rearrangement.[7] Epstein-Barr virus (EBV) is virtually always present in endemic BL and in 25% to 40% of sporadic and immunodeficiency-associated cases.[8] The pathogenetic role that EBV plays in the disease is poorly understood. Virtually all cases of BL harbor a *MYC* translocation, typically between the long arm of chromosome 8, the site of the *MYC* gene (8q24), and 1 of 3 immunoglobulin genes.[9] In more than 80% of cases, the translocation partner in the *MYC* breakpoint is the immunoglobulin heavy chain (IgH) gene on chromosome 14; in the remaining cases translocations involve the kappa (15%) and lambda (5%) light-chain loci on chromo-somes 2 and 22. *MYC* breakpoints can vary in location between sporadic and endemic cases, suggesting distinct pathogenetic mechanisms.[10,11] Recently RNA sequencing studies identified other genes apart from *MYC* that are involved in BL. In approxi-mately 70% of cases there are mutations in *TCF3* or its negative regulator ID3, which encodes a protein that blocks *TCF3* activity. Thirty-eight percent of sporadic BL cases harbor a mutation in *CCDN3*, which is activated by *TCF3*, and encodes cyclin D3,

Table 1
Comparison of endemic, sporadic, and human immunodeficiency virus–associated Burkitt lymphoma

	Endemic	Sporadic	HIV-Associated
Epidemiology	Equatorial Africa, South America, Papua New Guinea	Worldwide	Worldwide
Incidence	5–10 cases/100,000	2–3 cases/1,000000	6 cases/1000
Age/Gender	4–7 y	Median age: 30 y	Median age: 44 y
EBV +	100%	25%–40%	25%–40%
Clinical Presentation	Jaw and facial bones: approx. 50%. Ileo-cecum and gonads. Increased risk of CNS disease.	Ileo-cecum most common. Other sites may include bone marrow, ovaries, kidneys, and breasts. Increased risk of CNS disease.	Nodal presentation most common. Bone marrow sometimes involved. Increased risk of CNS dissemination.

Abbreviations: CNS, central nervous system; EBV, Epstein–Barr virus.
Adapted from Dunleavy K, Little RF, Wilson WH. Update on Burkitt Lymphoma. Hematol Oncol Clin North Am 2016; 30(6): 1334; with permission.

which promotes cell cycle progression. *TCF3* and/or *ID3* mutations are also found in 40% of endemic cases of BL.[12–14]

Some recent studies have identified lymphomas that resemble BL morphologically and by gene expression profiling but lack *MYC*-translocation negative. These have a chromosome 11q alteration and in the revised 2016 classification are provisionally included in a new entity called "Burkitt-like Lymphoma with 11q aberration." Although they are more complex karyotypically than other *MYC*-rearranged (MYC-R) BL, albeit small numbers, they have a good outcome.

Clinical Presentation and Workup

Clinical presentation varies according to the epidemiologic variant as well as additional factors. In the United States, sporadic and immunodeficiency-associated BL are the subtypes that are encountered, and in both, the ileo-cecum is the most common site of involvement. Central nervous system (CNS) involvement (typically lepto-meningeal rather than parenchymal) may occur at presentation especially in advanced stage disease. Because of the high proliferation rate of BL, there is a high risk of tumor lysis syndrome (TLS) developing after instituting of therapy (or before ["auto" tumor lysis]), and TLS prophylaxis should be considered and instituted as appropriate. In diagnosing BL, the distinction from other (non-BL) B-cell lymphomas that harbor a *MYC* translocation is important and can sometimes be challenging. In addition to routine laboratory and imaging studies (including screening for HIV and hepatitis), a bone marrow biopsy should be performed and cerebrospinal fluid analyzed for tumor cells by cytology and flow cytometry. The Ann Arbor classification is widely used for staging in adults. There is no validated prognostic score in BL but population-based studies have identified prognostic factors such as age, black race, advanced stage, performance stage, and elevated lactate dehydrogenase (LDH).[15–18] Many studies have identified a low-risk category of BL characterized by normal LDH; Eastern Cooperative Oncology Group performance status 0 or 1; Ann Arbor stage 1 or II plus no mass size greater than 7 or 10 cm.[19,20]

Treatment of Burkitt Lymphoma

Because BL is a systemic disease, chemotherapy is needed for all stages. Early therapeutic strategies were modeled on acute lymphoblastic leukemia (ALL) approaches in pediatrics, and although highly effective in young patients, toxicity limited efficacy in older patients. Today, there remains a therapeutic challenge in older and immunocompromised patients with BL due to poor tolerability of intensive approaches—risk-adapted therapy (where lower-risk patients receive less intensive regimens) has been helpful in some studies but there remains an unmet need to develop optimal approaches that maintain high cure rates with low toxicity in these populations.[21] The development of tumor lysis syndrome is an important consideration in initial BL therapeutics and to mitigate the risk of this, several regimens incorporate a pretreatment phase in which low-dose cyclophosphamide and prednisone is administered initially. The high risk of CNS disease is typically addressed by using methotrexate and cytarabine—CNS prophylaxis is also typically used to reduce the risk of CNS relapse.[22]

Current therapeutic approaches in adults can be broadly categorized as follows (**Table 2**): intensive, short-duration, combination chemotherapy (eg, R-CODOX-M/IVAC, CALGB 9251); ALL-like therapy with stepwise induction, consolidation, and maintenance phases (eg, CALGB 8811, R-HyperCVAD [cyclophosphamide, vincristine, doxorubicin, and dexamethasone]); and infusional regimens such as EPOCH-R. Risk-adapted therapy is used commonly in low-risk patients receiving modifications of these approaches. CODOX-M/IVAC (cyclophosphamide, doxorubicin, vincristine, methotrexate/ifosfamide, cytarabine and etoposide)—the "Magrath regimen"—has been one of the most widely used approaches, and during its initial development, patients were risk stratified according to clinical presentation and LDH level.[23] Low-risk patients received 3 cycles of CODOX-M, whereas high-risk patients received 4 cycles of alternating CODOX-M with IVAC. In the initial report, 41 patients (median age: 25 years) were evaluated and the 2-year event-free survival rate

Table 2
Selected published regimens in Burkitt and high-grade B-cell lymphoma

Regimen	Pt N	Median Age yrs (Range)	Stage (%)	Survival
CODOX-M/IVAC[23]	21 (peds) 20 (adult)	12 (3–17) 25 (18–59)	III–IV 78%	EFS 85% (peds) and 100% (adults) @ 2 y
dmCODOX-M/IVAC[20]	53	37 (17–76)	III–IV 76%	PFS 64% @ 2 y
Hyper-CVAD[24]	26	58 (17–79)	N/A	OS 49% @ 3 y
R-Hyper-CVAD[25]	31	46 (17–77)	N/A	EFS 80% @ 3 y
GMALL-B-ALL/NHL 2002[30]	363	42 (16–85)	III–IV 71%	PFS 71% @ 5 y
DA-EPOCH-R SC-EPOCH-RR[27]	19 11	25 (15–88) 44 (24–60)	III–IV 58% III–IV 82%	FFP 95% @ 7 y FFP 100% @ 6 y
LMB ± R[29]	260	N/A	III–IV 62%	EFS 75% vs 62% (+R vs −R) @ 3 y
AMC 048. Modified R-CODOX-M/IVAC[32]	34	42 (19–55)	III–IV 74%	PFS 69% @ 1 y
RA-DA-EPOCH-R[28]	113	49 (18–86)	III–IV 64%	PFS 86% @ 3 y
DA-EPOCH-R[44] (MYC-R DLBCL)	53	61 (29–80)	III–IV 81%	EFS 71% @ 4 y

Abbreviations: EFS, event-free survival; OS, overall survival; PFS, progression-free survival.

(EFS) was 92%. Other groups have confirmed the efficacy of this regimen albeit with lower survival rates. In one prospective, nonrandomized trial of 53 patients treated with risk-adjusted, dose-modified CODOX-M/IVAC, 2-year progression free survival (PFS) and overall survival (OS) were 64% and 67%, respectively.[20] Hyperfractionated CVAD was based on a modification of a pediatric L3 ALL regimen. In the initial report, 26 adults with newly diagnosed BL were treated and complete remission was seen in 81% and the 3-year OS was 49%.[24] A subsequent study looked at the addition of rituximab to this regimen and this augmented OS to 89%.[25] Dose-adjusted (DA) EPOCH-R (etoposide, prednisone, vincristine, cyclophosphamide, doxorubicin, and rituximab) is an intermediate intensity strategy that was tested in BL, due to its high efficacy in DLBCL and its hypothetical ability to overcome high tumor proliferation.[26,27] An early small single-center study testing the strategy in 30 patients demonstrated a freedom from progression rate of greater than 90% with low toxicity and very low rates of tumor lysis syndrome. Recently, early multicenter results of this approach were reported where low-risk patients received 3 cycles of therapy and high-risk received 6. In 113 patients, PFS was 100% and greater than 80% in low-risk and high-risk groups, respectively at more than 2 years follow-up.[28] Older age or HIV status had no significant impact on outcome. The group with CNS involvement at diagnosis fared poorly compared with those who were CNS negative, but it is not clear how much overlap there was with other high-risk characteristics and an analysis is ongoing to further investigate this. To compare this approach to "standard" therapy, a randomized trial comparing DA-EPOCH-R with R-CODOX-M/R-IVAC is currently ongoing.

One hundred twelve of 116 planned patients have been enrolled; 110 who completed at least 1 cycle of therapy are included in this analysis. Characteristics include median (range) age 48 (19–86) years with 53 (48%) patients aged 50 years or older and 29 (26%) patients aged 60 years or older: male sex 86 (78%); stage III or IV disease 76 (69%); elevated LDH 73 (66%); CNS involvement 11 (10%); and HIV positive 29 (26%). The frequency of bone marrow disease is under evaluation. Thirteen (12%) and 97 (88%) patients were classified as LR and HR, respectively. There were 6 deaths in the hazard ratio (HR) arm not attributed to disease progression/relapse: 2 deaths due to infection and 1 death each attributed to respiratory failure, second malignancy, myocardial infarction, and unknown. All other reported toxicities were expected toxicities of DA-EPOCH-R. With a median follow-up of 34 months, the progression-free survival (PFS) for all patients beyond 10.2 months is 84.6% (95% confidence interval [CI]: 75.6%–90.4%), time-to-progression is 91.1% (95% CI: 82.8%–95.4%), and OS is 84.7% (95% CI: 75.4%–90.7%). Age (>40 years vs <40 years) and HIV status did not affect survival (see **Table 2**). PFS for low-risk patients was 100% and 82% for high-risk patients. Notably, only 1 patient who progressed after DA-EPOCH-R was successfully salvaged and is still alive.

Incorporation of Rituximab

The success of rituximab in DLBCL prompted its testing in BL. Several small single-arm studies suggested that adding rituximab may improve outcomes and this was confirmed in a multicenter, randomized phase 3 trial—260 adults with previously untreated HIV-negative BL were randomly assigned to receive dose-dense chemotherapy with or without rituximab and at 38-month follow-up, adding rituximab improved EFS from 62% to 75% with no differences in adverse event rate.[29] Further support for rituximab comes from nonrandomized trials—one of the largest was a prospective, multicenter German study in which 363 patients were treated with short-duration intensive combination chemotherapy with rituximab. OS and PFS were

80% and 71%, respectively.[30] Recent evidence from pediatric group studies also supports the use of rituximab in BL.[31]

HIV-Associated Burkitt Lymphoma

Historically and particularly in the preantiretroviral era, HIV-associated BL was approached less aggressively than HIV-negative BL. As a result, outcomes were inferior for this population of patients. Today most people who develop BL in the setting of HIV do not have advanced immunosuppression and should receive similar therapy to HIV-negative counterparts. Recently outcomes have been similar irrespective of HIV status.[21,32]

Relapsed/refractory BL is uncommon and is usually associated with very short survival. There is no standard approach for these patients and clinical trials should be considered.

HIGH-GRADE B-CELL LYMPHOMA ± MYC AND BCL2 AND/OR BCL6 REARRANGEMENTS

It has long been appreciated that DLBCL are molecularly heterogeneous in terms of cell of origin (COO), oncogenic mutations, and deregulated signaling pathways.[33–35] Although most cases of DLBCL can be classified according to their COO (activated B-cell [ABC] versus germinal center B-cell [GCB]) and this has prognostic implications, it is clear that biological factors other than COO may also predict worse outcomes in aggressive B-cell lymphomas. In particular, rearrangements of *MYC* alone or in combination with secondary hits like *BCL2* and/or *BCL6* (double-hit and triple-hit lymphomas) are associated with inferior survivals.[36,37] There are also highly aggressive lymphomas that morphologically are intermediate between DLBCL and BL but without the aforementioned rearrangements, and this group also likely do worse but have not been extensively studied. In this respect, the new category as per the 2016 revision "HGBL with or without *MYC*, *BCL2* and/or *BCL6* rearrangements" is very helpful in defining a group of aggressive B-cell lymphomas with poorer biology and more adverse outcomes (**Fig. 1**). It is important to identify these rearrangements in addition to predicting a more aggressive course, they may have better outcomes with more intensive therapies than R-CHOP and are associated with a high risk of CNS involvement.[38] Although dual translocated cases (*MYC* with *BCL2* and/or *BCL6*) do particularly poorly with standard therapy, albeit controversial, many studies suggest that MYC-R alone "single-hit" cases, also have an inferior outcome compared with other DLBCLs (these are not included in the 2016 revised category).[39–41]

Treatment Approach for High-grade B-cell Lymphomas

Several algorithms have been proposed in an attempt at limiting FISH testing, including testing lymphomas of the GCB subtype by IHC, testing lymphomas with very high proliferation indices (Ki-67), or testing lymphomas that express MYC by IHC.[42] However, limiting testing to those subsets may lead to underrecognition. Currently, it is recommended that all large cell lymphomas be evaluated for double-hit status by FISH if resources permit. If resources preclude this approach, an acceptable but inferior alternative is to limit testing to those lymphomas of the GCB subtype that express MYC by IHC.[38] All patients should undergo routine staging procedures as per other aggressive B-cell lymphomas. Given the statistically higher risk of CNS involvement in patients with HGBLs, it is also recommended that patients undergo a lumbar puncture to exclude leptomeningeal disease.[38]

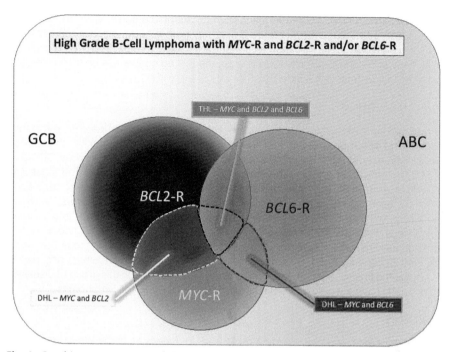

Fig. 1. Graphic representation of the new category of aggressive B-cell lymphomas, "HGBL with MYC and BCL2 and/or BCL6 rearrangements," described in the 2016 revision to the WHO Classification of Tumors of Hematopoietic and Lymphoid Tumors (2008). Most cases with MYC and BCL2 rearrangements are of GCB origin, whereas most cases with BCL6 rearrangements are of ABC origin. This category includes double-hit lymphomas that involve MYC and BCL2 or MYC and BCL6 and triple hit lymphomas that involve MYC, BCL2, and BCL6. (*Modified from* Dunleavy K. Aggressive B cell Lymphoma: Optimal Therapy for MYC-positive, Double-Hit, and Triple-Hit DLBCL. Curr Treat Options Oncol 2015; 16(12): 58; with permission.)

Numerous retrospective studies have demonstrated that patients with HGBL with translocations involving *MYC*, *BCL2*, and or *BCL6* do poorly with conventional chemo-immunotherapy (R-CHOP).[43] The inferior prognosis of these lymphomas following R-CHOP and improved outcome (in retrospective studies) following more intensive approaches prompted the recommendation of more aggressive approaches (than R-CHOP) as outlined in the National Comprehensive Cancer Network guidance (version 4.2018). It is unclear what the optimal "more intensive" strategy is for these patients, but regimens that are used in BL are favored by many. As in the treatment of BL, tolerability must be carefully considered in selecting up-front therapy, as most of these patients are in their seventh and eighth decade of life. The NCI/US intergroup just completed the first prospective single-arm study of DA-EPOCH-R therapy in 53 patients with MYC-R aggressive B-cell lymphomas.[44] Of those, 19 patients had a single MYC rearrangement "single hit" and 23 patients had rearrangements also involving *BCL2* and or *BCL6* "double hit." At a median follow-up of 55.6 months, the 48-month EFS and OS for patients with MYC-R aggressive B-cell lymphomas was 71% and 77%, respectively. Similarly, in patients with "double-hit" lymphomas the EFS and OS were 73.4% and 82%, respectively. Patients with MYC-R alone had a marginally worse outcome compared with those with "double-hit" lymphomas.[45] All patients in this study received CNS prophylaxis. In addition, it is recommended that patients be considered for CNS pro-phylaxis with intrathecal methotrexate if they have extra nodal disease, an elevated LDH, or have other CNS risk factors.[46] For those NOS tumors that are high grade without any *MYC* and *BCL2* rearrangements, there is no consensus on their manage-ment and clinical trials are needed.

FUTURE DIRECTIONS

Although young patients with BL have excellent outcomes with standard BL regimens, treatment-related toxicity (even with "risk adaptation" using less intensive therapy for low-risk disease) curtails the routine use of standard approaches such as CODOX-M/IVAC in many adult groups. Therefore, new approaches are needed and these are being developed. In BL, key molecular aberrations other than *MYC* continue to be discov-ered and present interesting targets for new drugs such as PI3 kinase inhibitors, inhibitors of *CDK6*, and inhibitors of *MYC*. Ultimately, as novel agents are incorporated into up-front BL regimens, they offer the possibility of curative strategies with less reliance on highly toxic agents. The recent separate categorization of HGBLs including those that have *MYC* and *BCL2* and/or *BCL6* rearrangements is a welcome advancement and paves the way for the investigation of new strategies and novel agents in this group of diseases that currently have a worse outcome than other aggressive B-cell lymphomas.

REFERENCES

1. Swerdlow SH, Campo E, Pileri SA, et al. The 2016 revision of the World Health Or-ganization classification of lymphoid neoplasms. Blood 2016;127(20):2375–90.
2. Burkitt D. A sarcoma involving the jaws in African children. Br J Surg 1958; 46(197):218–23.
3. Magrath I. Epidemiology: clues to the pathogenesis of Burkitt lymphoma. Br J Haematol 2012;156(6):744–56.
4. Armitage JO, Weisenburger DD. New approach to classifying non-Hodgkin's lym-phomas: clinical features of the major histologic subtypes. Non-Hodgkin's Lym-phoma Classification Project. J Clin Oncol 1998;16(8):2780–95.
5. Guech-Ongey M, Simard EP, Anderson WF, et al. AIDS-related Burkitt lymphoma in the United States: what do age and CD4 lymphocyte patterns tell us about eti-ology and/or biology? Blood 2010;116(25):5600–4.
6. Campo E, Swerdlow SH, Harris NL, et al. The 2008 WHO classification of lymphoid neoplasms and beyond: evolving concepts and practical applications. Blood 2011;117(19):5019–32.
7. Falini B, Fizzotti M, Pileri S, et al. Bcl-6 protein expression in normal and neoplastic lymphoid tissues. Ann Oncol 1997;8(Suppl 2):101–4.
8. Kelly GL, Rickinson AB. Burkitt lymphoma: revisiting the pathogenesis of a virus-associated malignancy. Hematology Am Soc Hematol Educ Program 2007;1:277–84.
9. Dalla-Favera R, Bregni M, Erikson J, et al. Human c-myc onc gene is located on the region of chromosome 8 that is translocated in Burkitt lymphoma cells. Proc Natl Acad Sci U S A 1982;79(24):7824–7.
10. Lenze D, Leoncini L, Hummel M, et al. The different epidemiologic subtypes of Burkitt lymphoma share a homogenous micro RNA profile distinct from diffuse large B-cell lymphoma. Leukemia 2011;25(12):1869–76.
11. Piccaluga PP, De Falco G, Kustagi M, et al. Gene expression analysis uncovers similarity and differences among Burkitt lymphoma subtypes. Blood 2011; 117(13):3596–608.

12. Schmitz R, Young RM, Ceribelli M, et al. Burkitt lymphoma pathogenesis and therapeutic targets from structural and functional genomics. Nature 2012;490(7418):116–20.

13. Love C, Sun Z, Jima D, et al. The genetic landscape of mutations in Burkitt lymphoma. Nat Genet 2012;44(12):1321–5.

14. Richter J, Schlesner M, Hoffmann S, et al. Recurrent mutation of the ID3 gene in Burkitt lymphoma identified by integrated genome, exome and transcriptome sequencing. Nat Genet 2012;44(12):1316–20.

15. Castillo JJ, Nadeem O. Improving the accuracy in prognosis for Burkitt lymphoma patients. Expert Rev Anticancer Ther 2014;14(2):125–7.

16. Castillo JJ, Winer ES, Olszewski AJ. Population-based prognostic factors for survival in patients with Burkitt lymphoma: an analysis from the Surveillance, Epidemiology, and End Results database. Cancer 2013;119(20):3672–9.

17. Wasterlid T, Brown PN, Hagberg O, et al. Impact of chemotherapy regimen and rituximab in adult Burkitt lymphoma: a retrospective population-based study from the Nordic Lymphoma Group. Ann Oncol 2013;24(7):1879–86.

18. Wasterlid T, Jonsson B, Hagberg H, et al. Population based study of prognostic factors and treatment in adult Burkitt lymphoma: a Swedish Lymphoma Registry study. Leuk Lymphoma 2011;52(11):2090–6.

19. Mead GM, Sydes MR, Walewski J, et al. An international evaluation of CODOX-M and CODOX-M alternating with IVAC in adult Burkitt's lymphoma: results of United Kingdom Lymphoma Group LY06 study. Ann Oncol 2002;13(8):1264–74.

20. Mead GM, Barrans SL, Qian W, et al. A prospective clinicopathologic study of dose-modified CODOX-M/IVAC in patients with sporadic Burkitt lymphoma defined using cytogenetic and immunophenotypic criteria (MRC/NCRI LY10 trial). Blood 2008;112(6):2248–60.

21. Dunleavy K. Approach to the diagnosis and treatment of adult Burkitt's lymphoma. J Oncol Pract 2018;14(11):665–71.

22. Sariban E, Edwards B, Janus C, et al. Central nervous system involvement in American Burkitt's lymphoma. J Clin Oncol 1983;1(11):677–81.

23. Magrath I, Adde M, Shad A, et al. Adults and children with small non-cleaved-cell lymphoma have a similar excellent outcome when treated with the same chemotherapy regimen. J Clin Oncol 1996;14(3):925–34.

24. Thomas DA, Cortes J, O'Brien S, et al. Hyper-CVAD program in Burkitt's-type adult acute lymphoblastic leukemia. J Clin Oncol 1999;17(8):2461–70.

25. Thomas DA, Faderl S, O'Brien S, et al. Chemoimmunotherapy with hyper-CVAD plus rituximab for the treatment of adult Burkitt and Burkitt-type lymphoma or acute lymphoblastic leukemia. Cancer 2006;106(7):1569–80.

26. Wilson WH, Dunleavy K, Pittaluga S, et al. Phase II study of dose-adjusted EPOCH and rituximab in untreated diffuse large B-cell lymphoma with analysis of germinal center and post-germinal center biomarkers. J Clin Oncol 2008;26(16):2717–24.

27. Dunleavy K, Pittaluga S, Shovlin M, et al. Low-intensity therapy in adults with Burkitt's lymphoma. N Engl J Med 2013;369(20):1915–25.

28. Dunleavy K, Little RF, Wilson WH. Update on Burkitt lymphoma. Hematol Oncol Clin North Am 2016;30(6):1333–43.

29. Ribrag V, Koscielny S, Bosq J, et al. Rituximab and dose-dense chemotherapy for adults with Burkitt's lymphoma: a randomised, controlled, open-label, phase 3 trial. Lancet 2016;387(10036):2402–11.

30. Hoelzer D, Walewski J, Dohner H, et al. Improved outcome of adult Burkitt lymphoma/leukemia with rituximab and chemotherapy: report of a large prospective multicenter trial. Blood 2014;124(26):3870–9.
31. Dunleavy K, Gross TG. Management of aggressive B-cell NHLs in the AYA population: an adult vs pediatric perspective. Blood 2018;132(4):369–75.
32. Noy A, Lee JY, Cesarman E, et al. AMC 048: modified CODOX-M/IVAC-rituximab is safe and effective for HIV-associated Burkitt lymphoma. Blood 2015;126(2): 160–6.
33. Alizadeh AA, Eisen MB, Davis RE, et al. Distinct types of diffuse large B-cell lymphoma identified by gene expression profiling. Nature 2000;403(6769):503–11.
34. Rosenwald A, Wright G, Chan WC, et al. The use of molecular profiling to predict survival after chemotherapy for diffuse large-B-cell lymphoma. N Engl J Med 2002;346(25):1937–47.
35. Wright GW, Wilson WH, Staudt LM. Genetics of diffuse large B-cell lymphoma. N Engl J Med 2018;379(5):493–4.
36. Scott DW, King RL, Staiger AM, et al. High-grade B-cell lymphoma with MYC and BCL2 and/or BCL6 rearrangements with diffuse large B-cell lymphoma morphology. Blood 2018;131(18):2060–4.
37. Barrans S, Crouch S, Smith A, et al. Rearrangement of MYC is associated with poor prognosis in patients with diffuse large B-cell lymphoma treated in the era of rituximab. J Clin Oncol 2010;28(20):3360–5.
38. Friedberg JW. How I treat double-hit lymphoma. Blood 2017;130(5):590–6.
39. Niitsu N, Okamoto M, Miura I, et al. Clinical features and prognosis of de novo diffuse large B-cell lymphoma with t(14;18) and 8q24/c-MYC translocations. Leukemia 2009;23(4):777–83.
40. Landsburg DJ, Falkiewicz MK, Petrich AM, et al. Sole rearrangement but not amplification of MYC is associated with a poor prognosis in patients with diffuse large B cell lymphoma and B cell lymphoma unclassifiable. Br J Haematol 2016; 175(4):631–40.
41. Kuhnl A, Cunningham D, Counsell N, et al. Outcome of elderly patients with diffuse large B-cell lymphoma treated with R-CHOP: results from the UK NCRI R-CHOP14v21 trial with combined analysis of molecular characteristics with the DSHNHL RICOVER-60 trial. Ann Oncol 2017;28(7):1540–6.
42. Ennishi D, Mottok A, Ben-Neriah S, et al. Genetic profiling of MYC and BCL2 in diffuse large B-cell lymphoma determines cell-of-origin-specific clinical impact. Blood 2017;129(20):2760–70.
43. Savage KJ, Johnson NA, Ben-Neriah S, et al. MYC gene rearrangements are associated with a poor prognosis in diffuse large B-cell lymphoma patients treated with R-CHOP chemotherapy. Blood 2009;114(17):3533–7.
44. Dunleavy K, Fanale MA, Abramson JS, et al. Dose-adjusted EPOCH-R (etoposide, prednisone, vincristine, cyclophosphamide, doxorubicin, and rituximab) in untreated aggressive diffuse large B-cell lymphoma with MYC rearrangement: a prospective, multicentre, single-arm phase 2 study. Lancet Haematol 2018; 5(12):e609–17.
45. Lai C, Roschewski M, Melani C, et al. MYC gene rearrangement in diffuse large B-cell lymphoma does not confer a worse prognosis following dose-adjusted EPOCH-R. Leuk Lymphoma 2018;59(2):505–8.
46. Schmitz N, Zeynalova S, Nickelsen M, et al. CNS international prognostic index: a risk model for CNS relapse in patients with diffuse large B-cell lymphoma treated with R-CHOP. J Clin Oncol 2016;34(26):3150–6.

Central Nervous System Lymphoma

Ugonma N. Chukwueke, MD[a,b], Lakshmi Nayak, MD[a,b,*]

KEYWORDS

- Non-Hodgkin lymphoma • Central nervous system • Diffuse large B-cell lymphoma
- Methotrexate • Extranodal

KEY POINTS

- Primary central nervous system lymphoma (PCNSL) is a rare subtype of extranodal non-Hodgkin lymphoma (NHL).
- Approximately 90% of PCNSL cases are diffuse large B-cell lymphoma, with a smaller percentage consisting of T-cell lymphoma.
- Other types of PCNSL include the following: primary vitreoretinal lymphoma, primary leptomeningeal lymphoma, primary intramedullary spinal lymphoma, neurolymphomatosis, and intravascular large cell lymphoma.
- Involvement of the central nervous system in systemic NHL varies in frequency based on the subtype of disease and typically presents in the relapsed setting of systemic NHL.

INTRODUCTION

Primary central nervous system lymphoma (PCNSL) is a rare but aggressive subtype of extranodal, non-Hodgkin lymphoma (NHL), accounting for 4% of all primary brain tumors with approximately 1500 new cases annually.[1] It is a multicompartment disease, involving all aspects of the central nervous system (CNS), including the brain, eyes, spine, and leptomeninges, in the absence of systemic NHL. Ninety percent of PCNSL cases are diffuse large B-cell lymphoma (DLBCL), with a smaller population of disease representing T-cell lymphoma, Burkitt lymphoma, or poorly characterized low-grade lymphoma.[2] Despite efforts extending survival and reducing neurotoxicity of therapy, less than 50% of patients will achieve a durable remission, and mitigating late effects of treatment remain of paramount concern.

Disclosures: L. Nayak: Consulting for Bristol-Myers Squibb.
[a] Department of Medical Oncology, Center for Neuro-Oncology, Dana-Farber Cancer Institute, 450 Brookline Avenue, Boston, MA 02215, USA; [b] Department of Neurology, Brigham and Women's Hospital, Harvard Medical School, Boston, MA, USA
* Corresponding author. Department of Medical Oncology, Center for Neuro-Oncology, Dana-Farber Cancer Institute, 450 Brookline Avenue, Boston, MA 02215.
E-mail address: Lakshmi_Nayak@dfci.harvard.edu

Hematol Oncol Clin N Am 33 (2019) 597–611
https://doi.org/10.1016/j.hoc.2019.03.008
hemonc.theclinics.com
0889-8588/19/© 2019 Elsevier Inc. All rights reserved.

CNS involvement of systemic NHL may present at the time of initial diagnosis, however occurs more commonly at the time of disease relapse. The frequency of CNS involvement of systemic NHL varies on factors including the histologic subtype and aggressiveness of underlying disease.[3]

EPIDEMIOLOGY

Historically, the primary risk factor for development of PCNSL has been acquired or congenital immune deficiency. During the peak period of human immunodeficiency virus (HIV) and AIDS during the 1980s and 1990s, the peak incidence of PCNSL was primarily attributed to the rising incidence among men, aged 20 to 64 years.[4] Since then, there has been stabilization of the overall incidence of PCNSL in the United States, likely owing to the introduction and use of highly active antiretroviral therapy in this population. Beyond HIV/AIDS, other immunodeficient states that predispose to PCNSL include the following: iatrogenic immune suppression and congenital immunodeficient syndromes, such as ataxia-telangiectasia and severe combined immunodeficiencies, conferring a 4% risk of developing PCNSL.[4] Patients with autoimmune diseases such as Sjogren disease, systemic lupus erythematosus, sarcoidosis, and other vasculitic diseases have been reported to develop PCNSL either secondary to disease-modifying therapies or the underlying disease itself.[5] In patients who have undergone solid organ transplantation, primary CNS posttransplant proliferative disease is the second most common malignancy to be diagnosed following skin cancers, typically monomorphic and Epstein-Barr virus (EBV)-positive disease of B-cell origin.[6] In comparison to the immunodeficient patients, the incidence of PCNSL in the immunocompetent population has slowly increased, with elderly patients (aged >65 years) largely accounting for this increase.[4]

PATHOGENESIS

The pathogenesis of PCNSL is poorly understood, particularly in immunocompetent patients.[5,7] Because the CNS lacks B cells, the site of malignant transformation is unknown, whether within the CNS and its lymphocytes or in systemic lymphocytes with a propensity for the CNS dissemination mediated by chemokines and cell-adhesion molecules, such as *MUM1*, *CXCL13*, and *CHI3L1*.[8,9] In immunocompromised hosts, the role of EBV as an oncogenic virus has been speculated as a potential mechanism for disease because PCNSL cells have been found to have detectable levels of EBV present. EBV genomic DNA has not been identified, however, within tumors of immunocompetent tumors.

Comprehensive molecular genetic analysis has revealed that PCNSL is distinct from systemic DLBCL. On histopathology, PCNSL demonstrates malignant B cells with a high proliferative index, in an angiocentric pattern. Expression of pan-B-cell markers, including BD20, CD79a, and others, such as BCL6, CD10, and BCL2, has been noted. Most PCNSL cases are considered to be activated B-cell-like/non-germinal center subtype based on gene-expression profiling.[10,11] Other molecular features of PCNSL are related to adhesion and extracellular matrix molecules, such as CD44 and the transmembrane receptor protein Fas (CD95), which are thought to be involved in spreading of lymphoid cells within the CNS.[12,13] Immunoglobulin heavy (IgH) gene chain rearrangement is present in all PCNSL cells with high somatic mutation rates, suggesting their origins in mutated germinal center B cells, which ultimately hone to the CNS by way of cell adhesion molecules.[11] Activation of B-cell receptor signaling pathway with its downstream target nuclear factor kappa B is thought to contribute to proliferation of malignant B cells. PCNSL exhibit oncogenic Toll-like receptor (TLR) signaling as a result of myeloid differentiation primary response 88 (*MYD88*) mutations and concurrent BCR signaling and *CD79B* mutations.[14,15] The molecular alterations have therapeutic implications for PCNSL because ibrutinib, a first-in-class oral inhibitor of Bruton tyrosine kinase (BTK), which integrates BCR and TLR, has shown activity in patients with relapsed/recurrent PCNSL.[10] More recently, gain at chromosome 9p24.1, which includes the locus for programmed death ligand 1 and 2, has been identified potentially representing a mechanism for immune evasion and modulation in PCNSL.[16]

CLINICAL PRESENTATION

In contrast to systemic NHL, patients with PCNSL typically do not present with B symptoms (night sweats, fever, weight loss).[17] The initial presenting symptoms of PCNSL are determined by and vary based on the compartment of the CNS, which is involved by disease. In most patients, behavioral and neurocognitive concerns are the presenting symptoms, often delaying the diagnosis due to the nonspecific qualities.[18] Because the cerebral cortex tends to be spared by disease, with largely subcortical and deep structure involvement, seizures less often herald a diagnosis of PCNSL as compared with other primary or metastatic brain tumors.[18] Similar to intracranial space-occupying lesions, symptoms reflective of elevated intracranial pressure may be present and should prompt timely diagnostic evaluation. Fifteen percent to 25% of PCNSL patients will develop ocular manifestations of disease, often characterized by decreased acuity, blurry vision, or floaters.[19] In a patient with intramedullary spinal involvement of PCNSL, symptom burden may vary based on location within the spine of disease, although the thoracic cord is a typical location.[20] If cerebrospinal fluid (CSF) dissemination is present with parenchymal involvement, symptoms are typical of leptomeningeal disease in the context of other malignancies.[21] It should be noted that involvement of these compartments in the absence of parenchymal brain disease is rare and discussed in subsequent sections.

DIAGNOSIS

Timely diagnosis of PCNSL requires a high index of suspicion, because presenting symptoms may be nonspecific. In parallel with thorough history, physical examination, and neurologic examination, the International PCNSL Collaborative Group (IPCG) has developed guidelines for evaluation of extent of disease, including imaging, CSF analysis, serum testing, ophthalmologic examination, and testicular examination, primarily for older men (**Box 1**).[22] The gold standard for diagnosis is by pathology.

Imaging Features

Gadolinium-enhanced MRI remains the primary preferred imaging modality for suspected PCNSL; if contraindications to MRI, contrast-enhanced computed tomography (CT) may be obtained, although there are limitations to what may be detected on CT. The characteristic appearance of PCNSL on MRI is an isointense to hypointense lesion on T1-weighted images with homogenous gadolinium contrast enhancement, typically solitary in focus, involving the deep white matter and periventricular in location. PCNSL lesions are not typically associated with hemorrhage, calcifications, necrosis, or ring enhancement, with exception of in immunocompromised patients.[23,24] Diffusion-weighted imaging sequences may also demonstrate increased

---

Box 1
Extent of disease and comorbidity evaluation for treatment of primary central nervous system lymphoma

Physical examination

Lymph node evaluation

Testicular examination

Comprehensive neurologic examination

Laboratory studies

Complete blood count with differential

Comprehensive metabolic panel

Lactate dehydrogenase level

Serologic testing for HIV

CSF

Cell count

Protein

Glucose

Cytology

Flow cytometry

IgH gene rearrangement

Bone marrow assessment

Bone marrow aspirate and biopsy

Full ophthalmologic testing

Slit-lamp testing

Imaging

MR imaging: brain and spine (if clinical symptoms)

Combined CT/ PET: chest, abdomen, and pelvis

Testicular ultrasound

Cognitive/functional assessments

Karnofsky Performance Status or Eastern Cooperative Oncology Group

Mini-Mental State Examination

---

cellularity characterized by hyperintensity, with accompanying hypointensity on apparent deficient coefficient sequences (**Fig. 1**).[25]

Cerebrospinal Fluid Analysis

CSF analysis may aid in the diagnosis of PCNSL because malignant cells may be present in up to 40% of PCNSL patients. Evaluation of the CSF should include cell count, protein, glucose, cytology, flow cytometry, and IgH gene rearrangement testing. The typical CSF profile demonstrates elevated protein, normal glucose, and lymphocytic predominant pleocytosis. The diagnosis of leptomeningeal involvement of PCNSL can be made by the presence of IgH gene rearrangement and identification of a clonal B-cell population in the CSF. Diagnosis of primary leptomeningeal lymphoma is discussed in later sections.

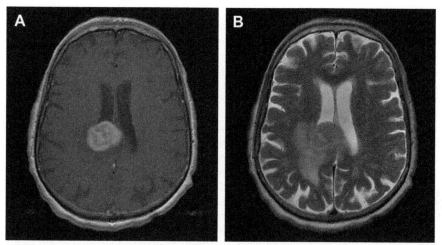

Fig. 1. (A) Brain MRI showing contrast-enhancing lesion on postcontrast T1-weighted image and (B) surrounding hyperintense signal change on T2-weighted image.

PATHOLOGY

Tissue is required for definitive diagnosis and should not be delayed in patients with suspected PCNSL with surgically accessible lesions. Stereotactic biopsy is the preferred surgical approach, given the likelihood of achieving tissue diagnosis and avoiding neurologic morbidity and mortality. Historically, it was thought no survival benefit has been established with more extensive resection; additionally, given the deep location of most PCNSL lesions, gross total resection is often not feasible.[26,27] This assertion is currently being challenged, with some benefit noted in higher-performing and lower-surgical-risk patients to facilitate timely introduction of systemic therapy and for symptom control.[28,29]

If possible and safe, corticosteroids should be avoided in order to maximize the diagnostic yield of biopsy. The lymphocytotoxic properties of corticosteroids have been well described and short courses of treatment have been shown to cause disappearance of the lesions.[23,30,31]

TREATMENT FOR NEWLY DIAGNOSED PRIMARY CENTRAL NERVOUS SYSTEM LYMPHOMA

For newly diagnosed disease, treatment continues to be offered in 2 stages: induction and consolidation. Treatment of PCNSL contributes to prolonged survival; however, cure is not achieved in most patients. Untreated PCNSL progresses rapidly with overall survival (OS) of 6 weeks. Several factors have been identified that influence outcome and survival, with age and performance status being the most predictive of patient outcome. Two prognostic scoring systems have been used since its inception, from International Extranodal Lymphoma Study Group (IELSG) and Memorial Sloan Kettering.[32] In addition to these scoring systems, BCL6 rearrangements and deletion of 6q22 are associated with shorter OS.[33]

Induction

Standard induction therapy regimen for newly diagnosed PCNSL includes high-dose methotrexate-based chemotherapy. The exact choice of therapy often varies based on institutional preferences and standards. Historically, whole-brain radiation therapy (WBRT) was used in the induction phase for treatment of newly diagnosed PCNSL; however, given the established cytotoxicity of high-dose methotrexate and with quality of life and preservation of neurocognitive function of paramount concern, the role of WBRT is less defined at present, although it still remains as a potential modality for salvage or palliative benefit.[34] To date, a regimen incorporating intravenous high-dose methotrexate (in combination with other cytotoxic therapy) remains the most effective and best supported induction course, with multiple phase 2 studies suggesting efficacy as well as safety and survival benefit.[34,35] There is, however, considerable debate around the optimal "high dose," which ranges in from 1 to 8 g/m^2. Prior work has established that peak serum methotrexate concentrations and adequate CSF concentrations are reached with doses greater than or equal to 3 g/m^2.[36–38]

The activity of the induction regimen of high-dose methotrexate, rituximab, and temozolomide was investigated in a phase 2, multicenter trial, CALGB 50202, of 44 patients.[35] High-dose methotrexate was dosed at 8 g/m^2 and is administered with rituximab and temozolomide, followed by consolidation with etoposide and cytarabine after complete response (CR) had been achieved. At median follow-up of 4.9 years, 29 of 44 patients had achieved CR and were recommended for consolidation, with median progression-free survival (PFS) of 2.4 years. Neurocognitive testing was not performed in this study. A follow-up phase 2 trial was conducted by the IELSG-32, comparing 3 induction regimens: methotrexate/cytarabine, methotrexate/cytarabine/rituximab, and methotrexate/cytarabine/rituximab/thiotepa or MATRIx.[39] MATRIx was found to be superior to the alternate regimens with respect to overall response, although also associated with higher toxicity.[39] High-dose methotrexate in combination with rituximab, procarbazine, and vincristine has been studied prospectively in multicenter, phase 2 trials.[40,41] Sixty percent of patients achieved a CR and were ultimately treated with low-dose WBRT for consolidation. Median PFS and OS were 3.3 and 6.6 years.[40]

The goal of the induction phase of treatment is to achieve a radiographic CR, characterized as complete resolution of all enhancing disease on MRI in the absence of corticosteroid use for at least 2 weeks before imaging, before proceeding with consolidation therapy. If disease was noted in other CNS compartments, CR is similarly defined by the absence of disease in this space. Consensus criteria for disease response were established by the IPCG, defined as the following: CR, unconfirmed complete response (CRu), partial response (PR), stable disease, or progressive disease.[22] CR is achieved in approximately 30% to 60% of patients who received high-dose methotrexate.[42]

Consolidation

Although almost 60% of patients who receive high-dose methotrexate as part of their induction regimen are able to achieve CR, there still remains a need for further treatment given the risk for disease relapse. Approaches to consolidation include WBRT, additional chemotherapy, or high-dose chemotherapy followed by autologous stem cell transplantation (ASCT).

In 2 phase 2 prospective trials, patients were treated following induction with carmustine/thiotepa with ASCT with or without WBRT. Survival rates were comparable between the 2 groups; however, all patients who developed subsequent neurotoxicity had received WBRT.[43] In a separate phase 2 study, 79 patients received induction therapy with high-dose methotrexate, cytarabine, thiotepa, and rituximab, followed by high-dose carmustine/thiotepa with ASCT, if CR was achieved. In this population, the overall response rate was 91% with 2-year survival of 87%.[44] There are several trials investigating the efficacy of consolidative high-dose chemotherapy with ASCT as compared with WBRT or chemotherapy alone (**Table 1**).

Although PCNSL is radiation sensitive, given the potential for neurocognitive decline following WBRT, several studies are investigating whether this modality should be included in consolidation regimens. In a multicenter, phase 3 trial, 551 patients with newly diagnosed PCNSL were treated with either chemotherapy alone (high-dose methotrexate with or without ifosfamide) or chemotherapy followed by WBRT.[45] Of 320 patients included in the per-protocol treatment analysis, those who were randomized to receive WBRT showed an increase in PFS of 18 months versus 12 months, however, without any increase in OS.[46] In addition, those who received WBRT were found to have higher rates of neurotoxicity and cognitive decline.[47] The second randomization of the IESLG-32 trial compared the efficacy of thiotepa-based myeloablative chemotherapy and ASCT to WBRT. The early results of this study demonstrated both treatments were effective with no significant difference in 2-year PFS. As expected, hematologic toxicity was higher with ASCT, and cognitive impairment was noted with WBRT in patients who underwent neuropsychological assessment. Although the late effects of cranial irradiation remain a risk following WBRT, in specific clinical contexts, such as in patients with contraindications to systemic treatment, consolidative low-dose WBRT may be a consideration.[40]

RELAPSED/RECURRENT PRIMARY CENTRAL NERVOUS SYSTEM LYMPHOMA

Following completion of initial therapy with CR, guidelines exist for disease surveillance with clinical and imaging follow-up at 3 months for the first 2 years, every 6 months for the following 3 years, and then annually for at least 5 years (National Comprehensive Cancer Network). Surveillance of other CNS compartments is based on initial site of disease and symptoms. Unfortunately, despite aggressive induction and consolidation regimens, most patients will have recurrence of disease, with most relapses occurring 5 years after treatment.[48] Survival is worse in patients who experience relapse within 1 year of completing treatment.[49] In the setting of relapsed

Table 1
Summary of ongoing randomized trials for consolidation of primary central nervous system lymphoma

Clinical Trial	Phase	Treatment Arms
NCT01011920 (IELSG 32)	2	Arm 1: WBRT Arm 2: HDT/ASCT
NCT00863460 (ANOCEF-GOELAMS)	2	Arm 1: HDT/ASCT Arm 2: WBRT
NCT01399372 (RTOG 1114)	2	Arm 1: Low-dose WBRT followed by cytarabine Arm 2: Cytarabine
NCT01511562 (Alliance 51101)	2	Arm 1: HDT/ASCT Arm 2: Etoposide, Cytarabine
MATRix/IELSG 43	2	Arm 1: HDT/ASCT Arm 2: Dexamethasone, Ifosfamide, etoposide, Carboplatin (DEViC)

Abbreviations: ANOCEF, Association des Neuro-Oncologue d'Expression Francaise; GOELAMS, Groupe Ouest Est d'Etude des Leucemies et Autres Maladies due Sang; HDT, high-dose chemotherapy; NCT, National Clinical Trial; RTOG, Radiation Therapy Oncology Group.

disease, it is recommended to repeat extent of disease evaluation for the CNS and systemically.[30]

Treatment options for relapsed disease largely depend on the time of relapse, site, prior therapies, and age. Rechallenge with high-dose methotrexate can be considered, particularly in those who previously responded well to this therapy and had a reasonably durable response.[50] Thiotepa-based conditioning followed by ASCT may be an option in patients who did not undergo autologous transplant during their initial treatment course.[51] Additional systemic salvage options may include high-dose cytarabine and pemetrexed. Novel targeted agents, including BTK inhibitors like ibrutinib, and immunomodulatory drugs like lenalidomide and pomalidomide,[52] have demonstrated encouraging results. As discussed in the earlier section on pathogenesis, mutations in the TLR domain of MYD88 occur quite frequently in PCNSL, more so than systemic DLBCL, thus potentially conferring sensitivity to ibrutinib in this population. Sensitivity to ibrutinib has been observed in patients with previously treated Waldenstrom macroglobulinemia, where MYD88 mutations are highly prevalent.[53] Immune checkpoint inhibitors, such as pembrolizumab and nivolumab, are being investigated in the relapsed/refractory setting. In specific clinical contexts, WBRT or stereotactic radiosurgery may be a treatment option.[54]

OTHER SUBTYPES OF PRIMARY CENTRAL NERVOUS SYSTEM LYMPHOMA
Primary Vitreoretinal Lymphoma

Primary vitreoretinal lymphoma (PVRL), a high-grade, B-cell type primary intraocular lymphoma, is a rare subtype of PCNSL that presents solely in the eye, in the absence of parenchymal brain disease, with a tropism for the posterior segments of the eye (choroid, vitreous, and retina). Because of a lack of central database for disease, annual incidence is challenging to estimate.[19] Up to 90% of PVRL patients will develop CNS disease.[19] Because presenting symptoms are often nonspecific (floaters, blurry vision, decreased acuity), there may be delays to achieving definitive diagnosis of PVRL. On ophthalmologic testing, findings include vitreous cell infiltration and subretinal tumor infiltration. Diagnostic confirmation is achieved by identification of malignant lymphoid cells in the eye, using any manner of methods for cytology and histopathology, including aspiration, vitrectromy, or retinal biopsy. The optimal treatment regimen for PVRL is yet to be established and may include direct local treatment (intravitreal therapy, ocular radiation) or systemic therapy. In a retrospective study of 78 immunocompetent patients with PVRL, 31 were treated with local therapy, 21 with systemic chemotherapy, and 23 with combination. CNS lymphoma developed in 36% of all patients, and the 5-year cumulative survival rate was similar among all treatment groups. In this series, systemic therapy did not prevent CNS relapse.[55]

Primary Leptomeningeal Lymphoma

Although 40% of PCNSL patients may have leptomeningeal involvement at the time of diagnosis, less than 10% of patients will present with isolated leptomeningeal disease in the absence of parenchymal brain involvement.[56] Symptoms of primary leptomeningeal lymphoma are consistent with other causes of leptomeningeal disease, in which headaches, cranial nerve palsies, meningismus, and radiculopathies may be present. CSF profile may be notable for malignant lymphocytes on cytology and IgH gene rearrangement. On imaging, there may be enhancing nodules on lumbar nerve roots. Retrospective series have shown efficacy of systemic chemotherapy with high-dose methotrexate in achieving response, although the optimal regimen for this entity has yet to be confirmed.[56]

Primary Intramedullary Spinal Cord Lymphoma

Primary spinal involvement by DLBCL is rare with characterization of this entity limited predominantly to case series. In comparison to spinal involvement of systemic NHL, where there may be leptomeningeal or dural-based disease, in primary spinal disease, intramedullary lesions are more prominent. Given the site of disease involvement, myelopathy may be a presenting symptom, with cauda equina or conus medullaris syndrome also possible.

Neurolymphomatosis

Neurolymphomatosis is a rare process in which there is lymphomatous invasion of the cranial or spinal nerves. Symptom presentation varies on location of disease and may include upper cranial nerve dysfunction or cauda dysfunction with asymmetric weakness of the lower extremities.[57,58]

Intravascular Large B-Cell Lymphoma

In this rare form of large B-cell lymphoma (intravascular large B-cell lymphoma [IVLBCL]), symptoms vary based on geographic region with CNS involvement in up to 40% of patients at the time of diagnosis.[59,60] Other than CNS, the skin is also most frequently involved in disease. Cerebral ischemia may occur in approximately 50% of cases. Diagnosis of CNS involvement of IVLBCL is achieved with biopsy. Similar to PCNSL, a methotrexate-based regimen is recommended for treatment of both systemic and CNS disease.[59]

CENTRAL NERVOUS SYSTEM INVOLVEMENT OF SYSTEMIC NON-HODGKIN LYMPHOMA
Introduction

CNS involvement of systemic NHL can occur either at the time of initial diagnosis, or more commonly, in the setting of disease relapse. The true incidence of CNS involvement may vary based on the histologic subtype of systemic NHL, with more aggressive subtypes more likely to experience CNS involvement at some point in their disease course.[3] The incidence of CNS involvement in patients with Burkitt lymphoma and lymphoblastic lymphoma may be as high as 50%, which may inform which patient populations may benefit from CNS prophylaxis.[61] There has also been consideration given to the primary site of disease as a factor in CNS relapse. The testes, nasal/paranasal sinuses, and bulky retroperitoneal involvement have been associated with increased risk of CNS disease.[62,63]

The International Prognostic Index (IPI) is a scoring tool that was developed to evaluate clinical variables that may predict survival in patients with systemic DLBCL, in which points are assigned based on factors including age, lactate dehydrogenase level, performance status, and presence of extranodal disease.[64] The CNS-IPI was subsequently developed and validated as a risk model for predicting CNS relapse of systemic DLBCL in patients treated with rituximab, cyclophosphamide, doxorubicin, vincristine, and prednisone. The CNS-IPI score consists of IPI, plus evidence of involvement of kidneys or the adrenal glands.[65] The groups are stratified by risk of CNS relapse, with low-risk patients carrying a less than 1% risk and high-risk population with a 10% risk of CNS relapse, in which case CNS prophylaxis may be considered.[65] Furthermore, patients with systemic DLBCL, with dual expression of *BCL2* and *MYC* ("double-hit lymphoma"), have been associated with worse prognosis and higher risk of CNS relapse.[65] Although CNS-IPI does not currently integrate gene-expression profiling, there is a separate effort in which the combination of CNS-IPI and cell of origin is used to predict risk of CNS relapse.[66]

Clinical Presentation

Systemic NHL can also involve any compartment of the central or peripheral nervous system. Similar to PCNSL, clinical symptoms are determined by the location of disease involvement. Leptomeningeal metastatic disease is common in systemic NHL and may occur as early as within the first year of diagnosis in up to 10% of patients.[67] Cranial nerve palsies and symptoms of hydrocephalus are manifestations of leptomeningeal spread. Intramedullary spinal cord and neurolymphomatosis may also occur in systemic NHL. As in PCNSL, gadolinium-enhanced MRI is the most sensitive imaging modality for evaluation of CNS disease.

Treatment and Prophylaxis

For CNS disease in this setting, high-dose systemic therapy, namely with high-dose methotrexate or cytarabine, has known CNS penetration and distribution throughout the neuroaxis. Extrapolating from the evidence for its use in the PCNSL population, rituximab may be combined with high-dose methotrexate.[68,69] A specific consideration in secondary CNS lymphoma, which is less of a factor in PCNSL, is the cumulative systemic toxicity of treatment, because patients with systemic NHL have received prior cytotoxic therapy. Although intrathecal (IT) and radiation therapy are local therapies that may mitigate the risk for systemic toxicity, CNS toxicity of these modalities must also be weighed, particularly if CNS disease is bulky, rendering IT treatments more neurotoxic. Targeted agents and immunotherapeutic approaches have been tried in the context of case reports.[70–72]

CNS prophylaxis has been considered for patients with high-risk features.[73–75] Specific NHL subtypes have been identified, including indolent NHL, highly aggressive NHL, and aggressive NHL. For high-risk patients, systemic high-dose methotrexate, dosed at 3.5 g/m^2, may be preferred in some practices, given the ability to achieve higher therapeutic levels in the CNS with better treatment tolerability, in comparison to IT chemotherapy, which has been used more commonly historically.[76] A retrospective single-institution study of 65 patients with DLBCL in high-risk patients was performed, investigating the safety and CNS recurrence rates with systemic, high-dose methotrexate.[77] Median follow-up was 33 months with PFS and OS rates of 76% and 78%, respectively; CNS recurrence rate was 3%.[77] Methotrexate-induced renal injury leading to discontinuation of treatment occurred in 14% of patients, with 12% of patients experiencing delays in subsequent treatment due to toxicity; 1 patient died related to complication from treatment, including nephrotoxicity and pancytopenia.[77] IT methotrexate may still be favored in specific instances, namely, in the setting of poor tolerability of systemic therapy.

SUMMARY

PCNSL and its subtypes are uncommon variants of extranodal NHL, which can involve any compartment within the CNS. As symptoms of disease may be nonspecific, a high index of clinical suspicion is necessary in order to conduct pretreatment evaluation and to initiate treatment in a timely manner. Similarly, secondary CNS lymphoma is a rare manifestation of systemic NHL, which may present at the time of initial diagnosis, however more commonly at the time of disease relapse. Although the optimal treatment regimens have yet to be defined, high-dose methotrexate is an important and well-established component of therapeutic regimens. With advances in collective understanding of the molecular and genetic mechanisms of pathogenesis, there is emerging use of novel therapies that may soon be incorporated into management of both primary and secondary CNS lymphoma.

REFERENCES

1. Ostrom QT, Gittleman H, Liao P, et al. CBTRUS statistical report: primary brain and other central nervous system tumors diagnosed in the United States in 2010-2014. Neuro Oncol 2017;19(suppl_5):v1–88.
2. Swerdlow SH, Campo E, Pileri SA, et al. The 2016 revision of the World Health Organization classification of lymphoid neoplasms. Blood 2016;127(20):2375–90.
3. Bernstein SH, Unger JM, Leblanc M, et al. Natural history of CNS relapse in patients with aggressive non-Hodgkin's lymphoma: a 20-year follow-up analysis of SWOG 8516 – the Southwest Oncology Group. J Clin Oncol 2009;27(1):114–9.
4. O'Neill BP, Decker PA, Tieu C, et al. The changing incidence of primary central nervous system lymphoma is driven primarily by the changing incidence in young and middle-aged men and differs from time trends in systemic diffuse large B-cell non-Hodgkin's lymphoma. Am J Hematol 2013;88(12):997–1000.
5. Bhagavathi S, Wilson JD. Primary central nervous system lymphoma. Arch Pathol Lab Med 2008;132(11):1830–4.
6. Cavaliere R, Petroni G, Lopes MB, et al, International Primary Central Nervous System Lymphoma Collaborative Group. Primary central nervous system post-transplantation lymphoproliferative disorder: an International Primary Central Nervous System Lymphoma Collaborative Group Report. Cancer 2010;116(4):863–70.
7. Ponzoni M, Issa S, Batchelor TT, et al. Beyond high-dose methotrexate and brain radiotherapy: novel targets and agents for primary CNS lymphoma. Ann Oncol 2014;25(2):316–22.
8. Kadoch C, Treseler P, Rubenstein JL. Molecular pathogenesis of primary central nervous system lymphoma. Neurosurg Focus 2006;21(5):E1.
9. Smith JR, Braziel RM, Paoletti S, et al. Expression of B-cell-attracting chemokine 1 (CXCL13) by malignant lymphocytes and vascular endothelium in primary central nervous system lymphoma. Blood 2003;101(3):815–21.
10. Grommes C, Pastore A, Palaskas N, et al. Ibrutinib unmasks critical role of bruton tyrosine kinase in primary CNS lymphoma. Cancer Discov 2017;7:1018–29.
11. Camilleri-Broët S, Crinière E, Broët P, et al. A uniform activated B-cell-like immunophenotype might explain the poor prognosis of primary central nervous system lymphomas: analysis of 83 cases. Blood 2006;107:190–6.
12. Aho R, Kalimo H, Salmi M, et al. Binding of malignant lymphoid cells to the white matter of the human central nervous system: role of different CD44 isoforms, beta 1, beta 2 and beta 7 integrins, and L-selectin. J Neuropathol Exp Neurol 1997;56(5):557–68.
13. Baiocchi RA, Khatri VP, Lindemann MJ, et al. Phenotypic and functional analysis of Fas (CD95) expression in primary central nervous system lymphoma of patients with acquired immunodeficiency syndrome. Blood 1997;90(5):1737–46.
14. Ngo VN, Young RM, Schmitz R, et al. Oncogenically active MYD88 mutations in human lymphoma. Nature 2011;470(7332):115–9.
15. Montesinos-Rongen M, Godlewska E, Brunn A, et al. Activating L265P mutations of the MYD88 gene are common in primary central nervous system lymphoma. Acta Neuropathol 2011;122:791–2.

16. Chapuy B, Roemer MG, Stewart C, et al. Targetable genetic features of primary testicular and primary central nervous system lymphomas. Blood 2016;127(7): 869–81.

17. Grommes C, DeAngelis LM. Primary CNS lymphoma. J Clin Oncol 2017;35(21): 2410–8.

18. Bataille B, Delwail V, Menet E, et al. Primary intracerebral malignant lymphoma: report of 248 cases. J Neurosurg 2000;92(2):261–6.

19. Chan CC, Rubenstein JL, Coupland SE, et al. Primary vitreoretinal lymphoma: a report from an International Primary Central Nervous System Lymphoma Collaborative Group symposium. Oncologist 2011;16(11):1589–99.

20. Grommes C, Rubenstein JL, DeAngelis LM, et al. Comprehensive approach to diagnosis and treatment of newly diagnosed primary CNS lymphoma. Neuro Oncol 2018. [Epub ahead of print].

21. Balmaceda C, Gaynor JJ, Sun M, et al. Leptomeningeal tumor in primary central nervous system lymphoma: recognition, significance, and implications. Ann Neurol 1995;38(2):202–9.

22. Abrey LE, Batchelor TT, Ferreri AJ, et al, International Primary CNS Lymphoma Collaborative Group. Report of an international workshop to standardize baseline evaluation and response criteria for primary CNS lymphoma. J Clin Oncol 2005; 23(22):5034–43.

23. Rock JP, Cher L, Hochberg FH, et al. Primary CNS lymphoma. In: Yomans JR, editor. Neurological surgery. 4th edition. Philadelphia: WB Saunders; 1996. p. 268.

24. Bühring U, Herrlinger U, Krings T, et al. MRI features of primary central nervous system lymphomas at presentation. Neurology 2001;57(3):393–6.

25. Haldorsen IS, Espeland A, Larsson EM. Central nervous system lymphoma: characteristic findings on traditional and advanced imaging. AJNR Am J Neuroradiol 2011;32(6):984–92.

26. Jahr G, Da Broi M, Holte H Jr, et al. The role of surgery in intracranial PCNSL. Neurosurg Rev 2018;41(4):1037–44.

27. Holdhoff M. Role of surgical resection in primary CNS lymphoma: a resurrected discussion. Oncology (Williston Park) 2014;28(7):641–2.

28. Rae AI, Mehta A, Cloney M, et al. Craniotomy and survival for primary central nervous system lymphoma. Neurosurgery 2019;84(4):935–44.

29. Weller M, Martus P, Roth P, et al, German PCNSL Study Group. Surgery for primary CNS lymphoma? Challenging a paradigm. Neuro Oncol 2012;14(12): 1481–4.

30. Miller DC, Hochberg FH, Harris NL, et al. Pathology with clinical correlations of primary central nervous system non-Hodgkin's lymphoma. The Massachusetts General Hospital experience 1958-1989. Cancer 1994;74(4):1383–97.

31. Hochberg FH, Miller DC. Primary central nervous system lymphoma. J Neurosurg 1988;68(6):835–53.

32. Ferreri AJ, Blay JY, Reni M, et al. Prognostic scoring system for primary CNS lymphomas: the International Extranodal Lymphoma Study Group experience. J Clin Oncol 2003;21(2):266–72.

33. Cady FM, O'Neill BP, Law ME, et al. Del(6)(q22) and BCL6 rearrangements in primary CNS lymphoma are indicators of an aggressive clinical course. J Clin Oncol 2008;26(29):4814–9.

34. Batchelor T, Carson K, O'Neill A, et al. Treatment of primary CNS lymphoma with methotrexate and deferred radiotherapy: a report of NABTT 96-07. J Clin Oncol 2003;21(6):1044–9.

35. Rubenstein JL, Hsi ED, Johnson JL, et al. Intensive chemotherapy and immunotherapy in patients with newly diagnosed primary CNS lymphoma: CALGB 50202 (Alliance 50202). J Clin Oncol 2013;31(25):3061–8.

36. Glantz MJ, Cole BF, Recht L, et al. High-dose intravenous methotrexate for patients with nonleukemic leptomeningeal cancer: is intrathecal chemotherapy necessary? J Clin Oncol 1998;16(4):1561–7.

37. DeAngelis LM, Seiferheld W, Schold SC, et al, Radiation Therapy Oncology Group Study 93-10. Combination chemotherapy and radiotherapy for primary central nervous system lymphoma: Radiation Therapy Oncology Group Study 93-10. J Clin Oncol 2002;20(24):4643–8.

38. Ferreri AJ, Guerra E, Regazzi M, et al. Area under the curve of methotrexate and creatinine clearance are outcome-determining factors in primary CNS lymphomas. Br J Cancer 2004;90(2):353–8.

39. Ferreri AJ, Cwynarski K, Pulczynski E, et al. International Extranodal Lymphoma Study Group (IELSG). Chemoimmunotherapy with methotrexate, cytarabine, thiotepa, and rituximab (MATRix regimen) in patients with primary CNS lymphoma: results of the first randomisation of the International Extranodal Lymphoma Study Group-32 (IELSG32) phase 2 trial. Lancet Haematol 2016;3(5):e217–27.

40. Morris PG, Correa DD, Yahalom J, et al. Rituximab, methotrexate, procarbazine, and vincristine followed by consolidation reduced-dose whole-brain radiotherapy and cytarabine in newly diagnosed primary CNS lymphoma: final results and long-term outcome. J Clin Oncol 2013;31(31):3971–9.

41. Shah GD, Yahalom J, Correa DD, et al. Combined immunochemotherapy with reduced whole-brain radiotherapy for newly diagnosed primary CNS lymphoma. J Clin Oncol 2007;25(30):4730–5.

42. Reni M, Ferreri AJ, Guha-Thakurta N, et al. Clinical relevance of consolidation radiotherapy and other main therapeutic issues in primary central nervous system lymphomas treated with upfront high-dose methotrexate. Int J Radiat Oncol Biol Phys 2001;51(2):419–25.

43. Kasenda B, Schorb E, Fritsch K, et al. Prognosis after high-dose chemotherapy followed by autologous stem-cell transplantation as first-line treatment in primary CNS lymphoma–a long-term follow-up study. Ann Oncol 2012;23(10):2670–5.

44. Illerhaus G, Kasenda B, Ihorst G, et al. High-dose chemotherapy with autologous haemopoietic stem cell transplantation for newly diagnosed primary CNS lymphoma: a prospective, single-arm, phase 2 trial. Lancet Haematol 2016;3(8): e388–97.

45. Thiel E, Korfel A, Martus P, et al. High-dose methotrexate with or without whole brain radiotherapy for primary CNS lymphoma (G-PCNSL-SG-1): a phase 3, randomised, non-inferiority trial. Lancet Oncol 2010;11(11):1036–47.

46. Korfel A, Thiel E, Martus P, et al. Randomized phase III study of whole-brain radiotherapy for primary CNS lymphoma. Neurology 2015;84(12):1242–8.

47. Herrlinger U, Schäfer N, Fimmers R, et al. Early whole brain radiotherapy in primary CNS lymphoma: negative impact on quality of life in the randomized G-PCNSL-SG1 trial. J Cancer Res Clin Oncol 2017;143(9):1815–21.

48. Wang N, Gill C, Betensky R, et al. Relapse patterns in primary CNS diffuse large B-cell lymphoma. Neurology 2015;84(14 Supplement). P3.147.

49. Langner-Lemercier S, Houillier C, Soussain C, et al. Primary CNS lymphoma at first relapse/progression: characteristics, management, and outcome of 256 patients from the French LOC network. Neuro Oncol 2016;18(9):1297–303.

50. Plotkin SR, Betensky RA, Hochberg FH, et al. Treatment of relapsed central nervous system lymphoma with high-dose methotrexate. Clin Cancer Res 2004; 10(17):5643–6.

51. Soussain C, Hoang-Xuan K, Taillandier L, et al. Intensive chemotherapy followed by hematopoietic stem-cell rescue for refractory and recurrent primary CNS and intraocular lymphoma: Société Française de Greffe de Moëlle Osseuse-Thérapie Cellulaire. J Clin Oncol 2008;26(15):2512–8.

52. Grommes C, Nayak L, Tun HW, et al. Introduction of novel agents in the treatment of primary CNS lymphoma. Neuro Oncol 2018. [Epub ahead of print].

53. Treon SP, Tripsas CK, Meid K, et al. Ibrutinib in previously treated Waldenström's macroglobulinemia. N Engl J Med 2015;372(15):1430–40.

54. Chao ST, Barnett GH, Vogelbaum MA, et al. Salvage stereotactic radiosurgery effectively treats recurrences from whole-brain radiation therapy. Cancer 2008; 113(8):2198–204.

55. Riemens A, Bromberg J, Touitou V, et al. Treatment strategies in primary vitreoretinal lymphoma: A 17-center european collaborative study. JAMA Ophthalmol 2015;133:191–7.

56. Taylor JW, Flanagan EP, O'Neill BP, et al. Primary leptomeningeal lymphoma: International Primary CNS Lymphoma Collaborative Group report. Neurology 2013; 81(19):1690–6.

57. Da Silva AN, Lopes MB, Schiff D. Rare pathological variants and presentations of primary central nervous system lymphomas. Neurosurg Focus 2006;21(5):E7.

58. Levin N, Soffer D, Grissaru S, et al. Primary T-cell CNS lymphoma presenting with leptomeningeal spread and neurolymphomatosis. J Neurooncol 2008;90(1): 77–83.

59. Shimada K, Murase T, Matsue K, et al, IVL Study Group in Japan. Central nervous system involvement in intravascular large B-cell lymphoma: a retrospective analysis of 109 patients. Cancer Sci 2010;101(6):1480–6.

60. Kebir S, Kuchelmeister K, Niehusmann P, et al. Intravascular CNS lymphoma: successful therapy using high-dose methotrexate-based polychemotherapy. Exp Hematol Oncol 2012;1(1):37.

61. Hill QA, Owen RG. CNS prophylaxis in lymphoma: who to target and what therapy to use. Blood Rev 2006;20(6):319–32.

62. Liang R, Chiu E, Loke SL. Secondary central nervous system involvement by non-Hodgkin's lymphoma: the risk factors. Hematol Oncol 1990;8(3):141–5.

63. MacKintosh FR, Colby TV, Podolsky WJ, et al. Central nervous system involvement in non-Hodgkin's lymphoma: an analysis of 105 cases. Cancer 1982; 49(3):586–95.

64. International Non-Hodgkin's Lymphoma Prognostic Factors Project. A predictive model for aggressive non-Hodgkin's lymphoma. N Engl J Med 1993;329(14): 987–94.

65. Schmitz N, Zeynalova S, Nickelsen M, et al. CNS International prognostic index: a risk model for CNS relapse in patients with diffuse large B-cell lymphoma treated with R-CHOP. J Clin Oncol 2016;34(26):3150–6.

66. Klanova M, Sehn LH, Bence-Bruckler I, et al. Integration of cell of origin into the clinical CNS International Prognostic Index improves CNS relapse prediction in DLBCL. Blood 2019;133(9):919–26.

67. Mead GM, Kennedy P, Smith JL, et al. Involvement of the central nervous system by non-Hodgkin's lymphoma in adults. A review of 36 cases. Q J Med 1986; 60(231):699–714.

68. Batchelor TT, Grossman SA, Mikkelsen T, et al. Rituximab monotherapy for patients with recurrent primary CNS lymphoma. Neurology 2011;76(10):929–30.
69. Wong ET, Tishler R, Barron L, et al. Immunochemotherapy with rituximab and temozolomide for central nervous system lymphomas. Cancer 2004;101(1):139–45.
70. Nayak L, Iwamoto FM, LaCasce A, et al. PD-1 blockade with nivolumab in relapsed/refractory primary central nervous system and testicular lymphoma. Blood 2017;129(23):3071–3.
71. Abramson JS, McGree B, Noyes S, et al. Anti-CD19 CAR T cells in CNS diffuse large-B-cell lymphoma. N Engl J Med 2017;377(8):783–4.
72. Bernard S, Goldwirt L, Amorim S, et al. Activity of ibrutinib in mantle cell lymphoma patients with central nervous system relapse. Blood 2015;126(14): 1695–8.
73. Kridel R, Dietrich PY. Prevention of CNS relapse in diffuse large B-cell lymphoma. Lancet Oncol 2011;12(13):1258–66.
74. El-Galaly TC, Villa D, Michaelsen TY, et al. The number of extranodal sites assessed by PET/CT scan is a powerful predictor of CNS relapse for patients with diffuse large B-cell lymphoma: an international multicenter study of 1532 patients treated with chemoimmunotherapy. Eur J Cancer 2017;75:195–203.
75. Savage KJ, Zeynalova S, Kansara RR, et al. Validation of a prognostic model to assess the risk of CNS disease in patients with aggressive B-cell lymphoma. Blood 2014;124(21):394 (abstract).
76. Cheung CW, Burton C, Smith P, et al. Central nervous system chemoprophylaxis in non-Hodgkin lymphoma: current practice in the UK. Br J Haematol 2005; 131(2):193–200.
77. Abramson JS, Hellmann M, Barnes JA, et al. Intravenous methotrexate as central nervous system (CNS) prophylaxis is associated with a low risk of CNS recurrence in high-risk patients with diffuse large B-cell lymphoma. Cancer 2010; 116(18):4283–90.

Mantle Cell Lymphoma
Current and Emerging Treatment Strategies and Unanswered Questions

Benjamin Diamond, MD[a,b,*], Anita Kumar, MD[a,c]

KEYWORDS

- Mantle cell lymphoma • Novel agents • Minimal residual disease • Risk stratification
- Personalized medicine • Ibrutinib • Cytarabine

KEY POINTS

- There is no firmly established standard of care for treatment of mantle cell lymphoma.
- An evolving understanding of its biology, ontogeny, and molecular pathology has facilitated an increased ability to prognosticate and select increasingly individualized treatment.
- Applications for minimal residual disease assays are being tested, and may potentially find use in guiding de-escalation, intensification, and cessation of therapy.
- Novel agents can be added to current treatment paradigms. In some cases, they supplant older, chemotherapy-based approaches.

INTRODUCTION

Mantle cell lymphoma (MCL) is a B-cell non-Hodgkin lymphoma (NHL) historically grouped with indolent lymphomas given its mature cell of origin; however, it is best described as an aggressive, generally incurable lymphoma with formerly poor long-term survival. An evolving understanding of the biology, ontogeny, and molecular pathology of the disease has been the underlying driver underpinning our ability to prognosticate and select increasingly individualized treatment plans with improved outcomes.

Disclosure Statement: B. Diamond has nothing to disclose. A. Kumar was on an advisory board for Celgene and has received research funding from Abbvie Pharmaceuticals, Adaptive Biotechnologies, Celgene, Pharmacyclics, and Seattle Genetics.
[a] Lymphoma Department, MSKCC, 1275 York Avenue, Box 468, New York, NY 10065, USA; [b] Department of Medicine, Medical Oncology, New York, NY, USA; [c] Department of Medicine, Lymphoma Service, New York, NY, USA
* Corresponding author. Lymphoma Department, MSKCC, 1275 York Avenue, Box 468, New York, NY 10065.
E-mail address: diamondb@mskcc.org

Given its status as a relatively rare lymphoma with heterogeneous presentations, comprising roughly 5% of all NHL with an incidence of 0.5 per 100,000 in Western countries,[1] there is no established standard of care for treatment. The median age at diagnosis is 68 and predominantly found in men at a ratio of 3:1.[2]

MCL often presents with advanced-stage disease, typically with involvement of the lymph nodes, bone marrow, spleen, and/or gastrointestinal tract at the time of diagnosis. The defining activating mutation in most MCLs is the translocation of the proto-oncogene CCND1, the encoder of cyclin D1, to the immunoglobulin heavy chain (IgH). T(11;14) results in the constitutive activation of cyclin D1, a key mediator in cell-cycle progression from G1 to S phase not normally expressed in B lymphocytes.[3] Alternatively, point mutations can also result in truncated CCND1 mRNA, which can lead to increased protein levels.

Overexpression of cyclins D1, 2, or 3 may be necessary, but not sufficient for lymphomagenesis as demonstrated in mouse models.[4,5] Secondary mutations and alterations facilitate lymphomagenesis and can lead to the development of more aggressive MCL subtypes, such as transformation to blastic or blastoid MCL that is often associated with TP53 mutation. NOTCH1/2 mutations have been reported in approximately 5% to 10% of MCLs, and are associated with an inferior prognosis in few retrospective series.[6] Several integral cellular pathways, including phosphatidylinositol 3-kinase (PI3K)/protein kinase B (AKT)/mammalian target of rapamycin (mTOR) and nuclear factor κB (NF-κB), are often affected.[7] In addition, a recently implicated gene, SOX11, can account for some of the variability in the spectrum of presentation of MCL. A principal target of SOX11 is PAX5, a key mediator in B-cell maturity and plasmacytic differentiation.[6] Although there are conflicting data, a high degree of expression is generally associated with "classical," aggressive MCL versus indolent leukemic phase MCL.[8]

The heterogeneous mutation profile of MCL is increasingly implicated in prognostic metrics for MCL and causes a diverse range of clinically important responses, from efficacy of intensive chemotherapy to resistance to ibrutinib. The focus of this review is the current landscape of current U.S. Food and Drug Administration (FDA)–approved treatment paradigms, and their inclusion in clinical trial platforms as they pertain to evolving data on MCL pathobiology and to enumerate yet-to-be answered questions that may transform our understanding and treatment of the disease.

OBSERVABLE AND LOCALIZED DISEASE

A subset of patients with MCL do not meet criteria for treatment. In a population-based study assessing outcomes in cases of deferred treatment, those placed on observation were more likely to have non-nodal disease, good performance status, low lactate dehydrogenase (LDH), nonbulky disease, nonblastoid morphology, and lower Ki67 values. Tumors also display hypermutation of IgH, low SOX11 expression, and a noncomplex karyotype. The clinical phenotype is generally manifested as non-nodal, leukemic phase disease with or without splenomegaly.[9] Gastrointestinal tract-only and low-volume nodal disease are also described. Median time to treatment in the observation group was 35 months and median overall survival (OS) was 72 versus 52.5 months in the early treatment group. Non-nodal presentation was the strongest factor associated with prolonged time to treatment and OS.[10]

Early-stage MCL is a clinically uncommon presentation and there is no clear standard of care; however, radiation therapy or combined modality therapy are considered appropriate options for localized disease.

TREATMENT APPROACH IN FIT PATIENTS

For young, fit patients, a standard treatment regimen is cytarabine-containing induction chemotherapy followed by consolidation with autologous stem cell transplant (ASCT). Recent data demonstrate that rituximab maintenance after ASCT is associated with superior progression-free survival (PFS) and OS.[11] Data from multiple centers confirm the superiority of cytarabine-containing regimens.[12–14] However, the only randomized studies demonstrating superior PFS (not OS) benefit for consolidative ASCT come from an era without modern therapy—before the establishment of cytarabine backbones as standard of care[15] and before routine use of rituximab.[16] In fact, there are emerging data challenging the role of transplantation in CR1 in certain biologic subtypes of the disease, particularly in patients with TP53 mutation.[17]

Early data emphasized the impressiveness of cytarabine with a modified R-hyper-CVAD (rituximab-cyclophosphamide, vincristine, doxorubicin, and dexamethasone) regimen, alternating with R-MC (rituximab-methotrexate, cytarabine). Ninety-seven percent of patients responded with complete response (CR) rates of 87% with 3-year OS rates of 82%. Toxicity was significant with 8 treatment-related deaths (8%).[12] Hyper-CVAD-based regimens have proven efficacious, as seen in a Southwest Oncology Group (SWOG) multicenter trial,[14] but have not been compared against less toxic regimens, such as R-DHAP (rituximab-dexamethasone, high-dose cytarabine, and cisplatin) or alternating R-CHOP/R-DHAP. In addition, the stellar response rates seen in the MDACC single-institution study were not replicated in the SWOG study. This may be, in part, because of the toxicity of the regimen and higher drop-out rates compared with the single-institution study.

The MCL Network's Younger trial provided phase III data for 6 cycles of R-CHOP compared with 6 alternating cycles of R-CHOP and R-DHAP. Both were followed by ASCT. With median follow-up of 6.1 years, time to treatment failure was 9.1 years in the cytarabine group compared with 3.9 years in the control group. There was more hematologic toxicity in the cytarabine group.[18] It is worth noting that minimal residual disease negativity was 79% versus 47% after induction in the cytarabine and control groups, respectively. This trend was maintained following transplant (85% vs 68%).[13]

Although traditionally seen as an option for older, transplant-ineligible induction (as discussed below), rituximab/bendamustine with alternating or sequential rituximab/cytarabine (RB/RC) have been evaluated for use in younger patients as a pretransplant regimen. The regimens are attractive given their safer toxicity profiles without much sacrifice in response rate. The Dana Farber Cancer Institute examined sequential therapy in a phase 2 study and produced CR rates of 96%, with PFS of 96% at 13 months. A total of 93% of evaluable patients had minimal residual disease (MRD)-negative remissions, and 21 of 23 proceeded to transplant.[19] When pooled with a Washington University at St. Louis protocol of alternating therapy and off-trial, retrospectively treated patients, CR rates were 92%, with 85% moving on to transplant. Pooled 24- and 48-month PFS rates were 88% and 82%, respectively.[20]

To further improve outcomes after ASCT, the phase III LyMa trial studied the role of maintenance therapy by comparing R-DHAP with or without maintenance rituximab for 3 years following ASCT. Event-free survival was higher in the rituximab group at 79% compared with 61% in the observation arm at 4 years.[11] Median PFS and OS were not reached but, based on current survival data, the regimen is poised to demonstrate superior long-term outcomes after ASCT—compared with other upfront transplant containing regimens, such as Nordic MCL2 (R-maxi-CHOP/high-dose Ara-C and transplant).[21] Of the 184 patients who received cisplatin in the first cycle, 27 switched to carboplatin and 38 switched to oxaliplatin with similar outcomes. These alternative platinum agents are commonly used given a more favorable toxicity profile.

Prognostication and High-Risk Disease

With improved understanding of MCL biology and the increasing array of novel targeted agents, new systems for prognostication are needed. Currently, the Mantle Cell Lymphoma International Prognostic Index (MIPI) score is the most widely used prognostication tool. It uses clinical parameters of age, LDH, leukocyte count, and performance status to divide patients into 3 groups: MIPI low, intermediate, and high risk. The most recent iteration, the MIPI-c, divides patients into 4 risk groups based on a Ki-67 cut-off of 30%.[22] It has improved on the lack of discrimination in lower-risk groups.

Irrespective of the MIPI, certain genetic and biologic factors have emerged as prognostically significant. Deletions in *CDKN2A* and *TP53* are independently associated with adverse outcomes.[23] In patients with high-risk biological features, the current paradigm of intensive chemoimmunotherapy arguably does not confer justifiable benefit, especially, for example, to those with *TP53* mutations. In the analysis of the 27% of patients with *TP53* mutations or deletions in the Nordic MCL2 and MCL3 trials by Eskelund and colleagues,[17] median OS was a dismal 1.8 years, with a 50% relapse rate at 1 year. Similar findings were reported in another analysis of the Younger trial, with combined *CDKN2A* and *TP53* aberrations yielding vastly inferior OS.[24] Scott and colleagues[25] recently reported data on a gene expression proliferation assay examining 35 genes that can identify patients who would still have poor outcomes despite intensified therapy.

NOTCH1 mutations have been implicated as a poor prognostic feature. The pathway is responsible for cell proliferation, cell death, and differentiation, among others. In an analysis of 121 patients with MCL, the mutation was found in 14. At a median follow-up of 47 months, patients with *NOTCH1* mutations had an OS of 1.4 years compared with 3.9 years in their wild-type counterparts.[6]

These data raise questions as to whether regimens could be added to, or even be supplanted by, novel agents given that the standard of care, including ASCT, may fail to provide worthwhile benefit with exposure to significant toxicity in certain high-risk subgroups. The WINDOW study (NCT02427620) is currently underway as a means to avoid transplant by treating young patients with newly diagnosed MCL with rituximab/ibrutinib until best response, followed by abbreviated consolidation with hyper-CVAD. Preliminary response rates to chemotherapy-free induction are quite promising.[26] Similarly, the TRIANGLE study compares outcomes in transplant-free induction and is discussed later.

TREATMENT APPROACH IN ELDERLY OR UNFIT PATIENTS

Alternatives to intensive immunochemotherapy and ASCT have been increasingly used in elderly or unfit patients, who make up most patients with MCL.[1] As the pathobiology of the disease is elucidated, tailored and more rational treatments aim to reduce toxicity. Current strategies, particularly in low-risk patients, favor bendamustine/rituximab (BR) over R-CHOP, as was reported in the noninferiority BRIGHT study.[27] Other phase III data display median PFS of 69.5 months (BR) to 31.2 months (R-CHOP) at median follow-up of 45 months.[28] Cytarabine can be added to the regimen (R-BAC) at the cost of additional hematologic toxicity with 2-year PFS rates of 95% and is still effective with dose reduction.[29]

Other regimens using a targeted agent include:

- VR-CAP, which replaces vincristine in R-CHOP with bortezomib, and yields CR rates of 53% versus 42% for R-CHOP and PFS of 24.7 to 14.4 months.[30] The regimen is not widely adopted because it was compared with a nonstandard of care therapy and has significant rates of neuropathy.
- Lenalidomide-BR, which has achieved a CR rate of 64% and median PFS of 42 months in a Nordic Group study.[31] Toxicity was substantial for these over 65-year-old patients.
- RiBVD (rituximab, bendamustine, bortezomib, and dexamethasone) yielding a CR rate of 75.5% and median PFS of 70% at 24 months[32] in a phase II LYSA study.
- R^2 (rituximab and lenalidomide) yielding CR rate of 64% and 2-year PFS of 85% in a phase II, multicenter study.[33] The omission of alkylating chemotherapy significantly curtails toxicity and makes the regimen particularly attractive for patients with multiple comorbidities.

MINIMAL RESIDUAL DISEASE

MRD assays can detect minute quantities of tumor cells or circulating tumor DNA. This technology has far-reaching implications for the disease. MRD assessment could potentially allow for risk-adapted treatment approaches, including de-escalation of therapy in MRD-negative patients or early initiation of therapy in MRD-positive patients. The prognostic value of MRD in MCL was demonstrated with the allele-specific oligonucleotide-polymerase chain reaction technology used to detect and amplify clonal rearrangements in IgH and t(11;14) in patients in clinical remission.[34,35] Since then, multiple techniques for determining MRD have been developed, including high-throughput sequencing of the immunoglobulin genes.

The Nordic Group's Younger and Elderly studies both demonstrated the importance of molecular remission as an independent predictor of clinical outcome by showing superior 2-year remission rates in patients who achieved it.[35] In fact, across MCL2 and MCL3, of the 86 patients who achieved molecular remission posttransplant, 76% were in clinical remission at 10 years.[36] The Nordic group took the concept further by arguing for the initiation of 4 doses of weekly rituximab at first sign of conversion to MRD positivity for patients in molecular remission following ASCT. They demonstrated that the vast majority of patients could return to a status of durable molecular remission lasting an average of 1.5 years.[21] Patients treated pre-emptively with rituximab on molecular relapse showed an average 55-month interval from molecular to clinical relapse and could return to molecular remission even with repeated courses of pre-emptive rituximab.[36]

Both LyMa and CALGB 50403 (bortezomib maintenance versus consolidation following high-dose immunochemotherapy and ASCT) demonstrated far superior PFS for patients who achieved molecular remission before ASCT.[11,37] The difference was profound in the Cancer and Leukemia Group B (CALGB) trial—with 5-year PFS rates of 51% in MRD-positive patients compared with 93% in those achieving molecular remission. This theme has been repeated across studies following induction therapy for elderly patients not fit for transplant.[32]

Most of the information pertaining to the use of MRD to guide prognostication in MCL comes from data in the pretransplant setting. An upcoming Eastern Cooperative Oncology Group trial (NCT03267433) will question the necessity of transplant (with rituximab maintenance) in MRD-negative patients following induction with intensive immunochemotherapy by comparing it with maintenance rituximab, alone. It is to be hoped that this will provide meaningful guidance regarding de-escalation of therapy in MRD-negative patients in the era of maintenance therapy.

The vast potential of MRD for multiple applications remains to be explored. Ongoing studies are evaluating its use to guide maintenance therapy and escalation/de-escalation (with regard to proceeding to transplant after an MRD-negative induction). Cessation of therapy remains a potential unstudied application. As an example, rituximab maintenance following transplant is currently used for a blanket 3 years using LyMa.[11] Perhaps an MRD assessment could guide a cessation strategy to avoid prolonged, unnecessary treatment (**Fig. 1**).

RELAPSE/REFRACTORY DISEASE AND NOVEL THERAPIES

Established chemotherapy programs for the treatment of relapse/refractory (RR) disease include R-GemOx (rituximab-gemcitabine, oxaliplatin) and R-DHAP. However, they have been seen to confer short median PFS of between 5 and 12 months.[38,39] The regimens are seldom used given the efficacy and tolerability of newer targeted agents. BR has also been studied in the R/R setting and has a superior overall response rate (ORR) of 75% to 92%, with a median PFS of about 18 months.[40] A tailored approach would typically involve selecting a regimen with agents that are non-cross resistant.

The development and implementation of novel therapies has transformed the therapeutic landscape for R/R disease, and understanding the rationale for their respective targets is valuable.

Proteasome Inhibition

The first novel agent to be approved in the R/R setting was bortezomib. Proteasome inhibition is active for many reasons including the inhibition of NF-κB by blockade of IκB and by causing oxidative and endoplasmic reticulum stress.[41] Its role in maintenance was exemplified by CALGB 50403,[37] which showed a PFS benefit with bortezomib maintenance and consolidation. However, the study was limited by its use of R-CHOP, now nonstandard, as induction therapy before transplant. Cytopenias and peripheral neuropathy are major dose limiting side effects. It maintains a small role in induction for older, less fit patient in VR-CAP[30] and RiBVD.[32]

Phosphatidylinositol 3-Kinase/Protein Kinase B/Mammalian Target of Rapamycin Pathway Inhibition

PI3K/AKT/mTOR dysregulation has been implicated in the oncogenesis of many cancers. Increased mTOR activity can drive cell-cycle progression, increase cell proliferation, and support tumor growth.[42] Constitutive activation of AKT correlates with expression of inactivated PTEN, a tumor suppressor.[43] Given the demonstration of the pathway's importance, it is an attractive target in MCL.

Temsirolimus, an mTOR inhibitor, has been evaluated both as a single agent and in combination with BR.[44] Similarly, the PI3Kδ inhibitor, idelalisib, has been examined in R/R MCL and showed a dose-dependent ORR of between 40% and 69%, although with an unsatisfactorily short median duration of response of 2.7 months.[45] This short duration suggests the rapid development of resistance to δ isomer inhibition, possibly through upregulation of the α isomer.[46] To circumvent this, copanlisib, a pan-class I PI3K inhibitor has been evaluated in a phase IIa trial for patients with R/R disease, with an ORR of 64% and a median duration of response of 5 months.[47]

Single-agent activity is notably modest, prompting the consideration of synergistic inhibition. In vitro studies have demonstrated superior inhibition of angiogenesis,

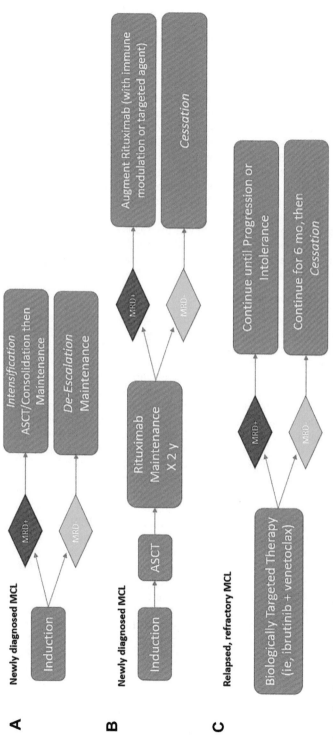

Fig. 1. (A–C) Future potential clinical applications of MRD testing in mantle cell lymphoma.

migration, and tumor invasiveness in MCL cells with dual inhibition of PI3K and mTOR as opposed to either alone.[48] A combination of buparlisib and ibrutinib was also examined in R/R disease. Of the 18 patients with MCL, the ORR was 88%, with 11 CRs.[49]

Immunomodulation

Lenalidomide had initially been tested in the R/R setting for patients who had progressed through bortezomib in the EMERGE trial and displayed ORR of 28% with relatively long-lasting efficacy in responders—leading to its FDA approval.[50] This was further validated in the European MCL Network's SPRINT trial, which compared it with the investigator's choice. With 254 patients randomized to either arm, there was a median PFS of 8.7 months compared with 5.2 months, favoring lenalidomide.[51] Lenalidomide exerts its effects, in part, by degrading lymphoid transcription factors (IKZF1 and IKZF3) via cereblon ubiquitin ligase.[52] Other lenalidomide-containing regimens that have been prospectively studied include the previously mentioned R^2 and lenalidomide-BR for induction.[31,33]

Further data will become available with the results of NCT01415752: a phase II, 4-arm study comparing variations of BR with lenalidomide consolidation. In addition, lenalidomide maintenance is currently under examination following high-dose sequential chemotherapy and ASCT in the MCL0208 trial.

B-Cell Receptor Pathway Inhibition

Ibrutinib, a small-molecule inhibitor of Bruton's tyrosine kinase, arrests aberrant B-cell receptor (BCR) signaling patterns that have been implicated in B-cell malignancy oncogenesis[53] and has shown promising activity in R/R MCL. Initially, PFS of 17.5 months were observed in an international phase II of single-agent ibrutinib in relapsed patients with MCL.[54] Notably, the median time to response was 1.9 months and the median time to CR was 5.5 months—longer than for most agents—with a reasonable interpretation that response deepens over time. This characteristic makes it attractive for use in maintenance. In addition, there seems to be emerging evidence that some patients with high-risk features can achieve remissions with ibrutinib therapy. In a head-to-head against temsirolimus, ibrutinib was clearly the superior therapy and had less toxicity, with a median PFS of 14.2 months compared with 6.2 months.[55]

In younger, fit patients who are transplant eligible, the randomized phase III TRIANGLE study is poised to challenge the well-established role of ASCT consolidation in CR1. The study will compare R-CHOP/R-DHAP with ASCT, R-CHOP + ibrutinib/R-DHAP with ASCT and ibrutinib maintenance, or R-CHOP + ibrutinib/R-DHAP (without ASCT) and ibrutinib maintenance. Preliminary data from the WINDOW study, using induction ibrutinib and rituximab, are promising as a means to avoid ASCT consolidation.[26] However, long-term follow-up data are needed to make a compelling case for a paradigm shift.

Results from other trials aiming to minimize toxicity, and also preserving efficacy, are on the horizon. For example, the results from the SHINE study, a phase III randomized clinical trial comparing ibrutinib/BR against BR alone for induction therapy in older, transplant-ineligible patients, are eagerly anticipated.

Mechanisms of ibrutinib resistance are being actively studied in MCL, such as upregulation of NF-κB signaling to overcome the BCR signaling inhibited by ibrutinib.[56] To overcome resistance, novel ibrutinib combinations are being tested with the aim of achieving higher CR rates and more durable remissions than with single-agent ibrutinib. The BCL-2 inhibitor, venetoclax, was recently combined with ibrutinib in a phase II trial of 24 patients with relapsed disease and achieved a CR rate of 42%.[57]

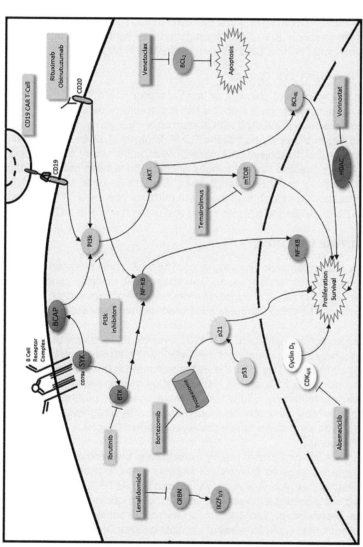

Fig. 2. Aberrant cellular pathways in MCL that may be targeted by novel agents. Synergistic combinations mentioned in the preceding text may be appreciated. AKT, protein kinase B; BCAP, B-cell adapter for PI3K; BCL2, B-cell lymphoma protein-2; BCLXL, B-cell lymphoma protein-extra large; BTK, Bruton's tyrosine kinase; CAR, chimeric antigen receptor; CDK4/6, cyclin-dependent kinase 4/6; CRBN, cereblon; HDAC, histone deactylase; IKZF1/3, Ikaros family zinc-finger protein 1/3; mTOR, mammalian target of rapamycin; NF-κB, nuclear factor κB; PI3K, phosphoinositide 3-kinase; SYK, spleen tyrosine kinase.

Cell-Cycle Inhibition

Cyclin D1 overexpression is a central tenet of MCL. The protein exerts its effects by complexing with CDK4/6 and phosphorylating Rb, a tumor suppressor, to allow progression through the cell cycle. Under study for multiple malignancies, single-agent efficacy in MCL with palbociclib has been demonstrated by Leonard and colleagues.[58] In 17 patients with R/R disease, 5 achieved PFS greater than 1 year with 1 CR and 2 partial responses. Palbociclib is currently being investigated in combination with ibrutinib (NCT03478514 and NCT02159755) and bortezomib (NCT01111188).

Two other CDK4/6 inhibitors are under investigation in a variety of malignancies: ribociclib and abemaciclib. Further data are needed for use in MCL.

Chimeric Antigen Receptor T-Cell Therapy

Given the established efficacy of chimeric antigen receptor (CAR) T-cell therapy in other B-cell NHLs, a multicenter phase II clinical trial is currently underway for patients with R/R MCL who have been pretreated with at least an anthracycline, or bendamustine, rituximab, and ibrutinib. It is hoped that the ZUMA-2 trial (NCT02601313) will yield another treatment approach to achieve durable responses. In the recent past, multiple variants of CAR T cells directed toward various antigens have been studied in the context of clinical trials for refractory lymphomas. Subsets of patients with MCL have generally been small, although responses are certainly observed.[59] The aforementioned ZUMA-2 trial will be the first dedicated trial of the therapy in MCL (**Fig. 2**).

SUMMARY AND FUTURE DIRECTIONS

MCL remains an incurable hematologic malignancy. The recent past has seen marked improvements made in our understanding and treatment of the disease. Longer-term follow-up of recent clinical trials will likely yield further practice-changing data, and the continued introduction of targeted therapies adds promise for responses and quality-of-life.

As our understanding of the pathobiology of MCL evolves, there is increasing interest in synergizing therapy to best counteract disease-driving pathways and to combat resistance to targeted therapy. This theme is well represented in the previous discussion of novel agents. Ibrutinib, for example, has been shown to have impressive activity in MCL but can be limited by failure to achieve a complete remission and by resistance—which inevitably develops on monotherapy. After progression, OS becomes dismal, with 1 retrospective analysis displaying median OS of 8.4 months after discontinuation of ibrutinib.[60]

As tumor sequencing becomes more readily available and biomarkers for response are elucidated, choosing targeted therapy will likewise become more tailored and patient-specific treatment approaches more widely applied. As MCL, and cancer, in general, are treated, the diseases evolves; they accrue more mutations, certain clones are more or less represented, and the tumor microenvironment changes. On-treatment biopsies (including liquid biopsies of circulating tumor DNA in the peripheral blood) at time of progression may offer us a chance to capture intrinsic biological changes and how best to target them. This approach has already elucidated mechanisms of resistance to BCR pathway inhibition using ibrutinib. It has also led to an understanding of resistance to immunomodulation via lenalidomide through decreased cereblon expression.[61]

Apart from novel therapies, we remain invested in minimizing toxicity while retaining favorable responses, particularly in this chronic disease, managed over many years, in an aging population, whereby quality-of-life concerns are paramount. Ongoing research in areas of maintenance therapy and MRD are identifying patients who may not require transplantation for durable response. Moreover, there are subsets of high-risk patients who do not benefit substantially from ASCT and for whom alternative, targeted approaches are being examined. It remains certain, however, that progress in this disease has been marked—and the future is bright.

REFERENCES

1. Zhou Y, Wang H, Fang W, et al. Incidence trends of mantle cell lymphoma in the United States between 1992 and 2004. Cancer 2008;113:791–8.
2. Armitage JO, Weisenburger DD. New Approach to classifying non-Hodgkin's lymphomas: clinical features of the major histologic subtypes. J Clin Oncol 1998;16(8):2780.
3. Rimokh R, Berger F, Delsol G, et al. Detection of the chromosomal translocation t(11;14) by polymerase chain reaction in mantle cell lymphomas. Blood 1994; 83(7):1871.
4. Lovec H, Grzeschiczek A, Kowalski MB, et al. Cyclin D1/bcl-1 cooperates with myc genes in the generation of B-cell lymphoma in transgenic mice. EMBO J 1994;13(15):3487.
5. Vegilante MC, Palomero J, Pérez-Galán P, et al. SOX11 regulates PAX5 expression and blocks terminal B-cell differentiation in aggressive mantle cell lymphoma. Blood 2013;121(12):2175–85.
6. Kridel R, Meissner B, Rogic S, et al. Whole transcriptome sequencing reveals recurrent NOTCH1 mutations in mantle cell lymphoma. Blood 2012;119:1963–71.
7. Perez-Galan P, Dreyling M, Wiestner A. Mantle cell lymphoma: biology, pathogenesis, and the molecular basis of treatment in the genomic era. Blood 2011;117: 26–38.
8. Nygren L, Baumgartner Wennerholm S, Klimkowska M, et al. Prognostic role of SOX11 in a population-based cohort of mantle cell lymphoma. Blood 2012; 119(18):4213–23.
9. Royo C, Navarro A, Clot G, et al. Non-nodal type of mantle cell lymphoma is a specific biological and clinical subgroup of the disease. Leukemia 2012;26: 1895–8.
10. Abrisqueta P, Scott DW, Slack GW, et al. Observation as the initial management strategy in patients with mantle cell lymphoma. Ann Oncol 2017;28(10):2489–95.
11. Le Gouill S, Hermine O, et al. Rituximab maintenance after autologous stem cell transplantation prolongs survival in younger patients with mantle cell lymphoma: final results of the randomized phase 3 LyMa trial of the LYSA/Goelams group. Blood 2016;128:145.
12. Romaguera JE, Fayad L, Rodriguez MA, et al. High rate of durable remissions after treatment of newly diagnosed aggressive mantle-cell lymphoma with rituximab plus hyper-CVAD alternating with rituximab plus high dose methotrexate and cytarabine. J Clin Oncol 2005;23(28):7013–23.
13. Hoster E, Rosenwald A, Berger F, et al. Prognostic value of Ki-67 index, cytology, and growth pattern in mantle cell lymphoma: results from randomized trials of the European Mantle Cell Lymphoma Network. J Clin Oncol 2016;34(12):1386–94.
14. Bernstein S, Epner E, Unger JM, et al. A phase II multicenter trial of hyperCVAD MTX/Ara-C and rituximab in patients with previously untreated mantle cell lymphoma: SWOG 0213. Ann Oncol 2013;24:1587–93.
15. Dreyling M, Lenz G, Hoster E, et al. Early consolidation by myeloablative radiochemotherapy followed by autologous stem cell transplantation in first remission

significantly prolongs progression-free survival in mantle-cell lymphoma: results of a prospective randomized trial of the European MCL Network. Blood 2005; 105:2677–84.

16. Geisler CH, Kolstad A, Laurell A, et al. Long-term progression-free survival of MCL after intensive front-line immunochemotherapy with in vivo-purged stem cell rescue: a randomized phase 2 multicenter study by the Nordic Lymphoma Group. Blood 2008;112:2687–93.

17. Eskelund CW, Gronbaek K, Hansen JW, et al. TP53 mutations identify younger mantle cell lymphoma patients who do not benefit from intensive chemoimmuno-therapy. Blood 2017;130:1903–10.

18. Hermine O, Hoster E, Walewski J, et al. Addition of high-dose cytarabine to immu-nochemotherapy before autologous stem cell transplantation in patients aged 65 years or younger with MCL (MCL Younger): a randomized, open-label, phase 3 trial of the European Mantle Cell Network. Lancet 2016;388(10044):565–75.

19. Armand P, Redd R, Bsat J, et al. A phase 2 study of rituximab-bendamustine and rituximab-cytarabine for transplant-eligible patients with mantle cell lymphoma. Br J Haematol 2016;173(1):89–95.

20. Merryman RW, Kahl BS. Rituximab/bendamustine and rituximab/cytarabine (RB/RC) induction chemotherapy for transplant-eligible patients with mantle cell lym-phoma: a pooled Analyis of two phase 2 clinical trials and off-trial Experience. Poster Presented at 2018 ASH. San Diego, CA, December, 2018.

21. Geisler CH, Kolstad A, Laurell A, et al. Nordic MCL2 trial update: six-year follow-up after intensive immunochemotherapy for untreated mantle cell lymphoma fol-lowed by BEAM or BEAC + autologous stem-cell support: still very long survival but late relapses do occur. Br J Haematol 2012;158(3):355–62.

22. Hoster E, Rosenwald A, Berger F, et al. Prognostic value of proliferation, cytology, and growth pattern in mantle cell lymphoma: results from randomized trials of the European MCL network. Hematol Oncol 2015;33:100–80.

23. Delfau-Larue M, Klapper W, Berger F, et al. CDKN2A and TP53 deletions predict adverse outcome in younger mantle cell lymphoma patients, independent of treatment and MIPI. Presented at the ASH Annual Meeting and Exposition. Or-lando, FL, December 5–8, 2015.

24. Delfau-Larue M-H, Hoster E, et al. CDKN2A and TP53 deletions predict adverse outcomes in younger mantle cell lymphoma patients, independent of treatment and MIPI. Presented at the ASH Annual meeting and Exposition. Orlando, FL, December 5–8, 2015.

25. Scott D, Abrisqueta D, Wright GW, et al. New molecular assay for the proliferation signature in mantle cell lymphoma applicable to formalin-fixed paraffin-embedded biopsies. J Clin Oncol 2017;35(15):1668–77.

26. Wang M, Romaguera J, et al. Chemotherapy-free induction with ibrutinib-rituximab followed by shortened cycles of chemo-immunotherapy consolidation in young, newly diagnosed mantle cell lymphoma patients: a phase II clinical trial. Blood 2016;128:147.

27. Flinn IW, van der Jagt R, Kahl BS, et al. Randomized trial of bendamustine-ritximab or R-CHOP/R-CVP in first line treatment of indolent NHL or MCL: the Bright study. Blood 2014;123(19):2944–52.

28. Rummel MJ, Niederle N, Maschmeyer G, et al. Bendamustine plus rituximab versus CHOP plus rituximab as first-line treatment for patients with indolent and mantle-cell lymphomas: an open-label, multicenter, randomized, phase 3 non-inferiority trial. Lancet 2013;381(9873):1203–10.

29. Visco C, Finotto S, Zambello R, et al. Combination of rituximab, bendamustine, and cytarabine for patients with mantle-cell non-Hodgkin lymphoma ineligible for intensive regimens or autologous transplantation. J Clin Oncol 2013;31(11): 1442–9.

30. Robak T, Huang H, Jin J, et al. Bortezomib-based therapy for newly diagnosed mantle-cell lymphoma. N Engl J Med 2015;372:944–53.

31. Albertsson-Lindblad A, Kolstad A, Laurell A, et al. Lenalidomide-bendamustine-rituximab in patients older than 65 years with untreated mantle cell lymphoma. Blood 2016;128:1814–20.

32. Gressin R, Callanan M, et al. Frontline therapy with RiBVD regimen elicits high clinical and molecular response rates and long PFS in elderly patients with mantle cell lymphoma; final results of a prospective phase II trial by the LYSA group. Blood 2014;124(21):148.

33. Ruan J, Rodriguez A, Svoboda J, et al. Lenalidomide plus rituximab as initial treatment for mantle-cell lymphoma. N Engl J Med 2015;373(19):1835–44.

34. Andersen NS, Donovan JW, Borus JS, et al. Failure of immunologic purging in mantle cell lymphoma assisted by polymerase chain reaction detection of minimal residual disease. Blood 1997;90(10):4212–21.

35. Pott C, Hoster E, Delfau-Larue MH, et al. Molecular remission is an independent predictor of clinical outcome in patients with mantle cell lymphoma after combined immunochemotherapy: a European MCL intergroup study. Blood 2010; 115:3215–23.

36. Kolstad A, Geisler CH, et al. Molecular monitoring and tailored strategy with preemptive rituximab treatment for molecular relapse: results from the Nordic mantle cell lymphoma studies (MCL2 and MCL3) with median follow-up of 8.5 years. Blood 2016;128:146.

37. Kaplan L, Cheson B, et al. Bortezomib maintenance versus consolidation following aggressive immunochemotherapy and autologous stem cell transplant for untreated mantle cell lymphoma: CALGB 50403. Blood 2015;126:337.

38. Rodriguez J, Gutierrez A, Palacios A, et al. Rituximab, gemcitabine, and oxaliplatin: an effective regimen in patients with refractory and relapsing mantle cell lymphoma. Leuk Lymphoma 2007;48:2172–8.

39. Witzig TE, Geyer SM, Kurtin PJ, et al. Salvage chemotherapy with rituximab DHAP for relapsed non-Hodgkin lymphoma: a phase II trial in the North Central Cancer Treatment Group. Leuk Lymphoma 2008;49:1074–80.

40. Robinson KS, Williams ME, van der Jagt RH, et al. Phase II multicenter study of bendamustine plus rituximab in patients with relapsed indolent B-cell and mantle cell non-Hodgkin's lymphoma. J Clin Oncol 2008;26:4473–9.

41. Pham LV, Tamayo AT, Yoshimura LC, et al. Inhibition of constitutive NF-KB activation in mantle cell lymphoma B-cells leads to induction of cell cycle arrest and apoptosis. J Immunol 2003;171:88–95.

42. Zoncu R, Sabatini DM. mTOR: from growth signal integration to cancer, diabetes, and ageing. Nat Rev Mol Cell Biol 2011;12(1):21–35.

43. Dal Col J, Zancai P, Terrin L, et al. Distinct functional significance of Akt and mTOR constitutive activation in mantle cell lymphoma. Blood 2008;111:5142–51.

44. Hess G, Keller U, Scholz CW, et al. Safety and efficacy of temsirolimus in combination with bendamustine and rituximab in relapsed mantle cell and follicular lymphoma. Leukemia 2015;29(8):1695–701.

45. Kahl BS, Spurgeon SE, Furman RR, et al. A phase 1 study of the PI3Kdelta inhibitor idelalisib in patients with relapsed/refractory mantle cell lymphoma. Blood 2014;123:3398–405.

46. Iyengar S, Clear A, Bödör C, et al. P110α-mediated constitutive PI3K signaling limited the efficacy of p110δ-selective inhibition in mantle cell lymphoma, particularly with multiple relapse. Blood 2013;121(12):2274–84.
47. Cunningham D, Dreyling M, et al. Results of the mantle cell lymphoma subset from a phase 2a study of copanlisib, a novel PI3K inhibitor, in patients with indolent and aggressive lymphoma. Blood 2015;126:3935.
48. Rosich L, Montraveta A, Xargay-Torrent S, et al. Dual PI3K/mTOR inhibition is required to effectively impair microenvironment survival signals in mantle cell lymphoma. Oncotarget 2014;5(16):6788–800.
49. Batlevi CL, Younes A, et al. Phase I/II clinical trial of ibrutinib and buparlisib in relapsed/refractory diffuse large B-cell lymphoma, mantle cell lymphoma, and follicular lymphoma. Presented at ASCO. Chicago, IL, June 4, 2018.
50. Goy A, Kalayoglu-Besisik S, Drach J, et al. Longer-term follow-up and outcome by tumour cell proliferation rate (Ki-67) in patients with relapsed/refractory mantle cell lymphoma treated with lenalidomide on MCL-001(EMERGE). Br J Haematol 2015;170(4):496–503.
51. Trněný M, Lamy T, Walewski J, et al. Lenalidomide versus investigator's choice in relapsed or refractory mantle cell lymphoma (MCL-002; SPRINT): a phase 2, randomised, multicentre trial. Lancet Oncol 2016;17(3):319–31.
52. Kronke J, Udeshi ND, Narla A, et al. Lenalidomide causes selective degradation of IKZF1 and IKZF3 in multiple myeloma cells. Science 2014;343:301–5.
53. Buggy JJ, Elias L. Bruton tyrosine kinase and its role in B-cell malignancy. Int Rev Immunol 2012;31:119–32.
54. Wang ML, Rule S, Martin P, et al. Targeting BTK with ibrutinib in relapsed or refractory mantle-cell lymphoma. N Engl J Med 2013;369(6):507–16.
55. Dreyling M, Jurczak W, Jerkeman M, et al. Ibrutinib versus temsirolimus in patients with relapsed or refractory mantle cell lymphoma: an international, randomized, open-label, phase 3 study. Lancet 2016;387(10020):770–8.
56. Woyach JA, Furman RR, Liu TM, et al. Resistance mechanisms for the Bruton's tyrosine kinase inhibitor ibrutinib. N Engl J Med 2014;370:2286–94.
57. Tam CS, Anderson MA, Pott C, et al. Ibrutinib plus venetoclax for the treatment of mantle cell lymphoma. N Engl J Med 2018;378(13):1211–23.
58. Leonard JP, LaCasce AS, Smith MR, et al. Selective CDK4/6 inhibition with tumor responses by PD0332991 in patients with mantle cell lymphoma. Blood 2012;119(20):4597–607.
59. Schuster S, June C, et al. Sustained remissions following chimeric antigen receptor modified T cells directed against CD19 (CTL019) in patients with relapsed or refractory lymphomas. Blood 2015;126:183.
60. Cheah CY, Chihara D, Romaguera JE, et al. Patients with mantle cell lymphoma failing ibrutinib are unlikely to respond to salvage chemotherapy and have poor outcomes. Ann Oncol 2015;26(6):1175–9.
61. Zhu Yx, Braggio E, Shi CX, et al. Cereblon expression is required for the antimyeloma activity of lenalidomide and pomalidomide. Blood 2011;118:4771–9.

Follicular Lymphoma
Redefining Prognosis, Current Treatment Options, and Unmet Needs

Karim Welaya, MBBCh, Carla Casulo, MD*

KEYWORDS

- Follicular lymphoma • Prognosis • Management • Unmet needs

KEY POINTS

- Follicular lymphoma is the most common indolent type of lymphoma with prolonged overall survival and durable response to initial treatment.
- Various prognostic biomarkers exist, including clinical, pathologic, treatment related, and genetic biomarkers. Among those, the ideal biomarker is still not well defined.
- Treatment of follicular lymphoma includes observation, immunotherapy, and chemoimmunotherapy.
- Despite the prolonged overall survival, there is a certain subset of patients with follicular lymphoma whose treatment is still not well defined.

INTRODUCTION

Follicular lymphoma (FL) is the most common indolent lymphoma in the United States with an incidence of 3.4 patients per 100,000 and an estimated 13,960 new patients diagnosed in 2016.[1] Over the past decades, there have been significant advances in the treatment of FL; the most effective was the introduction of rituximab, with a median overall survival (OS) now reaching 20 years.[2]

FL is a heterogeneous disease, with typically an indolent nature and durable response to initial treatment. However, subsets of patients have high rates of multiple relapses, short remission durations, and high rates of transformation. In this review, the authors discuss the prognosis of FL and various prognostic biomarkers used in stratifying patients with FL. They also discuss recent advances in front-line and relapsed FL treatment and review the unmet needs in patients with FL.

Disclosures and Conflict of Interest Statement: The authors have declared no conflicts of interest.

James P. Wilmot Cancer Institute, University of Rochester Medical Center, University of Rochester, 601 Elmwood Avenue Box 704, Rochester, NY 14642, USA
* Corresponding author.
E-mail address: carla_casulo@urmc.rochester.edu

Hematol Oncol Clin N Am 33 (2019) 627–638
https://doi.org/10.1016/j.hoc.2019.03.003
0889-8588/19/© 2019 Elsevier Inc. All rights reserved.

hemonc.theclinics.com

PROGNOSTIC INDICES
International Prognostic Index

There have been several prognostic biomarkers emerging over the past decades to predict survival for FL (**Table 1**). The International Prognostic Index (IPI) was among the first of these indices, first introduced in The International Non-Hodgkin Lymphoma Prognostic Factors Project study in patients with intermediate- and high-grade non-Hodgkin lymphoma (NHL) treated with anthracycline-based combination chemotherapy in the pre-rituximab era.[3] Although the IPI was predictive for progression-free survival (PFS) and OS, only 2% of FL patients were categorized in the high-risk group, and so a modified form of the IPI with more specific prognostic characteristics to FL was necessary.[4]

Follicular Lymphoma International Prognostic Index, Follicular Lymphoma International Prognostic Index-2, and PRIMA-Prognostic Index

The Follicular Lymphoma International Prognostic Index (FLIPI) emerged as a new prognostic model, including age ($\geq$60 years vs <60 years), Ann Arbor stage

Table 1
Prognostic markers for follicular lymphoma with predicated outcomes based on risk stratification

Prognostic Marker	Predicated Outcomes	
IPI[3]	CR rates: Low risk: 91% Low-intermediate risk: 71% High-intermediate risk: 56% High risk: 36%	5-y OS: Low risk: 73% Low-intermediate risk: 51% High-intermediate risk: 43% High risk: 26%
FLIPI[5]	5-y OS: Low risk: 91% Intermediate risk: 78% High risk: 52%	10-y OS: Low risk: 71% Intermediate risk: 51% High risk: 36%
FLIPI-2[6]	3-y PFS: Low risk: 91% Intermediate risk: 69% High risk: 51%	3-y OS: Low risk: 99% Intermediate risk: 96% High risk: 84%
PRIMA-PI[9]	5-y PFS: Low risk: 69% Intermediate risk: 55% High risk: 37%	
M7-FLIPI[18]	5-y FFS: Low risk: 77% High risk: 38%	5-y OS: Low risk: 90% High risk: 65%
Response to first-line therapy[13]	4-y PFS: Negative posttreatment FDG-PET: 63% Positive posttreatment FDG-PET: 23%	4-y OS: Negative posttreatment FDG-PET: 97% Positive posttreatment FDG-PET: 87%
TMTV[15]	5-y PFS: TMTV of <510 cm^3: 65% TMTV of >510 cm^3: 33%	5-y OS: TMTV of <510 cm^3 : 95% TMTV of >510 cm^3: 85%
POD24[17]	5-y OS: No POD24: 90% POD24: 50%	

(III–IV vs I–II), hemoglobin level (<120 g/L vs ≥120 g/L), number of nodal areas involved (>4 vs ≤4), and serum lactate dehydrogenase level (above normal vs normal or below). These pretreatment characteristics divided patients into 3 distinct groups: low- (0–1 risk factor), intermediate- (2 risk factors), and high-risk groups (≥3 risk factors) with a 5-year OS rate of 91%, 78%, and 52%, respectively. The model appeared to discriminate patient risk more accurately than the IPI.[5] FLIPI-2 arose as a newer prognostic index predicting PFS in the rituximab era. FLIPI-2 includes age greater than 60 years, bone marrow involvement, hemoglobin level less than 12.0 g/dL, greatest diameter of the largest involved node more than 6 cm, and serum β-2 micro-globulin (β2m) level greater than the upper limit of normal.[6] Based on these findings, FLIPI is the most broadly used prognostic tool in FL and has been extensively validated in the rituximab era.[7,8]

Bachy and colleagues[9] developed a new, yet simple prognostic tool based on the PRIMA study cohort. The PRIMA-PI is a 2-variable model score using only β2m and bone marrow involvement. It is composed of 3 risk categories, high with a β2m level greater than 3 mg/L, low with a β2m ≤3 mg/L without bone marrow involvement, and intermediate with a β2m ≤3 mg/L with bone marrow involvement. Despite the simplicity of the PRIMA-Prognostic Index (PI), further validation is warranted to use this prognostic tool in the everyday practice.

OTHER PROGNOSTIC FACTORS
Response to First-Line Therapy

Response to first-line therapy is also a strong predictor of outcome. Trotman and colleagues[10] evaluated the correlation between end of treatment ^{18}F fluorodeoxyglucose (FDG)-PET and survival in an analysis of 3 multicenter prospective studies,[11–13] including high tumor burden or advanced FL treated with rituximab-based systemic therapy. Posttreatment FDG-PET scan was evaluated using the 5-point Deauville scale. Patients with positive posttreatment FDG-PET scans (Deauville 4 or 5, about 17% of all patients) had significantly lower 4-year PFS (23% vs 63%, respectively) as well as 4-year OS (87% and 97%, respectively).[10] These findings indicate that achieving complete response (CR) to initial therapy is a strong favorable prognostic marker and maintaining CR to therapy is also being considered a surrogate marker of outcome in FL.[14]

Total Metabolic Tumor Volume

Assessing total metabolic tumor volume (TMTV) on a baseline FDG-PET is a unique approach in FL. Meignan and colleagues[15] evaluated the utility of the TMTV in the same cohort used by Trotman and colleagues.[10] In 185 patients with baseline scans suitable for TMTV calculations, median TMTV was 297 cm^3, and 510 cm^3 was identified as an optimal cutoff. A TMTV of greater than 510 cm^3 was associated with a significantly worse PFS and OS. The 5-year PFS and OS in patients with a TMTV of greater than 510 cm^3 were 33% and 85% compared with 65% and 95%, respectively, in patients with a TMTV less than 510 cm^3. In a multivariate analysis, TMTV as well as FLIPI2 score were independent predictors of PFS, and both could be combined to generate 3 different risk groups with significantly different outcomes.[15] Using the same cohort, Cottereau and colleagues[16] built a model that combined both the TMTV and the end of induction (EOI) FDG-PET. High TMTV was found in 28%, whereas 16% had a positive EOI FDG-PET. Both high TMTV and positive EOI PET were negative predictors of outcomes in terms of PFS and OS. Patients with high TMTV had a significantly higher rate of positive EOI FDG-PET compared with the patient with low TMTV (30% vs 11% in the high and low TMTV groups, respectively, $P = .008$). Although the TMTV seems to be a very promising prognostic tool, the TMTV calculations are not routinely available and used. With software advances, these calculations can be incorporated in the FDG-PET report, which would further add another prognostic parameter to further assist in personalizing treatment.

Duration of Response to Initial Therapy

One of the strongest prognostic markers is the duration of response to initial systemic therapy. An analysis of the National LymphoCare study that included more than 2700 patients with FL evaluated the outcomes in 588 patients with FL who received rituximab with cyclophosphamide, doxorubicin, vincristine, and prednisone (R-CHOP) as an initial treatment. Twenty percent of the patients developed progression of disease within 24 months (POD24) of initiating treatment. There was a statistically significant difference in the 5-year OS in patients who developed POD24 compared with patients who did not progress within the first 24 months (50% compared with 90%, respectively). These findings were validated in an analysis from the Iowa/Molecular Epidemiology Resource as well.[17] Unfortunately, none of the aforementioned prognostic tools can effectively identify patients who would progress within 24 months of initial treatment, which, as discussed, can significantly predict outcome. POD24 is now considered among the most robust predictors of poor survival in FL.

M7-Follicular Lymphoma International Prognostic Index

The m7-FLIPI is a newer prognostic score incorporating both clinical factors in addition to genetic alterations to create a clinicogenetic risk model of failure-free survival (FFS). It incorporates FLIPI, Eastern Collaborative Oncology Group performance status, and the mutational status of 7 genes (EZH2, ARID1A, MEF2B, EP300, FOXO1, CREBBP, and CARD11). The m7-FLIPI subdivided R-CHOP- or (rituximab with cyclophosphamide, vincristine, and prednisone) R-CVP-treated patients into high- and low-risk categories based on the sum of predictor values with a 5-year FFS of 38.29% in the high-risk group and 77.21% in the low-risk group. Based on the new risk category, 44% of the patients in the study cohort as well as 55% of patients in the validation cohort who were originally classified as high risk by FLIPI were reclassified as low risk by m7-FLIPI.[18] M7-FLIPI is a promising tool becoming more widely applied in FL research but remains to be validated prospectively.

Jurinovic and colleagues[19] found that the m7-FLIPI could identify some patients with future POD24, but had limitations. Patients with high-risk m7-FLIPI were more likely to develop early progression, yet 50% of the patients with early progression were in the low-risk m7-FLIPI group.[20] These findings suggest that the m7-FLIPI might need further adjustments to define true high-risk patients with FL. The POD24 prognostic index (POD24-PI) was a newer model incorporating the mutational status of only 3 genes, along with performance status and FLIPI. Similar to FLIPI, POD24-PI identified 78% of the patients with POD24 as high risk; however, 33% of the patients who did not progress within 24 months were still classified as high risk. Although more accurate when compared with FLIPI and m7-FLIPI in predicting early progressors, the POD24-PI requires validation.[19]

TREATMENT OPTIONS

The management of FL is based on the staging per the Revised Staging System for Primary Nodal Lymphomas (Lugano classification).[21] Treatment of early-stage FL includes radiotherapy, single-agent rituximab, systemic chemotherapy, or observation. In this review, the authors focus on treatment of advanced-stage FL grades 1, 2, and 3a.

FIRST-LINE TREATMENT
Observation and Single-Agent Rituximab

Although some patients can attain durable remission with first-line therapy, FL tends to recur with subsequent lines of therapy. Because of the indolent nature of FL, "watchful waiting" or observation has been a strategy in patients with advanced but low disease burden based on the Groupe d'Etude des Lymphomes Folliculaires (GELF) criteria.[22] Several studies in the pre-rituximab era failed to show a survival benefit for initiating treatment with chemotherapy versus observation in patients with low-burden FL.[22–24] As such for patients with limited stage or low tumor burden disease, observation or single-agent rituximab is an appropriate option.[25,26]

For patients requiring treatment, immunotherapy with an anti-CD20 monoclonal antibody whether as single agent or in combination with systemic chemotherapy has been the cornerstone for treating this subset of patients.

Chemoimmunotherapy

The addition of rituximab to systemic chemotherapy has significantly improved response rates, PFS, and OS in the front-line treatment of FL.[27–29] There are several chemoimmunotherapy regimens active as first-line treatment in advanced, symptomatic FL, evaluated in randomized studies. The phase 3 multicenter, randomized, non-inferiority StiL study compared bendamustine plus rituximab (BR) with R-CHOP in previously untreated advanced FL, marginal zone lymphoma, and mantle cell lymphomas. Median PFS was significantly longer in the BR arm compared with the R-CHOP arm (69.5 months vs 31.2 months), with benefit in all histologic subtypes. BR was also more tolerable than R-CHOP, with 19% of BR-treated patients developing serious adverse events compared with 29% in the R-CHOP arm.[30] In an updated report with a median follow-up of 113 months, the difference in PFS remained statically significant, without differences in OS (10-year OS rates were 71% and 66% for BR and R-CHOP, respectively).[31] The phase 3 randomized BRIGHT study of BR versus R-CHOP or R-CVP similarly showed no difference in CR (31% vs 25%, respectively) and overall response rates (ORR) (97% and 91%, respectively).[32] Updated long-term follow-up showed ongoing benefit to the BR arm (5-year PFS was 65% vs 56%, respectively) with similar OS.[33] Based on these 2 studies, BR is considered a widely accepted regimen for treating low-grade FL in the first-line setting. Neither the StiL nor the BRIGHT studies included patients with grade 3a, so in the authors' practice, they reserve R-CHOP as the treatment of choice for patients with grade 3a FL.

Obinutuzumab is a newer type II anti-CD20 monoclonal antibody with greater antibody-dependent cellular cytotoxicity and phagocytosis and lower complement-dependent cytotoxicity than rituximab. The GALLIUM study compared obinutuzumab- versus rituximab-based therapy, in combination with investigator's choice chemotherapy (BR, R-CHOP, or R-CVP), in first-line FL therapy with obinutuzumab or rituximab maintenance in responders. Three-year PFS for obinutuzumab-based therapy was significantly higher than that for the rituximab-based therapy (82% and 75% in the obinutuzumab-based therapy and the rituximab-based therapy, respectively), with similar ORR and CR rates and OS. Four percent and 3.4% of the patients had fatal events in the obinutuzumab and the rituximab arms, respectively. Patients who received bendamustine as their chemotherapy backbone had more fatal adverse events (4%) when compared with CHOP and CVP (both 2%). These fatal events were more common in the mainte-nance phase and in patients greater than the age of 70 years. Bendamustine had more deaths related to second malignancies and infections.[34,35] Obinutuzumab is gaining acceptance as a first-line treatment option in advanced FL. However, given the marginal improvement in the PFS, lack of OS benefit, and the relatively higher risk of death and second malignancies especially with the obinutuzumab plus bendamustine combination, use must be individualized based on patient age and comorbidity.

Maintenance After Chemoimmunotherapy

The phase 3 PRIMA study compared maintenance rituximab every 8 weeks for a total of 2 years in 1019 patients with previously untreated FL who responded to induction chemoimmunotherapy to observation. Maintenance rituximab significantly reduced progression when compared with observation (3-year PFS was 74.9% vs 57.6% in the maintenance arm and the observation arm, respectively).[11] In the 10-year follow-up report that was recently published, median PFS for the maintenance arms was reached at 10.49 years compared with 4.06 years in the observation group; how-ever, this was not translated to an OS benefit (10-year OS rate was 80% in both groups).[36] In the absence of improved OS, the authors believe maintenance should be used on an individual basis.

Lenalidomide and Rituximab

Emerging data suggest that rituximab plus lenalidomide (R^2) is a reasonable therapeu-tic alternative or frontline FL therapy. The phase 3 RELEVANCE study compared R^2 versus chemoimmunotherapy in 1030 patients with previously untreated advanced FL. Most patients in the chemoimmunotherapy arm received R-CHOP (72%), whereas BR and R-CVP were given in 23% and 5% of the patients, respectively. After 18 months of R^2, treatment was followed by 1 year of rituximab maintenance. At a me-dian follow-up of 3 years, both arms had similar rates of CR (48% and 53% in the R^2 and the chemoimmunotherapy arms, respectively). Three-year PFS and OS were also similar (PFS 77% and 78% in the R^2 and the chemoimmunotherapy arms, respec-tively; 3 year OS 94% in both arms), with similar rates of treatment discontinuation (31% vs 29%). Given the short follow-up and long treatment duration, and not insig-nificant toxicity of this regimen, it is still unclear whether it will be a widely accepted alternative to other chemoimmunotherapy regimens, such as BR and R-CHOP in the first-line setting.[37]

SECOND-LINE TREATMENT

Ultimately, most patients with FL will relapse, and almost 10% of patients will have re-fractory disease. Relapsed disease should be pathologically documented because the annual risk of histologic transformation (HT) in patients with FL in the rituximab era ranges between 2% and 3% per year.[38] These patients should be treated similarly to diffuse large B-cell lymphoma.

Observation remains a valid and widely accepted option in selected patients with relapsed FL. Indications to start treatment in the relapse setting, similar to the first-line setting, may be based on GELF criteria, time of relapse, and symptom burden. There are multiple treatment options for relapse/refractory FL, including observa-tion, rechallenging with first-line treatment, lenalidomide, phosphoinositide 3-kinase (PI3K) inhibitors, chemoimmunotherapy followed by high-dose chemotherapy, and autologous stem cell transplant. For the select patient, allogenic stem cell transplant is also an option.

BR and R-CHOP remain reasonable strategies at relapse.[39,40] The addition of lenalidomide to rituximab or obinutuzumab also demonstrates activity in the relapsed setting. The phase 2 Cancer and Leukemia Group B (Alliance) study randomized relapsed FL patients to rituximab, lenalidomide, or R[2]. The rituximab arm closed early. The study included 91 patients, and the ORR in patients who received R[2] was 76% compared with 53% in the lenalidomide arm (CR was 39% vs 20%). With a median follow-up of 2.5 years, the OS was similar in both groups.[41]

The GADOLIN study was an open-label, randomized, phase 3 study in 396 patients that compared obinutuzumab plus bendamustine (followed by maintenance) versus bendamustine alone in patients with relapse/refractory (and rituximab refractory) FL. Responding patients received obinutuzumab maintenance for up to 2 years. The PFS was significantly longer in the obinutuzumab plus bendamustine arm than with the bendamustine monotherapy arm (median not reached vs 14.9 months in the obinutuzumab plus bendamustine arm and the bendamustine monotherapy arm, respectively). Grade 3 to 5 adverse events were slightly higher in the obinutuzumab plus bendamustine and the bendamustine monotherapy arm (68% vs 62%).[42] In a more recent report with a median follow-up of 31.8 months, the median PFS in the obinutuzumab plus bendamustine arm was 25.8 months compared with 14.1 months in the bendamustine arm. Importantly, there was an OS benefit in the combination arm versus the monotherapy arms with 25.5% and 34.9% of the patients dying in the combination arm and bendamustine arm, respectively (hazard ratio, 0.67; 95% confidence interval, 0.47–0.96; $P = .0269$).[43]

Patients with Multiple Relapses

The optimal treatment option after multiple relapses remains undefined, and despite the large number of treatment options, the preferred order for using these treatment options is unclear. PI3K inhibitors are a new class of drugs that have showed activity in indolent NHL[44] and chronic lymphocytic leukemia.[45] Over the past 3 years, the Food and Drug Administration (FDA) has approved 3 PI3K inhibitors, idelalisib, copanlisib, and duvelisib, for treatment of FL in patients who have received at least 2 prior lines of therapy. Idelalisib, an oral PI3K inhibitor, was the first to gain FDA approval in 2014 based on a multicenter study of 125 patients with relapsed/refractory indolent NHL who had no response to rituximab and an alkylating agent, or had relapse within 6 months after receiving these treatments. The primary end point was ORR. The ORR for the entire cohort was 57% with 6% achieving CR with a median time to response of 1.9 months, and similar outcomes for FL. Median PFS was 11 months, and median OS was 20.3 months.[46]

Copanlisib is an intravenous pan-class I PI3K inhibitor that gained approval in 2017 for treatment of relapsed FL after 2 lines of therapy.[47] The approved inhibitor was based on a phase 2 study evaluating the efficacy and safety of copanlisib in 142 patients with indolent lymphoma; of those, 73% had FL. In patients with FL, the ORR was 59%, whereas 14% achieved CR; median duration of response was 12.2 months. The median PFS for the entire cohort was 11.2 months, whereas the median OS has not been reached. Almost 80% of the entire cohort experienced grade 3 or 4 toxicities, and the most common side effects were hyperglycemia, hypertension, lung infections, and neutropenia.[48] One of the downsides of copanlisib is that it requires a weekly intravenous infusion, a point to consider when choosing appropriate patients.

Recently, duvelisib, another PI3K dual inhibitor, was approved for the treatment of relapsed/refractory FL after at least 2 prior lines of therapy.[49] The approval was based on the DYNAMO study. The DYNAMO study was a phase 2 study that evaluated the efficacy of duvelisib in patients with refractory indolent NHL. The cohort included 83 patients with FL refractory to rituximab and/or chemotherapy with a median number of prior lines of 3. The ORR was 41% with 1 patient achieving CR. The most common adverse events reported were diarrhea, neutropenia, and skin rash.[50]

Despite these newly approved drugs, the response is not durable, and some of these agents are poorly tolerated. More randomized trials are needed to evaluate these drugs in this setting, with an emphasis on fixed duration of therapy and ways of sequencing treatments to minimize toxicity.

UNMET NEEDS

POD24 is one of the strongest predictors of OS in FL patients; with 50% OS at 5 years compared with patients without progression (50% vs 90%).[17] Not FLIPI, FLIPI-2, nor m7-FLIPI can reliably and reproducibly predict such high-risk patients early in the course of disease, although this knowledge could permit a risk-modified approach to front-line therapy. Another challenge in this high-risk patient population is the paucity of treatment options to offer when they relapse. The US intergroup designed the SWOG 1608 study, which is a phase 2 study that includes patients with FL who progressed within 24 months or were refractory to bendamustine- or CHOP-based therapy. Patients are randomized to obinutuzumab-based therapy with either umbralisib, a PI3K inhibitor, lenalidomide, or CHOP. An addition translational objective is validation of the m7-FLIPI through analyzing the original biopsies and to determine if it is a predictor of response to initial therapy.[51] The authors recommend that this high-risk group of patients be treated in the context of a clinical trial, given the expected poor outcome. Outside the context of a clinical trial, an appropriate treatment option would be high-dose chemotherapy followed by stem cell transplant. In a retrospective registry review of 349 patients with early relapse, patients who underwent autologous stem cell transplant (ASCT) within 1 year of disease progression had a statistically significant improvement in the 5-year OS compared with patients who did not receive ASCT (73% vs 60%, respectively).[52] Based on these data, the authors believe that this is a true indication for ASCT in patients with FL; other indications of ASCT are less well defined. Allogeneic stem cell transplant, on the other hand, is associated with higher treatment-related mortalities ranging between 25% and 40%. In a large trial, allogenic HCT was compared with ASCT following initial rituximab-based chemotherapy in patients with relapsed/refractory FL. ASCT had a lower rate of nonrelapse mortality with an inferior PFS as well as OS compared with allogenic HCT beyond 24 months; however, within the first 24 months, patients who underwent ASCT had a superior OS.[53] The authors usually preserve allogenic HCT to fit, otherwise healthy patients who were heavily pretreated in the past.

For the appropriate patient, consideration of high-dose chemotherapy with stem cell rescue is also appropriate.

Patients with multiply relapsed FL remain another treatment challenge and unmet need. Given the plethora of agents currently available, what is the best sequence of drugs, selection, and duration of therapy? Patients with HT, although outside the scope of this review, have inferior outcomes compared with those with low-grade disease. However, improved survival has been observed in the rituximab era when treated with anthracycline-based therapy.

SUMMARY

The heterogeneous nature of FL and generally favorable outcomes have led researchers to focus on patients with higher-risk disease and unmet medical need. As such, numerous prognostic factors have emerged to try to further define subsets of patients with more aggressive disease who may need different treatment. The future approach to FL should involve, when possible, the use of clinic-pathologic risk strategies, such as modified m7-FLIPI, or use of other gene signatures to classify patients into high- or low-risk groups, which are currently being studied.[54] This approach will facilitate precision, personalized treatment of poor-risk patients and the exposure to toxicity and cost of therapy for patients who will ultimately have excellent survival.

REFERENCES

1. Teras LR, DeSantis CE, Cerhan JR, et al. 2016 US lymphoid malignancy statistics by World Health Organization subtypes. CA Cancer J Clin 2016;66(6):443–59.
2. Tan D, Horning SJ, Hoppe RT, et al. Improvements in observed and relative survival in follicular grade 1-2 lymphoma over four decades: the Stanford University experience. Blood 2013;122(6):981–7.
3. International Non-Hodgkin's Lymphoma Prognostic Factors Project. A predictive model for aggressive non-Hodgkin's lymphoma. N Engl J Med 1993;329(14): 987–94.
4. Decaudin D, Lepage E, Brousse N, et al. Low-grade stage III-IV follicular lymphoma: multivariate analysis of prognostic factors in 484 patients—a study of the groupe d'Etude des lymphomes de l'Adulte. J Clin Oncol 1999;17(8):2499.
5. Solal-Céligny P, Roy P, Colombat P, et al. Follicular lymphoma international prognostic index. Blood 2004;104(5):1258–65.
6. Federico M, Bellei M, Marcheselli L, et al. Follicular lymphoma international prognostic index 2: a new prognostic index for follicular lymphoma developed by the international follicular lymphoma prognostic factor project. J Clin Oncol 2009; 27(27):4555–62.
7. Buske C, Hoster E, Dreyling M, et al. The Follicular Lymphoma International Prognostic Index (FLIPI) separates high-risk from intermediate-or low-risk patients with advanced-stage follicular lymphoma treated front-line with rituximab and the combination of cyclophosphamide, doxorubicin, vincristine, and prednisone (R-CHOP) with respect to treatment outcome. Blood 2006;108(5):1504–8.
8. Nooka A, Nabhan C, Zhou X, et al. Examination of the follicular lymphoma international prognostic index (FLIPI) in the National LymphoCare study (NLCS): a prospective US patient cohort treated predominantly in community practices. Ann Oncol 2012;24(2):441–8.
9. Bachy E, Maurer MJ, Habermann TM, et al. A simplified scoring system in de novo follicular lymphoma treated initially with immunochemotherapy. Blood 2018;132(1):49–58.
10. Trotman J, Luminari S, Boussetta S, et al. Prognostic value of PET-CT after firstline therapy in patients with follicular lymphoma: a pooled analysis of central scan review in three multicentre studies. Lancet Haematol 2014;1(1):e17–27.
11. Salles G, Seymour JF, Offner F, et al. Rituximab maintenance for 2 years in patients with high tumour burden follicular lymphoma responding to rituximab plus chemotherapy (PRIMA): a phase 3, randomised controlled trial. Lancet 2011;377(9759):42–51.
12. Dupuis J, Berriolo-Riedinger A, Julian A, et al. Impact of [18F] fluorodeoxyglucose positron emission tomography response evaluation in patients with high–tumor burden follicular lymphoma treated with immunochemotherapy: a prospective study from the Groupe d'Etudes des Lymphomes de l'Adulte and GOELAMS. J Clin Oncol 2012;30(35):4317–22.

13. Federico M, Luminari S, Dondi A, et al. R-CVP versus R-CHOP versus R-FM for the initial treatment of patients with advanced-stage follicular lymphoma: results of the FOLL05 trial conducted by the Fondazione Italiana Linfomi. J Clin Oncol 2013;31(12):1506–13.

14. Shi Q, Flowers CR, Hiddemann W, et al. Thirty-month complete response as a surrogate end point in first-line follicular lymphoma therapy: an individual patient-level analysis of multiple randomized trials. J Clin Oncol 2017;35(5):552–60.

15. Meignan M, Cottereau AS, Versari A, et al. Baseline metabolic tumor volume predicts outcome in high–tumor-burden follicular lymphoma: a pooled analysis of three multicenter studies. J Clin Oncol 2016;34(30):3618–26.

16. Cottereau AS, Versari A, Luminari S, et al. Prognostic model for high tumor burden follicular lymphoma integrating baseline and end induction PET: a LYSA/FIL study. Blood 2018;131(22):2449–53.

17. Casulo C, Byrtek M, Dawson KL, et al. Early relapse of follicular lymphoma after rituximab plus cyclophosphamide, doxorubicin, vincristine, and prednisone defines patients at high risk for death: an analysis from the National LymphoCare Study. J Clin Oncol 2015;33(23):2516.

18. Pastore A, Jurinovic V, Kridel R, et al. Integration of gene mutations in risk prognostication for patients receiving first-line immunochemotherapy for follicular lymphoma: a retrospective analysis of a prospective clinical trial and validation in a population-based registry. Lancet Oncol 2015;16(9):1111–22.

19. Jurinovic V, Kridel R, Staiger AM, et al. Clinicogenetic risk models predict early progression of follicular lymphoma after first-line immunochemotherapy. Blood 2016;128(8):1112–20.

20. Vindi J, Kridel R, Staiger AM, et al. A Clinicogenetic Risk Model (m7-FLIPI) Prospectively Identifies One-Half of Patients with Early Disease Progression of Follicular Lymphoma after First-Line Immunochemotherapy [abstract]. Blood 2015; 126. Abstract 333.

21. Cheson BD, Fisher RI, Barrington SF, et al. Recommendations for initial evaluation, staging, and response assessment of Hodgkin and non-Hodgkin lymphoma: the Lugano classification. J Clin Oncol 2014;32(27):3059.

22. Brice P, Bastion Y, Lepage E, et al. Comparison in low-tumor-burden follicular lymphomas between an initial no-treatment policy, prednimustine, or interferon alfa: a randomized study from the Groupe d'Etude des Lymphomes Folliculaires. Groupe d'Etude des Lymphomes de l'Adulte. J Clin Oncol 1997;15(3):1110–7.

23. Ardeshna K, Smith P, Norton A, et al. Long-term effect of a watch and wait policy versus immediate systemic treatment for asymptomatic advanced-stage non-Hodgkin lymphoma: a randomised controlled trial. Lancet 2003;362(9383): 516–22.

24. O'Brien M, Easterbrook P, Powell J, et al. The natural history of low grade non-Hodgkin's lymphoma and the impact of a no initial treatment policy on survival. Q J Med 1991;80(2):651–60.

25. Ardeshna KM, Qian W, Smith P, et al. Rituximab versus a watch-and-wait approach in patients with advanced-stage, asymptomatic, non-bulky follicular lymphoma: an open-label randomised phase 3 trial. Lancet Oncol 2014;15(4): 424–35.

26. Kahl BS, Hong F, Williams ME, et al. Rituximab extended schedule or Re-Treatment trial for low–tumor burden follicular lymphoma: eastern cooperative oncology group protocol E4402. J Clin Oncol 2014;32(28):3096.

27. Marcus R, Imrie K, Belch A, et al. CVP chemotherapy plus rituximab compared with CVP as first-line treatment for advanced follicular lymphoma. Blood 2005; 105(4):1417–23.

28. Marcus R, Imrie K, Solal-Celigny P, et al. Phase III study of R-CVP compared with cyclophosphamide, vincristine, and prednisone alone in patients with previously untreated advanced follicular lymphoma. J Clin Oncol 2008;26(28):4579–86.

29. Hiddemann W, Kneba M, Dreyling M, et al. Frontline therapy with rituximab added to the combination of cyclophosphamide, doxorubicin, vincristine, and predni-sone (CHOP) significantly improves the outcome for patients with advanced-stage follicular lymphoma compared with therapy with CHOP alone: results of a prospective randomized study of the German Low-Grade Lymphoma Study Group. Blood 2005;106(12):3725–32.

30. Rummel MJ, Niederle N, Maschmeyer G, et al. Bendamustine plus rituximab versus CHOP plus rituximab as first-line treatment for patients with indolent and mantle-cell lymphomas: an open-label, multicentre, randomised, phase 3 non-inferiority trial. Lancet 2013;381(9873):1203–10.

31. Rummel MJ, Maschmeyer G, Ganser A, et al. Bendamustine plus rituximab (B-R) versus CHOP plus rituximab (CHOP-R) as first-line treatment in patients with indolent lymphomas: Nine-year updated results from the StiL NHL1 study. J Clin Oncol 2017;35 (suppl; abstr 7501).

32. Flinn IW, van der Jagt R, Kahl BS, et al. Open-label, randomized, noninferiority study of bendamustine-rituximab or R-CHOP/R-CVP in first-line treatment of advanced indolent NHL or MCL: the BRIGHT study. Blood 2014.

33. Flinn I, van der Jagt R, Chang J, et al. First-line treatment of iNHL or MCL patients with BR or R-CHOP/R-CVP: results of the BRIGHT 5-year follow-up study. Hema-tol Oncol 2017;35:140–1.

34. Marcus R, Davies A, Ando K, et al. Obinutuzumab for the first-line treatment of follicular lymphoma. N Engl J Med 2017;377(14):1331–44.

35. Hiddemann W, Barbui A, Canales M, et al. Immunochemotherapy with obinutuzu-mab or rituximab for previously untreated follicular lymphoma in the GALLIUM study: influence of chemotherapy on efficacy and safety. J Clin Oncol 2018; 36(23):2395–404.

36. Salles G, Seymour JF, Feugier P, et al. Long term follow-up of the PRIMA study: half of patients receiving rituximab maintenance remain progression free at 10 years [abstract]. Blood 2017;130(suppl 1):486.

37. Morschhauser F, Fowler NH, Feugier P, et al. Rituximab plus lenalidomide in advanced untreated follicular lymphoma. N Engl J Med 2018;379(10):934–47.

38. Al-Tourah AJ, Gill KK, Chhanabhai M, et al. Population-based analysis of inci-dence and outcome of transformed non-Hodgkin's lymphoma. J Clin Oncol 2008;26(32):5165–9.

39. Robinson KS, Williams ME, van Der Jagt RH, et al. Phase II multicenter study of bendamustine plus rituximab in patients with relapsed indolent B-cell and mantle cell non-Hodgkin's lymphoma. J Clin Oncol 2008;26(27):4473–9.

40. van Oers MH, Van Glabbeke M, Giurgea L, et al. Rituximab maintenance treat-ment of relapsed/resistant follicular non-Hodgkin's lymphoma: long-term outcome of the EORTC 20981 phase III randomized intergroup study. J Clin Oncol 2010; 28(17):2853.

41. Leonard JP, Jung S-H, Johnson J, et al. Randomized trial of lenalidomide alone versus lenalidomide plus rituximab in patients with recurrent follicular lymphoma: CALGB 50401 (Alliance). J Clin Oncol 2015;33(31):3635.

42. Sehn LH, Chua N, Mayer J, et al. Obinutuzumab plus bendamustine versus bendamustine monotherapy in patients with rituximab-refractory indolent non-Hodgkin lymphoma (GADOLIN): a randomised, controlled, open-label, multicentre, phase 3 trial. Lancet Oncol 2016;17(8):1081–93.

43. Cheson BD, Chua N, Mayer J, et al. Overall survival benefit in patients with rituximab-refractory indolent non-Hodgkin lymphoma who received obinutuzumab plus bendamustine induction and obinutuzumab maintenance in the GADOLIN study. J Clin Oncol 2018;76:3656.

44. Benson DM, Kahl BS, Furman RR, et al. Final results of a phase I study of idelalisib, a selective inhibitor of PI3Kδ, in patients with relapsed or refractory indolent non-Hodgkin lymphoma (iNHL) [abstract]. J Clin Oncol 2013;31(Suppl):8526.

45. Flinn I, Brown J, Byrd J, et al. Final report of a phase I study of idelalisib (gs-1101) a selective inhibitor of Pi3kδ, in patients with relapsed or refractory Cll: 297. Hematol Oncol 2013;31:195.

46. Gopal AK, Kahl BS, de Vos S, et al. PI3Kδ inhibition by idelalisib in patients with relapsed indolent lymphoma. N Engl J Med 2014;370(11):1008–18.

47. Food and Drug Adminstration. FDA grants accelerated approval to copanlisib for relapsed follicular lymphoma 2017. Available at: https://www.fda.gov/drugs/informationondrugs/approveddrugs/ucm576098.htm. Accessed October 10, 2018.

48. Dreyling M, Santoro A, Mollica L, et al. Phosphatidylinositol 3-kinase inhibition by copanlisib in relapsed or refractory indolent lymphoma. J Clin Oncol 2017;35(35):3898–905.

49. Food and Drug Adminstration. duvelisib (COPIKTRA, Verastem, Inc.) for adult patients with relapsed or refractory chronic lymphocytic leukemia (CLL) or small lymphocytic lymphoma (SLL) 2018. Available at: https://www.fda.gov/Drugs/InformationOnDrugs/ApprovedDrugs/ucm621503.htm. Accessed October 10, 2018.

50. Flinn IW, van der Jagt R, Kahl BS, et al. Randomized trial of bendamustine-rituximab or R-CHOP/R-CVP in first-line treatment of indolent NHL or MCL: the BRIGHT study. Blood 2014;123(19):2944–52.

51. National Institute of Health. Obinutuzumab with or without umbralisib, lenalidomide, or combination chemotherapy in treating patients with relapsed or refractory grade I-IIIa follicular lymphoma 2018. Available at: https://www.clinicaltrials.gov/ct2/show/NCT03269669. Accessed October 10, 2018.

52. Casulo C, Friedberg JW, Ahn KW, et al. Autologous transplantation in follicular lymphoma with early therapy failure: a National LymphoCare Study and Center for International Blood and Marrow Transplant Research Analysis. Biol Blood Marrow Transplant 2018;24(6):1163–71.

53. Klyuchnikov E, Bacher U, Kröger NM, et al. Reduced-intensity allografting as first transplantation approach in relapsed/refractory grades one and two follicular lymphoma provides improved outcomes in long-term survivors. Biol Blood Marrow Transplant 2015;21(12):2091–9.

54. Huet S, Tesson B, Jais JP, et al. A gene-expression profiling score for prediction of outcome in patients with follicular lymphoma: a retrospective training and validation analysis in three international cohorts. Lancet Oncol 2018;19(4):549–61.

Lymphoplasmacytic Lymphoma and Marginal Zone Lymphoma

Luis M. Juárez-Salcedo, MD[a], Jorge J. Castillo, MD[b],*

KEYWORDS

- Lymphoplasmacytic lymphoma • Waldenstrom macroglobulinemia
- Marginal zone lymphoma • Extranodal marginal zone lymphoma
- Splenic marginal zone lymphoma • Nodal marginal zone lymphoma

KEY POINTS

- Lymphoplasmacytic lymphoma (LPL) and marginal zone lymphoma (MZL) are rare, indolent, and incurable subtypes of non-Hodgkin lymphoma.
- Mutations in MYD88 and CXCR4 are commonly detected in patients with LPL and mucosa-associated lymphoid tissue (MALT)1, NOTCH1, MYD88, and PTPRD mutations in patients with MZL.
- Alkylating agents, nucleoside analogues, proteasome inhibitors, anti-CD20 monoclonal antibodies, and BTK inhibitors are used to treat patients with LPL and MZL.
- Immunomodulating agents, BCL2 antagonists, PI3K inhibitors, and novel BTK inhibitors and monoclonal antibodies are undergoing clinical development in LPL and MZL.

LYMPHOPLASMACYTIC LYMPHOMA

Epidemiology

Lymphoplasmacytic lymphoma (LPL) is a B-cell disorder characterized by the malignant accumulation of clonally related B cells, lymphoplasmacytic cells, and plasma cells in the bone marrow and other tissues.[1] LPL is a rare disease, with an incidence of 1000 to 1500 new cases per year in the United States. The median age at diagnosis is 70 years, and fewer than 10% of patients are younger than 50 years.[2] More than 80% of LPL patients are white, and about 20% are of Ashkenazi Jewish descent. About 20% of patients have a positive family history of hematologic malignancy in first-degree relatives.

[a] Department of Hematology, Gregorio Marañon University Hospital, Calle del Dr. Esquerdo, 46, 28007, Madrid, Spain; [b] Bing Center for Waldenstrom Macroglobulinemia, Dana-Farber Cancer Institute, Harvard Medical School, 450 Brookline Avenue, Mayer 221, Boston, MA 02215, USA
* Corresponding author.
E-mail address: jorgej_castillo@dfci.harvard.edu

Hematol Oncol Clin N Am 33 (2019) 639–656
https://doi.org/10.1016/j.hoc.2019.03.004
0889-8588/19/© 2019 Elsevier Inc. All rights reserved.

Clinical Presentation

Although many LPL patients can be asymptomatic at the time of diagnosis, most patients will become symptomatic during the course of their disease. The most common symptoms in patients with LPL are fatigue and tiredness in the context of anemia (40% to 50%); constitutional symptoms such as drenching night sweats and unintentional weight loss (25% to 30%); neurologic symptoms, usually symmetric sensory neuropathy in lower extremities with evidence of demyelination in electromyography studies (20% to 25%); symptoms of hyperviscosity such as nosebleeds; blurred vision; and recurrent headaches (10% to 20%). A funduscopic examination should be performed in patients with typical symptoms, and if signs of hyperviscosity are seen (eg, increased tortuosity and sausaging of retinal vessels and retinal hemorrhages), plasmapheresis should be instituted urgently. Other presenting features include lymphadenopathy (10% to 15%) and hepatosplenomegaly (10% to 15%). Rare symptoms can be associated with cryoglobulinemia (eg, vasculitic rash or nonhealing ulcers in lower extremities), cold agglutinemia (eg, hemolysis or hemoglobinuria), and amyloidosis. Renal involvement and bone lytic lesions in LPL are rare, unlike in multiple myeloma.

Diagnosis

Over 95% of patients with LPL secrete an immunoglobulin M (IgM) monoclonal paraprotein, a condition known as Waldenstrom macroglobulinemia (WM). Less than 5% of LPL cases associate with non-IgM paraproteins, including IgG, IgA, kappa, or lambda, or are nonsecretory; these patients are not felt to have WM.

The diagnosis of LPL/WM is made based on findings in the bone marrow biopsy, serum protein electrophoresis (SPEP), and the clinical scenario. The following criteria must be met, based on the recommendations from the third International Workshop on Waldenstrom Macroglobulinemia (IWWM)[3]:

- A serum IgM monoclonal protein, of any size
- Involvement of the bone marrow by an intertrabecular infiltrate, of any size, of small lymphocytes, lymphoplasmacytoid forms, and plasma cells

The lymphocytic cells typically express surface IgM, CD19, CD20, and CD22. The plasmacytic cells express CD38 and CD138. The malignant cells typically do not express CD5, CD10, CD23, or cyclin D1. More than 90% of patients with WM carry the recurrent MYD88 L265P mutation, which can help secure the diagnosis.[4] MYD88 mutations can also be identified in the majority of patients with non-IgM LPL.[5,6] The MYD88 L265P mutation can be identified in about 50% of patients with IgM monoclonal gammopathy of undetermined significance and in 5% to 10% of patients with marginal zone lymphoma. MYD88 is constitutively activated in WM, promoting cell survival pathways through BTK upregulation.[7] This biologic observation provided the rationale of investigating BTK inhibitors in WM patients.

Initial Evaluation

The initial evaluation of patients with LPL/WM should include complete blood cell counts, liver and kidney function tests, SPEP and immunofixation, quantitative immunoglobulins and serum beta-2-microglobulin, free light chain, and lactate dehydrogenase (LDH) levels.[8] In special cases, the workup can include cryoglobulins, cold agglutinins, and von Willebrand disease screening (ie, von Willebrand antigen, ristocetin cofactor, and factor VIII levels). Bone marrow aspiration and biopsy and computed tomography (CT) scans of the chest, abdomen, and pelvis with intravenous contrast should be performed for confirmation of diagnosis and staging. Patients with predominantly sensory neuropathy should undergo nerve conduction and electromyography studies, and if demyelination is identified, then be tested for antimyelin-associated glycoprotein antibodies. Rarely, antiganglioside antibodies have been associated with axonal and motor neuropathy in patients with LPL/WM. Light chain (AL) amyloidosis is a rare complication in patients with WM, and can affect the kidneys, heart, peripheral nervous system, and the gastrointestinal (GI) tract. WM patients who present with nephrotic syndrome, shortness of breath, motor neuropathy, or intractable diarrhea should be evaluated for AL amyloidosis by means of an abdominal fat pad biopsy or suspected involved organ biopsy stained with Congo red.

Indications to Treat

Approximately 30% to 40% of patients with LPL/WM do not meet criteria for initiation of therapy at diagnosis. Immediate treatment is not needed in all LPL/WM cases given its incurability and also prolonged overall survival (OS). Criteria for initiation of therapy, based on recommendations from the second IWWM, are shown in **Table 1**. [9]

Response Criteria

Response to therapy is assessed using serum IgM levels, SPEP and immunofixation, bone marrow biopsy, and CT scans. The sixth IWWM response criteria are shown in **Table 2**. [10]

Prognostic Factors

A commonly used prognostic tool is the International Prognostic Scoring System for WM, which includes age greater than 65 years, hemoglobin less than or equal to 11.5 g/dL, platelet count less than or equal to 100×10^9/L, beta-2-microglobulin greater than 3 mg/dL, and serum IgM greater than 7000 mg/dL. Patients are stratified in low-, intermediate-, and high-risk categories, with 5-year survival rates from treatment initiation of 87%, 68%, and 36%, respectively.[11] However, the patients included in such a study were not treated with novel regimens.

Overall, the median survival of patients with LPL/WM in the United States has improved over the last decades.[12] A recent population-based study suggests the most important prognostic marker for OS is age at the time of diagnosis.[2] The median OS for patients aged 20 to 49, 50 to 59, 60 to 69, 70 to 79, and ≥80 years was not reached, 13, 10, 6 and 4 years, respectively.

More recently, there is mounting evidence that the MYD88 mutational status of patients with WM can have prognostic implications. An initial study showed that WM patients who do not have MYD88 mutations had shorter survival, with a median OS of 7 years versus greater than 15 years in WM patients with MYD88 L265P mutations.[13] More recently, a larger study evaluated the survival of WM patients without MYD88 L265P mutations, using a sensitive polymerase chain reaction (PCR) technique and adjusting for other clinical factors of importance, and concluded that these patients had a shorter survival than WM patients with MYD88 L265P mutations. [14]

Treatment Options

Therapy for LPL/WM should be reserved for patients with symptomatic disease.

There is no clear advantage for early therapy. Patients who are eligible for ASCT should not receive stem cell toxic drugs. In patients with symptomatic hyperviscosity, plasmapheresis should be instituted urgently and followed by definitive therapy directed at LPL/WM.

Table 1
Criteria for treatment initiation according to the second International Workshop for Waldenstrom Macroglobulinemia

Criteria	Comments
Constitutional symptoms	Recurrent fevers, night sweats, weight loss, and/or fatigue without other identifiable cause
Hyperviscosity	Recurrent nosebleeds, blurred vision, recurrent headaches, slow mentation, concerns with serum IgM >3000 mg/dL
Symptomatic extramedullary organ or tissue infiltration	Symptomatic lymphadenopathy, hepatomegaly and/or splenomegaly, pleural effusions, renal involvement, central nervous system involvement (Bing-Neel syndrome)
Moderate to severe peripheral neuropathy caused by LPL/WM	High likelihood of IgM-associated neuropathy in patients with length-dependent sensory deficit, demyelinating pattern in the nerve conduction studies, and high anti-MAG antibody titers
Cytopenias due to bone marrow infiltration	Hemoglobin less than or equal to 10 g/dL, platelet count <100 K/uL. Neutropenia is rare
Symptomatic cryoglobulinemia	Livedo reticularis, cold intolerance, nonhealing ulcers in low extremities, axonal/motor neuropathy
Symptomatic cold agglutinin anemia	Cold intolerance, hemolysis induced by exposure to cold
Systemic amyloidosis	Can affect kidneys (nephrotic syndrome), heart (restrictive cardiomyopathy), peripheral nerves (axonal/motor neuropathy), and GI tract (eg, diarrhea or malabsorption) Abdominal fat pad biopsy or organ biopsy for Congo Red stain can help diagnosis

From Kyle RA, Treon SP, Alexanian R, et al. Prognostic markers and criteria to initiate therapy in Waldenstrom's macroglobulinemia: consensus panel recommendations from the Second International Workshop on Waldenstrom's Macroglobulinemia. Semin Oncol 2003;30(2):116–20; with permission.

Most primary treatment regimens for LPL/WM are recommended based on single-arm prospective studies. Commonly used regimens include alkylators (bendamustine or cyclophosphamide) or proteasome inhibitors (bortezomib, carfilzomib, or ixazomib) in combination with the anti-CD20 monoclonal antibody rituximab.[15–21] In general terms, all these combinations have overall response rates between 80% and 90%, major response rates between 50% and 70%, and median progression-free survival times between 3 and 5 years, when used as frontline therapies. Alkylating agents can be associated with nausea, rash, cytopenias, increased risk of infections, and secondary cancers. Proteasome inhibitors can associate with neuropathy, cytopenias, and cardiac disorders. Rituximab can also be used as a single agent.[22,23] However, the response rate to single-agent rituximab is 40%, with a relatively short median progression-free survival of 12 to 18 months. Rituximab as a single agent can be used in patients not candidates for more intensive therapy. Rituximab should be used with caution in patients with LPL/WM and serum IgM levels greater than 4000 mg/dL, as in up to 40% of patients, rituximab therapy can be associated with an IgM flare that may be symptomatic.[24,25] Such an IgM flare does not represent progression of disease.

Table 2
Response criteria according to the sixth International Workshop for Waldenstrom Macroglobulinemia

Complete response	Normal serum IgM level, disappearance of monoclonal protein on immunofixation, resolution of extramedullary disease, and resolution of signs and symptoms attributed to WM
Very good partial response	At least 90% reduction in serum IgM, resolution of extramedullary disease, and resolution of signs and symptoms attributed to WM
Partial response	At least 50% but <90% decrease in serum IgM level and at least 50% decrease in extramedullary disease
Minor response	At least 25% but <50% reduction in serum IgM level
Stable disease	Neither minor response nor progressive disease
Progressive disease	Two measurements showing at least 25% increase in serum IgM level or progression of clinically significant cytopenias, extramedullary disease or constitutional symptoms, hyperviscosity, neuropathy, cryoglobulinemia, or amyloidosis

Adapted from Owen RG, Kyle RA, Stone MJ, et al. Response assessment in Waldenström macroglobulinaemia: update from the VIth International Workshop. Br J Haematol 2013;160(2):172; with permission.

About 7% of LPL/WM patients exposed to rituximab can become intolerant to it, and ofatumumab may be used in such cases. [26]

The Bruton tyrosine kinase inhibitor ibrutinib is the only US Food and Drug Administration (FDA)-approved agent in the frontline and relapsed settings for patients with LPL/WM. At least 3 prospective studies have evaluated the safety and efficacy of single-agent ibrutinib in patients with WM. In the pivotal phase II study including 63 previously treated patients with WM, ibrutinib was associated with an overall response rate (ORR) of 91%, a major response rate (MRR) of 73%, and a 2-year progression-free survival (PFS) rate of 69%.[27] A second study evaluated ibrutinib in 31 patients with rituximab-refractory WM, which was associated with similar results: ORR of 90%, MRR of 71%, and 18-month PFS rate of 86%.[28] Finally, a study on ibrutinib in 30 previously untreated WM patients showed ORR of 100%, MRR of 83%, and an estimated 18-month PFS rate of 92%.[29] Recently, a large randomized controlled study compared response and survival rates of patients with WM treated with ibrutinib and rituximab versus placebo and rituximab.[30] Previously treated and untreated patients were included in this study. The combination of ibrutinib and rituximab was superior than placebo and rituximab, with higher ORR (92% and 47%, respectively) and MRR rates (72% and 32%, respectively), as well as higher 30-month PFS rates (82% and 28%, respectively). Common adverse events associated with ibrutinib include rash, GI symptoms, bleeding, and atrial fibrillation. No studies have compared the combination of ibrutinib and rituximab versus ibrutinib alone.

All patients with LPL/WM will eventually relapse after primary therapy. Treatment options for relapsed disease include the same regimen used for primary therapy, another frontline regimen, clinical trials and, in selected cases, autologous stem cell transplantation. Other agents used in the relapsed setting include thalidomide, lenalidomide, everolimus, fludarabine, cladribine, and chlorambucil.

Future Therapies

Several novel agents are undergoing clinical development in patients with LPL/WM, including novel BTK inhibitors, BCL antagonists, anti-CD38 and anti-CXCR4 monoclonal antibodies, and phosphatidylinositol-3 kinase (PI3K) inhibitors.

The novel oral BTK inhibitors acalabrutinib and zanubrutinib have been shown to be safe and effective in patients with WM. These agents are more specific BTK inhibitors with a higher affinity for BTK than ibrutinib. Acalabrutinib is approved by the FDA for the treatment of relapsed and/or refractory mantle cell lymphoma (MCL). Data from a phase II study on over 100 patients with WM showed an ORR of 94%, with a VGPR rate of 32%.[31] Zanubrutinib has also shown safety and efficacy in an ongoing phase I/II study, with ORR of 92% and a VGPR rate of 43%.[32] A phase III study comparing zanubrutinib versus ibrutinib in patients with WM has recently completed accrual. Bleeding and atrial fibrillation are also associated with these BTK inhibitors.

A phase II study evaluating the BCL2 antagonist venetoclax has completed accrual in 30 patients with previously treated WM.[33] After a follow-up of 12 months, the ORR was 87% with a VGPR of 17%. Responses were seen in patients who were previously exposed to BTK inhibitors. The toxicity profile was acceptable, with neutropenia and diarrhea as common adverse events.

Clinical trials evaluating the anti-CD38 monoclonal antibody daratumumab, the anti-CXCR4 antibody ulocuplumab (in combination with ibrutinib), and the PI3K inhibitor umbralisib in WM patients are currently undergoing accrual.

MARGINAL ZONE LYMPHOMA
Introduction

Marginal zone lymphomas (MZLs) are indolent B-cell lymphomas that represent 5% to 10% of all non-Hodgkin lymphoma (NHL) in adults.[34] The incidence increases with age, and the median age at diagnosis 60 years, with a slight female predominance. [35]

MZL is characterized by the proliferation of B cells from the marginal zone of B-cell follicles found in mucosa-associated lymphoid tissue (MALT), lymph nodes, and the spleen. In the most recent World Health Organization (WHO) classification, this lymphoma comprises 3 different entities, extranodal MZL of MALT type (EMZL), splenic lymphoma (SMZL), and nodal MZL (NMZL).[35] These subtypes are heterogeneous and have clinical features and evolutionary presentation depending on the organ in which lymphoma has originated. Clinically, they behave indolently and have a prolonged course. Therefore, management strategies share similarly with other low-grade lymphomas, although specific biologic characteristics and particular pathophysiologic mechanism determine unique therapeutic approaches in some of the subtypes.

This article discusses the clinical features, diagnosis, and management of each subtype alongside the open questions that should be considered by the physicians who treat this complex disease.

Initial Evaluation

Excisional or incisional biopsies of an enlarged lymph node or suspicious mass are the gold standard for diagnosis of MZL.[36] A complete review of the sample for a pathologist with experience is essential to establish the diagnosis. CT or ultrasound-guided core needle biopsy is usually well tolerated and may be adequate for diagnosis. Fine-needle aspiration is not appropriate for diagnosis. In some cases, SMZL can present with lymphocytosis, in which case flow cytometry from peripheral blood can be diagnostic. Endoscopies are recommended in GI EMZL and are also helpful to stage EMZL affecting other sites, especially if there are abdominal symptoms. An adequate number of biopsies should be obtained during this procedure. Endoscopic ultrasound (EUS) could be an option to assess the depth of involvement in cases of GI EMZL. [37]

An exhaustive physical examination with special attention to peripheral lymph nodes and the abdomen should be performed. Laboratory evaluation should include complete blood count with a peripheral blood smear, as cytopenias may be a sign of bone marrow infiltration, and there could be circulating disease.[38] A basic biochemical study should include serum LDH level, as this parameter can have prognostic value and be an indicator of transformation to aggressive lymphoma. Beta-2-microglobulin (B2M) levels may also have a prognostic value. Serologic studies for detection of HCV are indicated, because of the association between MZL and HCV infection. Growing evidence indicates that HCV is closely correlated with the pathogenesis of MZL. The E2 glycoprotein of the HCV could interact with CD81 in B cells, thereby leading to chronic antigen stimulation and subsequent proliferation of B cells.[39] Obtaining an SPEP and serum immunoglobulins levels could be helpful in patients with MZL, as the presence of monoclonal gammopathy has been reported in up to 30% to 50% of patients with MZL. [40]

Staging of Marginal Zone Lymphoma

Chest, abdomen, and pelvis CT scans should be obtained to adequately stage MZL. Positron emission tomography (PET) scans may not be useful in MZL, because these lymphomas may have low fluorodeoxyglucose (18F-FDG) avidity. However, a meta-analysis reported a pooled detection rate for 18F-FDG-avid disease of 71% of patients with MZL, especially in extragastric presentation.[41] A bone marrow (BM) biopsy and aspirate are recommended in MZL cases, although it can be deferred if observations were to be the initial approach.

The Ann-Arbor system is a commonly most used staging method in lymphomas. Nonetheless, specific systems have been adopted for GI MZL. The Lugano staging system, which incorporates indices corresponding to depth of mucosal invasion and proximity of affected lymph nodes to the primary lesion, is shown in **Table 3**. [42]

EXTRANODAL MARGINAL ZONE LYMPHOMA OF MUCOSA-ASSOCIATED LYMPHOID TISSUE TYPE
Epidemiology and Presentation

EMZL, also called MALT lymphoma, is the most frequent of the MZL subtypes, and represents approximately 8% of all NHL cases. The median age at diagnosis is

Table 3
Lugano staging of primary gastrointestinal lymphoma

Stage	Extent of Lymphoma
I	Confined to GI tract (single primary, or multiple noncontiguous lesions)
II	Extending into abdomen from primary GI site II_1 = local nodal involvement II_2 = distant nodal involvement
IIE	Penetration of serosa to involve adjacent organ or tissues Specify site of involvement (eg, IIE [pancreas]) If both nodal involvement and involvement of adjacent organs, denote stage using both a subscript (1 or 2) and E, for example, II_1E (pancreas)
IV	Disseminated extranodal involvement or concomitant supradiaphragmatic nodal involvement

Adapted from Rohatiner A, d'Amore F, Coiffier B, et al. Report on a workshop convened to discuss the pathological and staging classifications of gastrointestinal tract lymphoma. Ann Oncol 1994;5(5):397–400; with permission.

60 years, with a slightly female predominance. EMZL frequently presents at a localized stage (40% of cases present with stage I and almost 30% with stage II disease). The most commonly affected primary site is the mucosa of the GI tract, in particular the stomach (44% of all EMZL cases), followed by the small intestine (7%). Ocular structures (orbit, conjunctiva, lacrimal glands, and eyelids), bronchial mucosa, skin, salivary glands, and thyroid gland can also be affected.[43] Signs and symptoms at presentation depend on the involved organ. In gastric EMZL, dyspepsia, epigastric pain, nausea, anorexia, and manifestation of GI bleeding are common symptoms. [44]

Pathogenesis

Pathogenesis of EMZL involves the continued proliferation of B cells and persistent stimulation of the B-cell receptor (BCR) signaling pathway. This stimulation seems to be induced by chronic antigenic stimulation as a result of either infectious or inflammatory causes. Gastric EMZL has a strong association with active *Helicobacter pylori* infection, cutaneous EMZL with *Borrelia burgdorferi*, ocular adnexa EMZL with *Chlamydophila psittaci*, small intestine EMZL with *Campylobacter jejuni*, and bronchial EMZL with *Achromobacter xylosoxidans*.[45,46] Chronic hepatitis C virus (HCV) infection has been implicated in the pathogenesis of all MZL subtypes and often associated with nongastric sites.[47,48] Autoimmune diseases also increase the risk of EMZL at various anatomic sites. For example, Sjogren syndrome associates with salivary gland EMZL, and Hashimoto thyroiditis associates with thyroid EMZL. [49]

Pathologic Features

EMZL is composed predominantly of morphologically heterogeneous malignant B cells. These resemble a spectrum spanning from small lymphocytes with scant cytoplasm to slightly larger cells with nuclei similar to those of centrocytes and having relatively abundant pale cytoplasm. These cells are located in the outer zone of reactive lymphoid follicles, extend into the interfollicular region, and may sometimes involve the germinal centers.[50] Plasmacytic differentiation is frequent and may pose diagnostic problems with lymphoplasmacytic lymphomas, especially in cases with associated paraproteinemia. In gastric EMZL, histology also plays an important role in establishing the diagnosis of *H pylori* infection.

EMZL cells display pan B-cell markers, such as CD19 and CD20. They are also positive for CD21 and CD35 (antigens shared with follicular dendritic cells) and also CD79a. The malignant cells have negative expression of CD5, CD10, CD23 and cyclin D1, which could help differentiating MZL from chronic lymphocytic leukemia/small lymphocytic lymphoma (CLL/SLL), follicular lymphoma (FL), and mantle cell lymphoma (MCL).

Specific chromosomal aberrations have been associated with EMZL, the frequency of which depends strongly on the primary site of disease. The most commonly observed abnormality is t(11;18) (q21;q21), which produce a fusion protein (native MALT1).[51] Expression of this protein leads to constitutive activations of the nuclear factor-*kappa* B (NF-kB) pathway, which in turn leads to resistance to apoptosis and uncontrolled proliferation. The presence of this mutation has been associated with worse response to antibiotics in *H pylori*-positive gastric EMZL.

A less frequently observed abnormality is the t(14;18) (q31;q21).[52] This translocation, different from that observed in FL, leads to the overexpression of MALT1 and subsequent activation of NF-kB. The t(1:14) (p22;q32) is also rare and causes overexpression of the BCL10 gene, which promotes the activation of MALT1. The t(3;14) (p14.1;q32) has been described in ocular, cutaneous, and thyroid EMZL, and involves the FOXP1 transcription factor and the heavy chain promoter. [53]

Prognostic Factors

A French study evaluated prognostic factors for PFS in 400 patients with EMZL, and identified stage III/IV, age older than 70 years, and serum LDH levels above the normal range as adverse prognostic factors.[54] Accordingly, 3 risk groups were identified with a median PFS of approximately 2.5 and 10 years for patients with high- and intermediate-risk disease. The median PFS was not reached in patients with low-risk disease. The 10-year PFS rate on these patients was approximately 75%. This score, the MALT-IPI, was also prognostic for OS, and patients with high-risk disease had a median OS of approximately 6 years, while the median OS in patients with low- and intermediate-risk disease was not reached at 10 years.

Treatment Options

In patients with gastric EMZL associated with *H pylori* infection, triple antibiotic therapy is the initial treatment option. Up to 75% of gastric EMZL patients with documented *H pylori* eradication will achieve remission of the lymphoma.[55] However, approximately 50% of patients will experience relapsed disease with antibiotic therapy alone and will require further therapy. A smaller proportion of *H pylori*-negative gastric EMZL patients and those with nongastric EMZL can respond to antibiotics.[56] Hence, it is reasonable to attempt antibiotic therapy as first-line therapy in most patients; however, most will require subsequent therapy. Until now, there have been no consensus guidelines regarding the optimal second-line treatment after initial therapy failure. Involved-field radiotherapy (IFRT) with a dose of 25 to 35 Gy is a reasonable first-line treatment for patients with localized disease with *H pylori*-negative EMZL or as second-line treatment in *H pylori*-positive cases who fail eradication therapy. IFRT has been associated with 5-year disease-free survival rates of 75% in a retrospective study.[57] Rituximab can be used alternatively if IFRT is not feasible. [58]

In asymptomatic patients with disseminated disease, observation may be an adequate initial approach. In symptomatic patients who require systemic treatment, rituximab alone or in combination has been studied. In 2013, a research group published the results of a study including previously untreated indolent lymphoma and compared rituximab, cyclophosphamide, doxorubicin, vincristine, and prednisone (R-CHOP) versus bendamustine and rituximab (Benda-R).[20] Benda-R had a similar progression-free survival (PFS) than R-CHOP with fewer adverse events (AEs). Thus, Benda-R is a reasonable treatment option in EMZL patients needing systemic therapy. More recently, the final results of the randomized multicenter IELSG-19 trial were published. This randomized trial focused specifically on frontline therapy for EMZL and included 3 arms, chlorambucil monotherapy, rituximab monotherapy, and chlorambucil plus rituximab.[59] There were no statistical differences in median OS between groups. However, the chlorambucil plus rituximab arm did provide significantly longer event-free survival (EFS) and PFS over chlorambucil or rituximab alone. Thus, chlorambucil and rituximab are an effective initial treatment option for EMZL. Single-agent rituximab has shown to be effective in the management of EMZL. There are series of patients with EMZL having reported overall response rates of 75%, with up to 50% CR in patients without previous therapy.[58,60,61] Rituximab single-agent seems to be more active in t(11;18)-negative than in t(11;118)-positive patients gastric MZL.[62] The therapeutic effect of the oral BTK inhibitor ibrutinib was evaluated in a prospective phase II study in 63 patients with relapsed and/or refractory MZL.[63] In this study, 32 patients (57%) had EMZL. The ORR to ibrutinib in this study was 48%; 45% attained partial response, and 3% attained complete response. In 30 patients with EMZL evaluable for response, the ORR was 50%. Ibrutinib is approved by the FDA for the treatment of patients with relapsed and/or refractory MZL.

High-dose chemotherapy followed by autologous stem cell rescue (ASCT) was evaluated in a retrospective, registry-based study that included 199 patients of whom 111 had EMZL.[64] The median age at transplantation was 56 years, and the median number of therapies prior to ASCT was 2 (range 1–8). The 5-year EFS and OS rates were 53% and 73%, respectively. Age 65 or older was independently associated with a shorter EFS and OS after ASCT. ASCT therefore may provide clinical benefit in MZL patients who have failed several prior lines of therapy.

SPLENIC MARGINAL ZONE LYMPHOMA
Epidemiology and Presentation

SMZL is a rare disease (<2% of all lymphomas) that arises predominantly from the marginal zone memory B cells located in the follicles of the spleen, splenic hilar lymph nodes, bone marrow, and peripheral blood.[65] SMZL represents approximately 20% of all MZL cases, and the median age at diagnosis is 69 years.[35] SMZL patients can be asymptomatic at the time of presentation or can present with anemia, thrombocytopenia, or lymphocytosis incidentally found on routine blood test. Anemia is seen in about 50% to 60% of the cases, and thrombocytopenia is seen in 20% of cases. Advanced stage SMZL, however, can present with massive splenomegaly, abdominal pain, and early satiety. Symptomatic cytopenias may be present, and imaging may show splenic hilar lymphadenopathy.[66] Up to 20% of patients can present with autoimmune manifestations, including hemolytic anemia, immune thrombocytopenia, and acquired coagulation disorders.[67] Although the association between HCV infection and SMZL has been described, there seems to be some geographic difference given the variation in seroprevalence between reported series.[68,69]

Pathology and Pathogenesis

The pathogenesis of SMZL has yet to be fully understood, but, similar to other subtypes of MZL, it likely involves the persistent stimulation of the BCR signaling pathway, with increasing proliferation and survival of malignant B cells.[70] Approximately 75% of cases with SMZL have an abnormal karyotype, with 7q deletions being the most frequently detected in 30% to 40% of the cases. Genomic profiling has detected recurring mutations that can be classified in 3 groups: NOTCH signaling, NF-kB pathway, and chromatin remodeling and cytoskeleton.[71] Specifically, mutations in KLF2, NOTCH1, NOTCH2, CARD11, and MYD88 have been described.[70,72,73] Unlike LPL, in which MYD88 mutations can be identified in about 90% of patients, this mutation can be identified in 5% to 10% of patients with MZL. Interestingly, mutations in the NOTCH and NF-kB pathways appear to be mutually exclusive.

A definitive diagnosis of SMZL can be made from histopathologic evaluation of the spleen, which shows a nodular lymphoid proliferation with a biphasic appearance effacing the white pulp, involving the red pulp in a patchy fashion, and infiltrating the vessel wall. The classic histology of SMZL includes a population of small lymphocytes that surrounds or replaces the germinal centers of the lymphoid follicles of the white pulp, progressively merging peripherally with larger cells. If histopathologic evaluation of the spleen is not possible, the diagnosis can be made by immunophenotyping of peripheral blood lymphocytes coupled with the histopathologic evaluation of the BM showing intrasinusoidal infiltration of CD20 + cells.[74,75]

Prognostic Factors

The Intergruppo Italiano Linfomi evaluated prognostic factors for cause-specific survival (CSS) in 309 patients with SMZL.[76] In a multivariate analysis, factors independently associated with a worse CSS were hemoglobin less than 12 g/dL, serum LDH greater than normal, and albumin less than 3.5 g/dL. Patients in the low- (no adverse factors), intermediate- (1 adverse factor), and high-risk (>1 adverse factor) group categories had 5-year CSS rates of 88%, 73%, and 50%, respectively. More recently, a multicenter study of 593 cases with SMZL identified hemoglobin and platelet counts as continuous variables, and elevated serum LDH and presence of extrahilar lymphadenopathy as adverse factors. [77]

Treatment Options

Asymptomatic patients with SMZL can undergo observation with routine clinical examinations and blood counts. Based on consensus guidelines, treatment for SMZL is indicated for constitutional symptoms, symptomatic splenomegaly, progressive nodal disease, and/or symptomatic cytopenias. Initial treatment options include splenectomy, rituximab alone, and chemotherapy combined with rituximab.[78–81] Conventionally, initial treatment for patients with symptomatic splenomegaly and/or cytopenias secondary to splenic sequestration was splenectomy, and patients could remain disease-free for many years after surgery. More recently, rituximab-based therapy has become a commonly used alternative to splenectomy, with outcomes comparable with splenectomy. A combination of rituximab and chemotherapy is indicated for those with disseminated disease, constitutional symptoms, and/or having signs of high-grade transformation, or in cases with inadequate or short response to rituximab as a first-line treatment option. HCV eradication therapy with interferon-α with or without ribavirin has induced responses in patients with HCV-associated MZL.[82] More recently, HCV eradication therapy with direct-acting antivirals such as sofosbuvir-based regimens has been associated with lymphoma responses in 75% of patients with HCV-associated MZL. [83]

Ibrutinib was evaluated prospectively in 14 patients with SMZL.[63] The ORR in 13 evaluable patients was 54%, providing a reasonable treatment option for patients with relapsed/refractory SMZL. A retrospective study evaluated the efficacy of high-dose chemotherapy followed by ASCT in 33 patients with SMZL.[64] SMZL patients who underwent ASCT had a median OS of 5 years, which appeared shorter than patients with EMZL, who had a median OS of approximately 17 years.

NODAL MARGINAL ZONE LYMPHOMA
Epidemiology and Presentation

NMZL is the least common subtype of MZL, representing between 1% and 2% of all NHL, and approximately 10% of all MZL.[35] The median age of patients diagnosed with NMZL is between 50 and 60 years. Similar to other indolent nodal lymphomas, such as SLL and FL, most patients with NMZL present with nonbulky disseminated peripheral, abdominal, and thoracic lymph node involvement.[84] B symptoms are rare, and diagnosis requires exclusion of splenic and other organ involvement to distinguish it from other subtypes of MZL. Although involvement of BM can occur in about one-third of patients, peripheral blood involvement and cytopenias are rare.

Pathogenesis

The molecular pathogenesis of NMZL is still incompletely described but likely involves constitutive BCR signaling, resulting in proliferation and survival of malignant B cells.[85]

A recent study combined whole exome and transcriptome sequencing as well as targeted sequencing of tumor-related genes and high-resolution single nucleotide polymorphism array analysis in 35 NMZL patients, and identified recurrent mutations in MLL2, PTPRD, NOTCH2, and KLF2.[86] Mutations in PTPRD were enriched in NMZL across other mature B-cell lymphomas.

Prognostic Factors

The follicular lymphoma international prognostic index (FLIPI) includes 5 adverse prognostic factors: age older than 60 years, serum LDH higher than the upper limit of normal, hemoglobin less than 12 g/dL, stage III/IV, and 4 or more involved nodal sites.[87] The FLIPI was prognostic for OS in patients with NMZL.[88] In this study, which included 32 patients with NMZL, patients with 0 to 2 adverse factors had a 5-year OS rate of 100% versus 70% in patients with 3 to 5 adverse factors.

Treatment Options

There are no treatment guidelines focusing specifically on NMZL. Treatment and management typically follow that of FL. In localized disease, targeted radiotherapy is appropriate. In both limited and advanced-stage disease, watchful waiting is followed in asymptomatic patients. In patients with advanced-stage and symptomatic disease requiring treatment, regimens combining rituximab plus chemotherapy with or without anthracycline are typically used. Ibrutinib was associated with an ORR of 41% in patients with NMZL,[63] and it is a reasonable option in the relapsed/refractory setting. ASCT appeared to be similarly effective in patients with NMZL as in patients with EMZL.[64] ASCT provides a treatment option to be considered in patients with multiply relapsed disease.

FUTURE THERAPIES

The therapeutic value of immunomodulators have been evaluated in patients with MZL. A prospective phase II study evaluated single-agent lenalidomide in 18 patients with relapsed/refractory EMZL, of whom 39% had ocular adnexal; 28% had gastric, and 17% had pulmonary sites of involvement.[89] The ORR was 61%, and the CR rate was 33%. Previously untreated patients had higher ORR at 73% than previously treated patients, who had an ORR of 34%. The combination of lenalidomide and rituximab was evaluated in 46 patients with relapsed/refractory EMZL.[90] In this study, sites of involvement included ocular adnexa in 26% of patients, stomach in 22% of patients, and lung in 11% of patients. The ORR and CR rate were 80% and 54%, respectively, with a median time to response of 3.6 months.

PI3K inhibitors and BCL2 antagonists have also been evaluated in a limited number of patients with MZL. A prospective study evaluated the PI3K-delta inhibitor idelalisib in 15 patients with relapsed/refractory MZL and found it was associated with an ORR of 47%.[91] The dual PI3K-alpha and delta inhibitor copanlisib was evaluated in 19 patients with MZL and induced a response in 13 patients, for an ORR of 68%.[92] The oral BCL2 antagonist venetoclax induced responses in 2 out of 3 patients with MZL treated in a phase I first-in-human prospective study. [93]

Several MZL-specific clinical trials evaluating novel agents and combinations such as the glycoengineered anti-CD20 monoclonal antibody obinutuzumab, the combination of copanlisib and rituximab, the combination of ibrutinib and rituximab, the combination of the proteasome inhibitor carfilzomib with or without rituximab, the mTOR inhibitor everolimus, and the novel BTK inhibitor zanuburitnib are ongoing.

REFERENCES

1. Swerdlow SH, et al, editors. WHO classification of tumours of haematopoietic and lymphoid tissues. Lyon (France): IARC; 2017.

2. Castillo JJ, Olszewski AJ, Kanan S, et al. Overall survival and competing risks of death in patients with Waldenstrom macroglobulinaemia: an analysis of the Surveillance, Epidemiology and End Results database. Br J Haematol 2015; 169(1):81–9.

3. Owen RG, Treon SP, Al-Katib A, et al. Clinicopathological definition of Waldenstrom's macroglobulinemia: consensus panel recommendations from the Second International Workshop on Waldenstrom's Macroglobulinemia. Semin Oncol 2003; 30(2):110–5.

4. Treon SP, Xu L, Yang G, et al. MYD88 L265P somatic mutation in Waldenstrom's macroglobulinemia. N Engl J Med 2012;367(9):826–33.

5. Itchaki G, Dubeau T, Keezer A, et al. Non-IgM secreting lymphoplasmacytic lymphoma - experience of a reference center for Waldenstrom macroglobulinemia. ASH Annual Meeting Abstracts. San Diego, December 2018: 2886.

6. King RL, Gonsalves WI, Ansell SM, et al. Lymphoplasmacytic lymphoma with a non-IgM paraprotein shows clinical and pathologic heterogeneity and may harbor MYD88 L265P mutations. Am J Clin Pathol 2016;145(6):843–51.

7. Yang G, Zhou Y, Liu X, et al. A mutation in MYD88 (L265P) supports the survival of lymphoplasmacytic cells by activation of Bruton tyrosine kinase in Waldenstrom macroglobulinemia. Blood 2013;122(7):1222–32.

8. Castillo JJ, Garcia-Sanz R, Hatjiharissi E, et al. Recommendations for the diagnosis and initial evaluation of patients with Waldenstrom macroglobulinaemia: a Task Force from the 8th International Workshop on Waldenstrom Macroglobulinaemia. Br J Haematol 2016;175(1):77–86.

9. Kyle RA, Treon SP, Alexanian R, et al. Prognostic markers and criteria to initiate therapy in Waldenstrom's macroglobulinemia: consensus panel recommendations from the Second International Workshop on Waldenstrom's Macroglobulinemia. Semin Oncol 2003;30(2):116–20.

10. Owen RG, Kyle RA, Stone MJ, et al. Response assessment in Waldenstrom macroglobulinaemia: update from the VIth International Workshop. Br J Haematol 2013;160(2):171–6.

11. Morel P, Duhamel A, Gobbi P, et al. International prognostic scoring system for Waldenstrom macroglobulinemia. Blood 2009;113(18):4163–70.

12. Castillo JJ, Olszewski AJ, Cronin AM, et al. Survival trends in Waldenstrom macroglobulinemia: an analysis of the Surveillance, Epidemiology and End Results database. Blood 2014;123(25):3999–4000.

13. Treon SP, Cao Y, Xu L, et al. Somatic mutations in MYD88 and CXCR4 are determinants of clinical presentation and overall survival in Waldenstrom macroglobulinemia. Blood 2014;123(18):2791–6.

14. Treon SP, Gustine J, Xu L, et al. MYD88 wild-type Waldenstrom macroglobulinaemia: differential diagnosis, risk of histological transformation, and overall survival. Br J Haematol 2018;180(3):374–80.

15. Dimopoulos MA, Garcia-Sanz R, Gavriatopoulou M, et al. Primary therapy of Waldenstrom macroglobulinemia (WM) with weekly bortezomib, low-dose dexamethasone, and rituximab (BDR): long-term results of a phase 2 study of the European Myeloma Network (EMN). Blood 2013;122(19):3276–82.

16. Ghobrial IM, Xie W, Padmanabhan S, et al. Phase II trial of weekly bortezomib in combination with rituximab in untreated patients with Waldenstrom Macroglobulinemia. Am J Hematol 2010;85(9):670–4.

17. Treon SP, Ioakimidis L, Soumerai JD, et al. Primary therapy of Waldenstrom macroglobulinemia with bortezomib, dexamethasone, and rituximab: WMCTG clinical trial 05-180. J Clin Oncol 2009;27(23):3830–5.

18. Treon SP, Tripsas CK, Meid K, et al. Carfilzomib, rituximab, and dexamethasone (CaRD) treatment offers a neuropathy-sparing approach for treating Waldenstrom's macroglobulinemia. Blood 2014;124(4):503–10.

19. Castillo JJ, Meid K, Gustine JN, et al. Prospective clinical trial of ixazomib, dexamethasone, and rituximab as primary therapy in waldenstrom macroglobulinemia. Clin Cancer Res 2018;24(14):3247–52.

20. Rummel MJ, Niederle N, Maschmeyer G, et al. Bendamustine plus rituximab versus CHOP plus rituximab as first-line treatment for patients with indolent and mantle-cell lymphomas: an open-label, multicentre, randomised, phase 3 non-inferiority trial. Lancet 2013;381(9873):1203–10.

21. Kastritis E, Gavriatopoulou M, Kyrtsonis MC, et al. Dexamethasone, rituximab, and cyclophosphamide as primary treatment of Waldenstrom macroglobulinemia: final analysis of a phase 2 study. Blood 2015;126(11):1392–4.

22. Dimopoulos MA, Zervas C, Zomas A, et al. Extended rituximab therapy for previously untreated patients with Waldenstrom's macroglobulinemia. Clin Lymphoma 2002;3(3):163–6.

23. Treon SP, Emmanouilides C, Kimby E, et al. Extended rituximab therapy in Waldenstrom's macroglobulinemia. Ann Oncol 2005;16(1):132–8.

24. Ghobrial IM, Fonseca R, Greipp PR, et al. Initial immunoglobulin M 'flare' after rituximab therapy in patients diagnosed with Waldenstrom macroglobulinemia: an Eastern Cooperative Oncology Group Study. Cancer 2004;101(11):2593–8.

25. Treon SP, Branagan AR, Hunter Z, et al. Paradoxical increases in serum IgM and viscosity levels following rituximab in Waldenstrom's macroglobulinemia. Ann Oncol 2004;15(10):1481–3.

26. Castillo JJ, Kanan S, Meid K, et al. Rituximab intolerance in patients with Waldenstrom macroglobulinaemia. Br J Haematol 2016;174(4):645–8.

27. Treon SP, Tripsas CK, Meid K, et al. Ibrutinib in previously treated Waldenstrom's macroglobulinemia. N Engl J Med 2015;372(15):1430–40.

28. Dimopoulos MA, Trotman J, Tedeschi A, et al. Ibrutinib for patients with rituximab-refractory Waldenstrom's macroglobulinaemia (iNNOVATE): an open-label substudy of an international, multicentre, phase 3 trial. Lancet Oncol 2017;18(2):241–50.

29. Treon SP, Gustine J, Meid K, et al. Ibrutinib monotherapy in symptomatic, treatment-naive patients with Waldenstrom macroglobulinemia. J Clin Oncol 2018;36(27):2755–61.

30. Dimopoulos MA, Tedeschi A, Trotman J, et al. Phase 3 trial of ibrutinib plus rituximab in Waldenstrom's macroglobulinemia. N Engl J Med 2018;378(25):2399–410.

31. Owen R, McCarthy H, Rule S, et al. Acalabrutinib in patients with Waldenström macroglobulinemia. EHA abstract. Stockholm, June 2018: S853.

32. Trotman J, Tam CS, Marlton P, et al. Improved depth of response with increased follow-up for patients (PTS) with Waldenström macroglobulinemia (WM) treated with Bruton's tyrosine kinase (BTK) inhibitor zanubrutinib. EHA abstract. Stockholm, June 2018. PS1186.

33. Castillo JJ, Gustine J, Meid K, et al. Prospective phase ii study of venetoclax (VEN) in patients (PTS) with previously treated Waldenstrom macroglobulinemia (WM). EHA abstract. Stockholm, June 2018: S854.

34. Swerdlow SH, Campo E, Pileri SA, et al. The 2016 revision of the World Health Organization classification of lymphoid neoplasms. Blood 2016;127(20):2375–90.

35. Olszewski AJ, Castillo JJ. Survival of patients with marginal zone lymphoma: analysis of the Surveillance, Epidemiology, and End Results database. Cancer 2013; 119(3):629–38.

36. Dreyling M, Thieblemont C, Gallamini A, et al. ESMO Consensus conferences: guidelines on malignant lymphoma. part 2: marginal zone lymphoma, mantle cell lymphoma, peripheral T-cell lymphoma. Ann Oncol 2013;24(4):857–77.

37. Caletti G, Fusaroli P, Togliani T, et al. Endosonography in gastric lymphoma and large gastric folds. Eur J Ultrasound 2000;11(1):31–40.

38. Horwitz SM, Zelenetz AD, Gordon LI, et al. NCCN guidelines insights: Non-Hodgkin's lymphomas, version 3.2016. J Natl Compr Canc Netw 2016;14(9):1067–79.

39. Arcaini L, Burcheri S, Rossi A, et al. Prevalence of HCV infection in nongastric marginal zone B-cell lymphoma of MALT. Ann Oncol 2007;18(2):346–50.

40. Wohrer S, Streubel B, Bartsch R, et al. Monoclonal immunoglobulin production is a frequent event in patients with mucosa-associated lymphoid tissue lymphoma. Clin Cancer Res 2004;10(21):7179–81.

41. Treglia G, Zucca E, Sadeghi R, et al. Detection rate of fluorine-18-fluorodeoxyglucose positron emission tomography in patients with marginal zone lymphoma of MALT type: a meta-analysis. Hematol Oncol 2015;33(3): 113–24.

42. Rohatiner A, d'Amore F, Coiffier B, et al. Report on a workshop convened to discuss the pathological and staging classifications of gastrointestinal tract lymphoma. Ann Oncol 1994;5(5):397–400.

43. Remstein ED, Dogan A, Einerson RR, et al. The incidence and anatomic site specificity of chromosomal translocations in primary extranodal marginal zone B-cell lymphoma of mucosa-associated lymphoid tissue (MALT lymphoma) in North America. Am J Surg Pathol 2006;30(12):1546–53.

44. Koch P, del Valle F, Berdel WE, et al. Primary gastrointestinal non-Hodgkin's lymphoma: I. Anatomic and histologic distribution, clinical features, and survival data of 371 patients registered in the German Multicenter Study GIT NHL 01/92. J Clin Oncol 2001;19(18):3861–73.

45. Zucca E, Bertoni F, Vannata B, et al. Emerging role of infectious etiologies in the pathogenesis of marginal zone B-cell lymphomas. Clin Cancer Res 2014;20(20): 5207–16.

46. Kuo SH, Cheng AL. Helicobacter pylori and mucosa-associated lymphoid tissue: what's new. Hematology Am Soc Hematol Educ Program 2013;2013:109–17.

47. Suarez F, Lortholary O, Hermine O, et al. Infection-associated lymphomas derived from marginal zone B cells: a model of antigen-driven lymphoprolifera-tion. Blood 2006;107(8):3034–44.

48. Bracci PM, Benavente Y, Turner JJ, et al. Medical history, lifestyle, family history, and occupational risk factors for marginal zone lymphoma: the InterLymph Non-Hodgkin Lymphoma Subtypes Project. J Natl Cancer Inst Monogr 2014;2014(48): 52–65.

49. Teixeira Mendes LS, Wotherspoon A. Marginal zone lymphoma: associated auto-immunity and auto-immune disorders. Best Pract Res Clin Haematol 2017; 30(1–2):65–76.

50. Kahl B, Yang D. Marginal zone lymphomas: management of nodal, splenic, and MALT NHL. Hematology Am Soc Hematol Educ Program 2008;1:359–64.

51. Dierlamm J, Baens M, Wlodarska I, et al. The apoptosis inhibitor gene API2 and a novel 18q gene, MLT, are recurrently rearranged in the t(11;18)(q21;q21) associated with mucosa-associated lymphoid tissue lymphomas. Blood 1999;93(11): 3601–9.

52. Murga Penas EM, Callet-Bauchu E, Ye H, et al. The t(14;18)(q32;q21)/IGH-MALT1 translocation in MALT lymphomas contains templated nucleotide insertions and a major breakpoint region similar to follicular and mantle cell lymphoma. Blood 2010;115(11):2214–9.

53. Streubel B, Vinatzer U, Lamprecht A, et al. T(3;14)(p14.1;q32) involving IGH and FOXP1 is a novel recurrent chromosomal aberration in MALT lymphoma. Leukemia 2005;19(4):652–8.

54. Thieblemont C, Cascione L, Conconi A, et al. A MALT lymphoma prognostic index. Blood 2017;130(12):1409–17.

55. Zullo A, Hassan C, Cristofari F, et al. Effects of *Helicobacter pylori* eradication on early stage gastric mucosa-associated lymphoid tissue lymphoma. Clin Gastroenterol Hepatol 2010;8(2):105–10.

56. Malfertheiner P, Megraud F, O'Morain C, et al. Current concepts in the management of *Helicobacter pylori* infection: the Maastricht III consensus report. Gut 2007;56(6):772–81.

57. Teckie S, Qi S, Lovie S, et al. Long-term outcomes and patterns of relapse of early-stage extranodal marginal zone lymphoma treated with radiation therapy with curative intent. Int J Radiat Oncol Biol Phys 2015;92(1):130–7.

58. Martinelli G, Laszlo D, Ferreri AJ, et al. Clinical activity of rituximab in gastric marginal zone non-Hodgkin's lymphoma resistant to or not eligible for anti-Helicobacter pylori therapy. J Clin Oncol 2005;23(9):1979–83.

59. Zucca E, Conconi A, Martinelli G, et al. Final results of the IELSG-19 randomized trial of mucosa-associated lymphoid tissue lymphoma: improved event-free and progression-free survival with rituximab plus chlorambucil versus either chlorambucil or rituximab monotherapy. J Clin Oncol 2017;35(17):1905–12.

60. Conconi A, Martinelli G, Thieblemont C, et al. Clinical activity of rituximab in extranodal marginal zone B-cell lymphoma of MALT type. Blood 2003;102(8): 2741–5.

61. Williams ME, Hong F, Gascoyne RD, et al. Rituximab extended schedule or retreatment trial for low tumour burden non-follicular indolent B-cell non-Hodgkin lymphomas: Eastern Cooperative Oncology Group Protocol E4402. Br J Haematol 2016;173(6):867–75.

62. Levy M, Copie-Bergman C, Amiot A, et al. Rituximab and chlorambucil versus rituximab alone in gastric mucosa-associated lymphoid tissue lymphoma according to t(11;18) status: a monocentric non-randomized observational study. Leuk Lymphoma 2013;54(5):940–4.

63. Noy A, de Vos S, Thieblemont C, et al. Targeting Bruton tyrosine kinase with ibrutinib in relapsed/refractory marginal zone lymphoma. Blood 2017;129(16): 2224–32.

64. Avivi I, Arcaini L, Ferretti VV, et al. High-dose therapy and autologous stem cell transplantation in marginal zone lymphomas: a retrospective study by the EBMT Lymphoma Working Party and FIL-GITMO. Br J Haematol 2018;182(6): 807–15.

65. Boveri E, Arcaini L, Merli M, et al. Bone marrow histology in marginal zone B-cell lymphomas: correlation with clinical parameters and flow cytometry in 120 patients. Ann Oncol 2009;20(1):129–36.
66. Starr AG, Caimi PF, Fu P, et al. Splenic marginal zone lymphoma: excellent outcomes in 64 patients treated in the rituximab era. Hematology 2017;22(7):405–11.
67. Thieblemont C, Felman P, Berger F, et al. Treatment of splenic marginal zone B-cell lymphoma: an analysis of 81 patients. Clin Lymphoma 2002;3(1):41–7.
68. Chuang SS, Liao YL, Chang ST, et al. Hepatitis C virus infection is significantly associated with malignant lymphoma in Taiwan, particularly with nodal and splenic marginal zone lymphomas. J Clin Pathol 2010;63(7):595–8.
69. Arcaini L, Paulli M, Boveri E, et al. Splenic and nodal marginal zone lymphomas are indolent disorders at high hepatitis C virus seroprevalence with distinct presenting features but similar morphologic and phenotypic profiles. Cancer 2004; 100(1):107–15.
70. Yan Q, Huang Y, Watkins AJ, et al. BCR and TLR signaling pathways are recurrently targeted by genetic changes in splenic marginal zone lymphomas. Haematologica 2012;97(4):595–8.
71. Martinez N, Almaraz C, Vaque JP, et al. Whole-exome sequencing in splenic marginal zone lymphoma reveals mutations in genes involved in marginal zone differentiation. Leukemia 2014;28(6):1334–40.
72. Clipson A, Wang M, de Leval L, et al. KLF2 mutation is the most frequent somatic change in splenic marginal zone lymphoma and identifies a subset with distinct genotype. Leukemia 2015;29(5):1177–85.
73. Rossi D, Trifonov V, Fangazio M, et al. The coding genome of splenic marginal zone lymphoma: activation of NOTCH2 and other pathways regulating marginal zone development. J Exp Med 2012;209(9):1537–51.
74. Matutes E, Oscier D, Montalban C, et al. Splenic marginal zone lymphoma proposals for a revision of diagnostic, staging and therapeutic criteria. Leukemia 2008;22(3):487–95.
75. Thieblemont C, Felman P, Callet-Bauchu E, et al. Splenic marginal-zone lymphoma: a distinct clinical and pathological entity. Lancet Oncol 2003;4(2): 95–103.
76. Arcaini L, Lazzarino M, Colombo N, et al. Splenic marginal zone lymphoma: a prognostic model for clinical use. Blood 2006;107(12):4643–9.
77. Montalban C, Abraira V, Arcaini L, et al. Risk stratification for Splenic Marginal Zone Lymphoma based on haemoglobin concentration, platelet count, high lactate dehydrogenase level and extrahilar lymphadenopathy: development and validation on 593 cases. Br J Haematol 2012;159(2):164–71.
78. Tsimberidou AM, Catovsky D, Schlette E, et al. Outcomes in patients with splenic marginal zone lymphoma and marginal zone lymphoma treated with rituximab with or without chemotherapy or chemotherapy alone. Cancer 2006;107(1): 125–35.
79. Olszewski AJ, Ali S. Comparative outcomes of rituximab-based systemic therapy and splenectomy in splenic marginal zone lymphoma. Ann Hematol 2014;93(3): 449–58.
80. Castelli R, Gidaro A, Deliliers GL. Bendamustine and rituximab, as first line treatment, in intermediate, high risk splenic marginal zone lymphomas of elderly patients. Mediterr J Hematol Infect Dis 2016;8(1):e2016030.
81. Kalpadakis C, Pangalis GA, Sachanas S, et al. Rituximab monotherapy in splenic marginal zone lymphoma: prolonged responses and potential benefit from maintenance. Blood 2018;132(6):666–70.

82. Kelaidi C, Rollot F, Park S, et al. Response to antiviral treatment in hepatitis C virus-associated marginal zone lymphomas. Leukemia 2004;18(10):1711–6.

83. Arcaini L, Besson C, Frigeni M, et al. Interferon-free antiviral treatment in B-cell lymphoproliferative disorders associated with hepatitis C virus infection. Blood 2016;128(21):2527–32.

84. Arcaini L, Lucioni M, Boveri E, et al. Nodal marginal zone lymphoma: current knowledge and future directions of an heterogeneous disease. Eur J Haematol 2009;83(3):165–74.

85. Thieblemont C, Molina T, Davi F. Optimizing therapy for nodal marginal zone lymphoma. Blood 2016;127(17):2064–71.

86. Spina V, Khiabanian H, Messina M, et al. The genetics of nodal marginal zone lymphoma. Blood 2016;128(10):1362–73.

87. Solal-Celigny P, Roy P, Colombat P, et al. Follicular lymphoma international prognostic index. Blood 2004;104(5):1258–65.

88. Heilgeist A, McClanahan F, Ho AD, et al. Prognostic value of the Follicular Lymphoma International Prognostic Index score in marginal zone lymphoma: an analysis of clinical presentation and outcome in 144 patients. Cancer 2013;119(1):99–106.

89. Kiesewetter B, Troch M, Dolak W, et al. A phase II study of lenalidomide in patients with extranodal marginal zone B-cell lymphoma of the mucosa associated lymphoid tissue (MALT lymphoma). Haematologica 2013;98(3):353–6.

90. Kiesewetter B, Willenbacher E, Willenbacher W, et al. A phase 2 study of rituximab plus lenalidomide for mucosa-associated lymphoid tissue lymphoma. Blood 2017;129(3):383–5.

91. Gopal AK, Kahl BS, de Vos S, et al. PI3Kdelta inhibition by idelalisib in patients with relapsed indolent lymphoma. N Engl J Med 2014;370(11):1008–18.

92. Dreyling M, Santoro A, Mollica L, et al. Phosphatidylinositol 3-kinase inhibition by copanlisib in relapsed or refractory indolent lymphoma. J Clin Oncol 2017;35(35):3898–905.

93. Davids MS, Roberts AW, Seymour JF, et al. Phase I first-in-human study of venetoclax in patients with relapsed or refractory Non-Hodgkin lymphoma. J Clin Oncol 2017;35(8):826–33.

Peripheral T-Cell Lymphoma
Moving Toward Targeted Therapies

Samuel Y. Ng, MD, PhD*, Eric D. Jacobsen, MD

KEYWORDS

- T-cell lymphoma • Targeted therapy • Jak/STAT pathway • DNA methylation

KEY POINTS

- Frontline therapy for peripheral T-cell lymphoma fails to produce durable remission in most patients.
- FDA-approved therapies to treat most cases of relapsed and/or refractory peripheral T-cell lymphoma have only modest activity.
- Brentuximab-vedotin demonstrates that agents with clear biomarkers that predict therapeutic efficacy can produce meaningful changes in clinical outcomes.
- Genomic profiling of peripheral T-cell lymphoma samples has revealed mutations that result in aberrant activity of T-cell receptor signaling, Jak/STAT signaling, and DNA methylation.
- Early-phase clinical trials suggest that agents targeting these pathways have activity in peripheral T-cell lymphoma.

INTRODUCTION

Meaningful therapeutic advances for peripheral T-cell lymphomas (PTCLs) have lagged behind their B-cell counterparts. Long-term overall survival (OS) is less than 35% for most subtypes of PTCLs. Most patients with PTCLs are treated with CHOP or CHOP-like chemotherapy, initially developed more than 30 years ago. With 1 notable recent exception discussed later, multiple efforts at dose-intensification or incorporation of novel therapeutic strategies have failed to improve OS. Treatments used in the relapsed and/or refractory (R/R) setting have a low response rate, and median OS is typically 6 months or less. The goal of this review is to address how recent biological insight into the pathogenesis of PTCLs might be used for drug development. The authors will review current clinical treatment paradigms and briefly revisit recently US Food and Drug Administration (FDA)–approved agents for PTCL. The authors will

Disclosure Statement: Dr S.Y. Ng has nothing to disclose. Dr E.D. Jacobsen receives research funding from Celgene, Merck, Janssen and honoraria from Bayer, Seattle Genetics.
Department of Medical Oncology, Dana-Farber Cancer Institute, 450 Brookline Avenue, Boston, MA 02215, USA
* Corresponding author.
E-mail address: samuel_ng@dfci.harvard.edu

Hematol Oncol Clin N Am 33 (2019) 657–668
https://doi.org/10.1016/j.hoc.2019.04.002
0889-8588/19/© 2019 Elsevier Inc. All rights reserved.

hemonc.theclinics.com

also summarize recent insights into PTCL biology and novel therapeutic approaches that attempt to capitalize on these insights.

SUMMARY AND RATIONALE FOR CURRENT TREATMENT PARADIGMS

The 2016 WHO Classification lists more than 15 subtypes of PTCL. This classification excludes cutaneous T-cell lymphomas (CTCLs) and natural killer cell lymphomas, which have different treatment paradigms. PTCL comprises approximately 10% to 15% of the 80,000 cases of non-Hodgkin lymphomas (NHL) diagnosed annually in the United States. The 3 most common PTCLs are peripheral T-cell lymphoma, not otherwise specified (PTCL-NOS), nodal lymphomas of follicular-helper T cell (T_{FH}) origin, of which angioimmunoblastic T-cell lymphoma (AITL) is the dominant subtype, and anaplastic large cell lymphoma (ALCL). Because of the rarity of these diseases, clinical studies of PTCL have typically combined these and other subtypes.

For a practical summary of PTCL treatment, the reader is referred to a review by Moskowitz and colleagues,[1] and to a series of subtype-specific reviews.[2-6] Most (approximately 85%) patients are treated with CHOP or CHOP-like therapy in the frontline.[7] The addition of etoposide to CHOP (CHOEP) can be considered for patients less than 60 years of age with normal lactate dehydrogenase based on an event-free survival benefit (75.4% vs 51.0%) or progression-free survival (PFS) benefit observed in retrospective analyses.[8,9] Several nonrandomized prospective studies have suggested that autologous stem cell transplant (auto-SCT) as consolidation following frontline treatment may confer a survival benefit. Perhaps the most widely cited is a Nordic lymphoma group trial of 180 patients treated with CHOP or CHOEP followed by auto-SCT in patients who responded to chemotherapy. On an intent-to-treat basis, the estimated 3-year PFS was 44% with an OS of 51%.[10] Approximately one-third of patients never proceeded to transplant due to lack of response to chemotherapy and, importantly, this trial also excluded patients with anaplastic lymphoma kinase-positive (ALK$^+$) ALCL, which generally has a much more favorable outcome than other TCLs.[7] The European multicenter AATT study compared allogeneic stem cell transplant (allo-SCT) with auto-SCT as consolidation for PTCL in first remission but was halted after interim analysis suggested that the statistical superiority of allo-SCT could not be demonstrated based on targeted trial enrollment.[11] Unfortunately, regardless of the frontline therapy used, most patients relapse. There is no consensus salvage therapy for R/R PTCL and the currently FDA-approved agents, with the exception of brentuximab-vedotin (BV) in ALCL, have low response rates. Also, aside from CD30 as a biomarker for BV, there are no validated methods to predict response to currently available agents.

FDA-APPROVED AGENTS FOR THE TREATMENT OF PERIPHERAL T-CELL LYMPHOMA

Four agents (pralatrexate, romidepsin, belinostat, and BV) are FDA approved to treat PTCL, with all except BV approved only in the R/R setting. These drugs are thought to target PTCLs through distinct mechanisms of action. Both pralatrexate and romidepsin were empirically found to have activity against CTCL and PTCL (TCLs) using efficacy analysis from subsets of patients enrolled on phase I trials. Pralatrexate was designed to have increased antitumor effects compared with methotrexate by increasing cellular internalization through the reduced folate carrier.[12] Given the established activity of methotrexate against NHL and encouraging results from preclinical models of lymphoma,[13] pralatrexate was tested in patients with R/R NHL and found to be primarily active in patients with TCL.[14] This led to the pivotal phase II PROPEL trial, which reported on 109 patients with R/R PTCL treated with single-agent pralatrexate. The overall response rate (ORR) was 29% and complete response (CR) rate was 11%, with the major grade 3 to 4 toxicities being mucositis and bone marrow suppression.[15] These phase II results led the FDA to grant accelerated approval for the use of pralatrexate in R/R PTCL. Histone deacetylase inhibitors (HDACi) prevent HDACs from removing acetyl groups from target substrates. This leads to a pleiotropic downstream set of effects including activation of cell death, cellular differentiation, and inhibition of angiogenesis.[16] HDACi initially were discovered to have activity against TCLs in phase I trials that included multiple tumor types.[17,18] Follow-up clinical trials confirmed activity of the class 1 HDACi romidepsin and the pan HDACi belinostat. In a pivotal phase II trial of romidepsin in 130 patients with R/R PTCLs, the ORR was 25%, including 15% CR.[19] Grade 3 toxicities primarily consisted of bone marrow suppression in each of these studies. A pivotal phase II trial of belinostat for patients with R/R PTCLs demonstrated an ORR 25% including 10.8% CRs.[20] Bone marrow suppression and infections were the most frequent adverse events (AEs). Both romidepsin and belinostat were granted accelerated approval by the FDA based on these pivotal trials. Nevertheless, in the case of each of these drugs, biomarkers for efficacy have not been established and, despite a small number of patients who remain in remission for years,[21] median PFS ranged from 1.8 to 4 months for participants on these trials.

BV is an antibody-drug-conjugate linking monomethylauristatin E to a monoclonal antibody against CD30, which thereby delivers a potent microtubule inhibitor to CD30$^+$ cells.[22] A phase I study of BV included 2 patients with ALCL, both of whom achieved CR.[23] This prompted a phase II trial in patients with R/R ALCL, most of whom (42/58) had ALK$^-$ disease.[24] The ORR was 86%, with 57% CRs with a median PFS of 13.3 months. Major toxicities included peripheral neuropathy and bone marrow suppression. A phase II study of BV in other CD30$^+$ PTCLs demonstrated an ORR of 41%.[25] Recent announcement of results from the phase III ECHELON-2 trial of CHP + BV versus CHOP chemotherapy assessing 452 patients with untreated CD30$^+$ PTCL demonstrated a PFS (hazard ratio [HR] = 0.71 with 95% CI, 0.54–0.93) and an OS advantage with CHP + BV (HR = 0.66 with CI, 0.46–0.95), resulting in a first-line FDA approval of this regimen.[26] As a result of regulatory concerns, 75% of patients enrolled in this study had ALCL, and in part because of the smaller numbers of patients enrolled, the benefit of this approach for treatment of PTCL-NOS and AITL is less certain. Nevertheless, this is the most significant advance in frontline PTCL treatment in decades. The success of BV suggests that, with properly targeted therapies, improvements in outcome can be made in PTCL.

Other attempts to use novel agents in combination with cytotoxic chemotherapy or with one another have met with limited success. A single-arm, phase II trial incorporating pralatrexate with a CHOP-like backbone that substituted etoposide for doxorubicin in frontline treatment of PTCLs failed to show improvement in 2-year PFS (39%) and OS (60%).[27] A phase Ib/II trial combined romidepsin with CHOP for frontline treatment of 37 patients with PTCLs demonstrated a 30-month PFS of 41% with OS 70.7%, albeit with more toxicity than would be expected from standard CHOP chemotherapy, including 2 with early cardiac events.[28] Nevertheless, because of the promising efficacy data, a phase III trial comparing CHOP + romidepsin with CHOP alone has enrolled 421 patients with primary endpoint analysis due in July 2019 (NCT01796002). In accordance with preclinical data demonstrating some synergy between the empiric combination of romidepsin and pralatrexate in TCL cell lines in vitro and in vivo,[29] a phase I trial combining these 2 in patients with R/R lymphomas has demonstrated an ORR of 71% including 29% CR among 14 patients with TCLs, although the median duration of response was 4.3 months. Grade 3 toxicities included primarily hematologic and infectious events. This trial continues to accrue patients treated with the recommended phase II dose of pralatrexate 25 mg/m^2 and romidepsin 12 mg/m^2 given every 2 weeks (NCT01947140). Thus, with the exception of BV, the efficacy of the FDA-approved agents for the treatment of PTCLs remains modest, and without a clear path to the establishment of biomarkers to identify exceptional responders, lasting benefit from these drugs for most patients remains elusive.

OTHER AGENTS WITH ACTIVITY IN T-CELL LYMPHOMAS

The immunologic consequences of T-cell ablation can be severe, underscored by the infectious toxicities observed during treatment of patients with PTCLs. For example, a clinical trial of frontline CHOP combined with alemtuzumab, a monoclonal antibody targeting CD52, which is broadly expressed on T cells and B cells, had to be stopped because of unacceptable infectious toxicities.[30] In addition, agents with efficacy in B-cell lymphomas have modest efficacy in patients with R/R TCLs, including gemcitabine,[31] bendamustine,[32] and lenalidomide.[33] Patients with R/R TCL treated with these drugs show ORRs of 36% to 51%, and PFS in the range of 3 months. Although some patients achieved durable responses, the vast majority of patients with R/R PTCLs are unlikely to derive benefit from such strategies.

MOLECULAR ADVANCES IN UNDERSTANDING PERIPHERAL T-CELL LYMPHOMAS

Genomic profiling studies of PTCLs have begun to reveal the landscape of recurrent molecular aberrancies that drive these diseases (**Table 1**). As a useful example of many reviews in the field, Van Arnam and colleagues[34] as well as Pizzi and colleagues,[35] have provided an excellent conceptual framework for initial classification of these aberrancies essentially based on how they would affect nonmalignant T-cell processes. These broadly include:

1. T-cell receptor (TCR) signaling pathways, including TCR-associated kinases, phosphatases, second messengers and G proteins, and costimulatory pathways;
2. Cytokine signaling and aberrant Jak/STAT activation; and
3. Epigenetic modifiers.

The TCR signaling complex mediates the epitope-specific antigen recognition that is fundamental to T-cell function, and downstream effects from full receptor engagement include T-cell activation, proliferation, cytokine production, and survival.[36] Recurrent ITK-SYK fusions, found in T$_{FH}$ lymphoma, result in aberrant localization of an active SYK kinase domain to the proximal TCR signaling complex. Expression of this fusion protein in T cells has experimentally been shown to drive T-cell transformation in mice,[37,38] providing compelling evidence that subversion of TCR signaling

Table 1
Current strategies to target known molecular aberrancies in T-NHL

T-Cell Pathway	Therapeutic Intervention	Current Clinical Trials
T-cell and costimulatory receptor signaling	PI3K γδ inhibition with duvelisib	NCT02783625: duvelisib + romidepsin NCT03372057: duvelisib
Jak/STAT signaling	Jak inhibition with ruxolitinib, cerdulatinib	NCT02974647: ruxolitinib
DNA methylation	DNA methylation inhibition with azacytidine	NCT03593018: azacytidine vs. romidepsin, bendamustine, or gemcitabine

drives lymphomagenesis. In addition, costimulatory signals, which use phosphatidyli-nositol 3-kinase (PI3K)/Akt signal transduction as a major effector, license a T cell for full activation.[39] In nonmalignant T cells, the absence of such a signal in the presence of strong TCR signaling produces a state of anergy in which T cells are unable to pro-liferate in response to proproliferative signals. Recent work by 3 groups demonstrated that the recurrent RHOA G17V mutation detected in approximately 60% of patients with AITL,[40–42] results in T-cell hyperactivation when TCR and costimulatory signals are provided, primarily through the PI3K/Akt/mammalian target of rapamycin (mTOR) signal transduction axis.[43–45] In addition, combination of RHOA G17V expres-sion with Ten-eleven translocation 2 (TET2) loss (see Discussion) results in T-cell lym-phomagenesis. Thus, inhibition of TCR or costimulatory signaling (via PI3K/Akt/mTOR inhibition) provides a plausible target for PTCL-directed therapy.

Many cytokine receptors that regulate T-cell proliferation and survival signal through the Janus kinase (Jak) family of cytoplasmic tyrosine kinases, which in turn use signal transducer and activation of transcription (STAT) proteins as second messengers that translocate into the nucleus to modulate gene expression. Almost the entire spectrum of PTCL subtypes demonstrates recurrent activating mutations in Jak and STAT family members, and there is often evidence of pathway upregulation, even in the absence of mutations, as was recently comprehensively reviewed by Waldmann and Chen.[46] The transforming potential of this pathway is underscored by the finding that multiple models of T-cell acute lymphoblastic leukemia can be driven by ectopic expression of Jak/STAT family members,[47,48] and that upregulation of JAK1 expression by retro-viral insertion is associated with mature T-cell transformation.[49] PTCLs do not require JAK/STAT mutations for dependence on this signaling pathway, as ALK-mediated proliferation of T cells is halted by loss of STAT3.[50] Thus, Jak/STAT signaling is a possible widely targetable pathway for treatment of PTCLs.

Epigenetic modifiers that would be expected to widely affect DNA methylation when their function is lost are found to be recurrently mutated in PTCLs. TET2 catalyzes the oxidation of 5-methylcytosine first to 5-hydroxymethylcytosine, and then 5-formylcy-tosine, and 5-carboxylcytosine, which are intermediates ultimately leading to deme-thylation of these bases in DNA.[51] DNMT3A acts as a de novo methyltransferase during cellular differentiation.[52] TET2 and DNMT3A mutations occur in approximately 80% and 30% of AITL cases, respectively.[53] In addition, TET2 loss of function can result in T-cell transformation[54,55] and combination with RHOA G17V mutation can accelerate this process.[44,45] DNMT3A can act as a haploinsufficient tumor suppressor in models of TCL[35] and when the dominant-negative DNMT3A (R882H) mutation is expressed in the setting of TET2 loss in mouse hematopoietic cells, an AITL-like phenotype is observed.[56] Thus, epigenetic modifiers are frequently mutated in PTCLs and can drive T-cell transformation.

RECENT CLINICAL FINDINGS FOR TARGETED THERAPY IN PERIPHERAL T-CELL LYMPHOMAS

The recent molecular findings in PTCLs have dovetailed with clinical findings in these diseases. Evidence for clinical efficacy from directly targeting TCR signaling came from a case series of 12 patient with AITL who were treated with cyclosporin A,[57] which is a calcineurin inhibitor that inhibits calcium efflux into T cells, abrogating TCR signaling effectors including activation of nuclear factor of activated T-cell tran-scription factors. Of the 12 patients treated, 8 responded, including 3 with CRs. Furthermore, T cells often require the PI3Kγ isoform in addition to the PI3Kδ isoform for full TCR-mediated activation.[58] A phase I study of duvelisib, an inhibitor of both the PI3Kγ and PI3Kδ isoforms, in 16 patients with R/R PTCL, demonstrated a 50% ORR including 3 CRs.[59] Grade 3 and 4 AEs among all patients (CTCL and PTCL) included increased alanine aminotransferase/aspartate aminotransferase, neutropenia, rash, and dyspnea/pneumonia. Studies performed on cell lines in vitro suggested that phosphorylated Akt could be used as a biomarker for sensitivity; however, clinical validation of this remains to be established. An ongoing phase Ib/II study combining either romidepsin or bortezomib with duvelisib (NCT02783625) reported an encouraging ORR of 55% (12/22 patients) and CR rate of 27% (6/22) in PTCL at the ASH 2018 conference.[60] At this point, as multiple subtypes are enrolled in this study, it is very unlikely that enough patients carrying RHOA G17V mutations will be enrolled to provide any statistical inference for efficacy in this population. However, the broader activity of this PI3Kγδ inhibitor suggests that PTCLs show a degree of addiction to this pathway across subtypes whether triggered by TCR costimulation or some other pathway. Duvelisib is currently being tested in a phase II registration study planned to enroll 120 patients with R/R PTCL (NCT03372057).

Both activating JAK and STAT mutations that are present in PTCLs can be targeted by JAK inhibitors because mutant STAT proteins require some Jak signaling for initiation of their activity.[61] Approximately 40% of T-cell large granular lymphocytic leukemia (T-LGL) harbor a STAT3 mutation.[62] Recently, a cohort of 9 patients with T-LGL and concomitant rheumatoid arthritis was treated with the JAK3 inhibitor tofacitinib for 6 weeks, with 6/9 patients, including all 4 who carried STAT3 mutations, achieving a hematologic response.[63] A phase IIa study of the dual Syk/Jak inhibitor cerdulatinib in R/R TCL reported an ORR of 35%, including 8 CRs, among 26 patients.[64] Grade 3+ AEs included neutropenia, diarrhea, elevated lipase, and pneumonia. Currently, a phase II study of ruxolitinib in patients with R/R TCL is enrolling a planned 52 patients, although no results are yet available (NCT02974647). Patients with and without JAK/STAT mutations will be included in the study and biomarker studies for this trial include markers of Jak/STAT pathway activation. Thus, inhibition of the Jak/STAT pathway using JAK inhibitors has shown initial promising results, although additional data describing the efficacy of these agents in PTCL are necessary to determine their role in the therapeutic armamentarium.

Because myeloid malignancies with TET2 mutations respond to therapy with hypomethylating agents,[65] investigators have studied their use in TCLs of T_{FH} derivation given the high frequency of such mutations in this subset. Recently, a retrospective case series of 12 patients with AITL treated with 7 days of azacitidine on 28-day cycles reported a 75% ORR including 50% CRs.[66] Genetic sequencing of patient samples revealed that all 12 patients treated carried at least 1 TET2 mutation, so no statistical inference about correlation between these mutations and response could be made. Nevertheless, the genetic and clinical data associated with TCLs of T_{FH} derivation has prompted initiation of a phase III trial comparing azacitidine with investigator's choice of romidepsin, bendamustine, or gemcitabine (NCT03593018). In addition, a phase Ib/II trial of romidepsin and azacitidine (NCT01998035) open to all lymphoma subtypes reported an ORR of 79% (11/14 patients) in TCL with 43% (6/14) CRs at the ASH 2018 conference.[67] Grade 3 to 4 toxicities included 39% with neutropenia or lymphopenia and 28% with thrombocytopenia. Direct comparison of these results with previous single-agent activity is difficult as this analysis included patients treated in the frontline; however, this report suggests that further clinical study of this combination is warranted.

IMMUNOTHERAPY IN PERIPHERAL T-CELL LYMPHOMAS

The excitement generated throughout oncology by the successful direction of the immune system to target malignancies through chimeric antigen receptor (CAR)-T-cell therapy[68] and checkpoint blockade[69] has generated enthusiasm to use these modalities in PTCLs. Following the success of targeting CD30 with BV, many groups have generated CAR-T cells targeting CD30$^+$ hematopoietic malignancies. One phase I trial of CD30-directed CAR-T-cell therapy reported results including 2 patients with ALCL, and, of these, 1 patient with ALK$^+$ ALCL had a dramatic response to treatment after the first infusion of CAR-T cells and achieved a CR of 9 months duration following a fourth infusion of CAR-T cells.[70] There is ongoing investigation of CD30-directed CAR-T cells from at least 7 international sites.[71] A recent study has provided proof of principle for a novel means to eliminate PTCL cells by targeting CAR-T cells against 1 of 2 isoforms of the TCRβ chain using the JOVI-1 antibody that recognizes approximately 35% of human αβ T cells.[72] Although this theoretically limits the potential efficacy of this reagent to 35% of PTCLs that maintain expression of an αβ TCR, there is the possible benefit of a reduction in toxicity by sparing a large portion nonmalignant T cells, although how the nonmalignant T-cell repertoire is represented across both TCRβ subtypes remains incompletely assessed. Concerns remain that targeting T-cell antigens with CAR-T cells might be precluded by fratricide within a CAR-T-cell product, although it has been experimentally demonstrated that use of CRISPR technology to eliminate CAR-T-cell targets in effector cells themselves is a possible means of addressing this issue.[73]

Checkpoint blockade has been explored in TCLs, with a phase I study of nivolumab in R/R NHL demonstrating partial responses in 2/5 patients with TCL.[74] Nevertheless, as programmed cell death 1 (PD-1) directly acts to inhibit TCR signaling,[75] there is mechanistic concern that abrogation of this process in TCLs might result in the unintentional exacerbation of lymphoma activity. PD-1 was identified by a genetic screen for tumor suppressors in the ITK-SYK model of PTCL, and even haploinsufficiency of PD-1 was sufficient to cause full development of lethal T-cell proliferation within 45 days of ITK-SYK expression.[76] These concerns have been amplified after a report that treatment with nivolumab has been associated with rapid progression of 3 previously indolent cases of acute T-cell leukemia lymphoma.[33] Thus, despite some indications that immunotherapy for treatment of PTCLs remains a promising approach, the unique circumstance of T cells acting as both target and effector must be carefully considered as these approaches are developed clinically.

FUTURE APPROACHES TO TREATMENT OF PERIPHERAL T-CELL LYMPHOMAS

Despite encouraging recent advances, there remains a significant need for more effective approaches to treat ptcl. However, the impulse to test multiple novel therapies needs to be balanced by the need to maximize the impact of these therapies in a limited patient population. Prioritizing therapeutic approaches based on a preclinical biologic rationale is necessary to improve clinical outcomes as rapidly and efficiently as possible.

The disappointing results with CHOP-based chemotherapy highlight the need to move newer treatments earlier in the treatment of PTCL, as demonstrated by the ECHELON-2 trial. However, the fact that there is a durable remission rate with frontline CHOP-based chemotherapy means that dispensing with CHOP completely could deprive a significant population of patients of such benefit. Therefore, trials seeking to supplant CHOP should be based on a strong preclinical rationale or tested in patients who are unfit for CHOP-based chemotherapy.

Given the limited single-agent activity of most new drugs, combining these agents either with each other or more conventional therapies will likely be necessary to produce meaningful changes. Recent analysis by Palmer and Sorger[77] suggests that the increased response rates of oncologic drug combinations over their single-agent components is primarily driven by activity in those patients who are cross-resistant to 1 component but not the other(s). Thus, in many combinations, tumors that are intrinsically resistant to single agents given sequentially derive no additional benefit from drugs delivered as a combination. These principles provide a possible explanation as to why previous empiric combination therapies in PTCL have had only limited activity in patients, but this limitation may be overcome by combinations that produce complementary inhibition of molecular vulnerabilities. Based on the widespread activity of the Jak/STAT pathway in TCL, combinations of Jak/STAT inhibitors with either PI3K inhibition in tumors with evidence of active TCR and costimulatory receptor signaling, or with hypomethylating agents in nodal lymphomas of T_{FH} origin that carry mutations affecting DNA methylation are promising possibilities. Although much work remains to be done, biologic insights into PTCLs have helped to distinguish targetable pathways distinct from B-cell NHL, and ongoing research into agents that modulate these pathways will hopefully be leveraged into novel therapeutic approaches for these diseases.

REFERENCES

1. Moskowitz AJ, Lunning MA, Horwitz SM. How I treat the peripheral T-cell lymphomas. Blood 2014;123(17):2636–44.
2. Al-Zahrani M, Savage KJ. Peripheral T-cell lymphoma, not otherwise specified: a review of current disease understanding and therapeutic approaches. Hematol Oncol Clin North Am 2017;31(2):189–207.
3. Chihara D, Fanale MA. Management of anaplastic large cell lymphoma. Hematol Oncol Clin North Am 2017;31(2):209–22.
4. Broccoli A, Zinzani PL. Angioimmunoblastic T-cell lymphoma. Hematol Oncol Clin North Am 2017;31(2):223–38.
5. Sud A, Dearden C. T-cell prolymphocytic leukemia. Hematol Oncol Clin North Am 2017;31(2):273–83.
6. Mehta-Shah N, Horwitz S. Uncommon variants of T-cell lymphomas. Hematol Oncol Clin North Am 2017;31(2):285–95.
7. Vose J, Armitage J, Weisenburger D, et al. International peripheral T-cell and natural killer/T-cell lymphoma study: pathology findings and clinical outcomes. J Clin Oncol 2008;26(25):4124–30.
8. Schmitz N, Trumper L, Ziepert M, et al. Treatment and prognosis of mature T-cell and NK-cell lymphoma: an analysis of patients with T-cell lymphoma treated in studies of the German High-Grade Non-Hodgkin Lymphoma Study Group. Blood 2010;116(18):3418–25.
9. Ellin F, Landstrom J, Jerkeman M, et al. Real-world data on prognostic factors and treatment in peripheral T-cell lymphomas: a study from the Swedish Lymphoma Registry. Blood 2014;124(10):1570–7.
10. d'Amore F, Relander T, Lauritzsen GF, et al. Up-front autologous stem-cell transplantation in peripheral T-cell lymphoma: NLG-T-01. J Clin Oncol 2012;30(25): 3093–9.
11. Schmitz N, Nickelsen M, Altmann B, et al. Allogenec or autologous transplantation as first-line therapy for younger patients with peripheral T-cell lymphoma—results of the interim analysis of the AATT trial. Hematol Oncol 2015;33(S1):8507.
12. DeGraw JI, Colwell WT, Piper JR, et al. Synthesis and antitumor activity of 10-propargyl-10-deazaaminopterin. J Med Chem 1993;36(15):2228–31.

13. Wang ES, O'Connor O, She Y, et al. Activity of a novel anti-folate (PDX, 10-propargyl 10-deazaaminopterin) against human lymphoma is superior to methotrexate and correlates with tumor RFC-1 gene expression. Leuk Lymphoma 2003;44(6): 1027–35.

14. O'Connor OA, Horwitz S, Hamlin P, et al. Phase II-I-II study of two different doses and schedules of pralatrexate, a high-affinity substrate for the reduced folate carrier, in patients with relapsed or refractory lymphoma reveals marked activity in T-cell malignancies. J Clin Oncol 2009;27(26):4357–64.

15. O'Connor OA, Pro B, Pinter-Brown L, et al. Pralatrexate in patients with relapsed or refractory peripheral T-cell lymphoma: results from the pivotal PROPEL study. J Clin Oncol 2011;29(9):1182–9.

16. New M, Olzscha H, La Thangue NB. HDAC inhibitor-based therapies: can we interpret the code? Mol Oncol 2012;6(6):637–56.

17. O'Connor OA, Heaney ML, Schwartz L, et al. Clinical experience with intravenous and oral formulations of the novel histone deacetylase inhibitor suberoylanilide hydroxamic acid in patients with advanced hematologic malignancies. J Clin Oncol 2006;24(1):166–73.

18. Piekarz RL, Robey R, Sandor V, et al. Inhibitor of histone deacetylation, depsipeptide (FR901228), in the treatment of peripheral and cutaneous T-cell lymphoma: a case report. Blood 2001;98(9):2865–8.

19. Coiffier B, Pro B, Prince HM, et al. Results from a pivotal, open-label, phase II study of romidepsin in relapsed or refractory peripheral T-cell lymphoma after prior systemic therapy. J Clin Oncol 2012;30(6):631–6.

20. O'Connor OA, Horwitz S, Masszi T, et al. Belinostat in patients with relapsed or refractory peripheral T-cell lymphoma: results of the pivotal phase II BELIEF (CLN-19) study. J Clin Oncol 2015;33(23):2492–9.

21. Coiffier B, Pro B, Prince HM, et al. Romidepsin for the treatment of relapsed/refractory peripheral T-cell lymphoma: pivotal study update demonstrates durable responses. J Hematol Oncol 2014;7:11.

22. Francisco JA, Cerveny CG, Meyer DL, et al. cAC10-vcMMAE, an anti-CD30-monomethyl auristatin E conjugate with potent and selective antitumor activity. Blood 2003;102(4):1458–65.

23. Younes A, Bartlett NL, Leonard JP, et al. Brentuximab vedotin (SGN-35) for relapsed CD30-positive lymphomas. N Engl J Med 2010;363(19):1812–21.

24. Pro B, Advani R, Brice P, et al. Brentuximab vedotin (SGN-35) in patients with relapsed or refractory systemic anaplastic large-cell lymphoma: results of a phase II study. J Clin Oncol 2012;30(18):2190–6.

25. Horwitz SM, Advani RH, Bartlett NL, et al. Objective responses in relapsed T-cell lymphomas with single-agent brentuximab vedotin. Blood 2014;123(20): 3095–100.

26. Horwitz S, O'Connor OA, Pro B, et al. Brentuximab vedotin with chemotherapy for CD30-positive peripheral T-cell lymphoma (ECHELON-2): a global, double-blind, randomised, phase 3 trial. Lancet 2019;393(10168):229–40.

27. Advani RH, Ansell SM, Lechowicz MJ, et al. A phase II study of cyclophosphamide, etoposide, vincristine and prednisone (CEOP) alternating with pralatrexate (P) as front line therapy for patients with peripheral T-cell lymphoma (PTCL): final results from the T-cell consortium trial. Br J Haematol 2016;172(4):535–44.

28. Dupuis J, Morschhauser F, Ghesquieres H, et al. Combination of romidepsin with cyclophosphamide, doxorubicin, vincristine, and prednisone in previously untreated patients with peripheral T-cell lymphoma: a non-randomised, phase 1b/2 study. Lancet Haematol 2015;2(4):e160–5.

29. Jain S, Jirau-Serrano X, Zullo KM, et al. Preclinical pharmacologic evaluation of pralatrexate and romidepsin confirms potent synergy of the combination in a murine model of human T-cell lymphoma. Clin Cancer Res 2015;21(9):2096–106.

30. Kim JG, Sohn SK, Chae YS, et al. Alemtuzumab plus CHOP as front-line chemotherapy for patients with peripheral T-cell lymphomas: a phase II study. Cancer Chemother Pharmacol 2007;60(1):129–34.

31. Zinzani PL, Venturini F, Stefoni V, et al. Gemcitabine as single agent in pretreated T-cell lymphoma patients: evaluation of the long-term outcome. Ann Oncol 2010; 21(4):860–3.

32. Damaj G, Gressin R, Bouabdallah K, et al. Results from a prospective, open-label, phase II trial of bendamustine in refractory or relapsed T-cell lymphomas: the BENTLY trial. J Clin Oncol 2013;31(1):104–10.

33. Toumishey E, Prasad A, Dueck G, et al. Final report of a phase 2 clinical trial of lenalidomide monotherapy for patients with T-cell lymphoma. Cancer 2015; 121(5):716–23.

34. Van Arnam JS, Lim MS, Elenitoba-Johnson KSJ. Novel insights into the pathogenesis of T-cell lymphomas. Blood 2018;131(21):2320–30.

35. Pizzi M, Margolskee E, Inghirami G. Pathogenesis of peripheral T cell lymphoma. Annu Rev Pathol 2018;13:293–320.

36. Brownlie RJ, Zamoyska R. T cell receptor signalling networks: branched, diversified and bounded. Nat Rev Immunol 2013;13(4):257–69.

37. Pechloff K, Holch J, Ferch U, et al. The fusion kinase ITK-SYK mimics a T cell receptor signal and drives oncogenesis in conditional mouse models of peripheral T cell lymphoma. J Exp Med 2010;207(5):1031–44.

38. Dierks C, Adrian F, Fisch P, et al. The ITK-SYK fusion oncogene induces a T-cell lymphoproliferative disease in mice mimicking human disease. Cancer Res 2010; 70(15):6193–204.

39. So T, Croft M. Regulation of PI-3-kinase and Akt signaling in T lymphocytes and other cells by TNFR family molecules. Front Immunol 2013;4:139.

40. Palomero T, Couronne L, Khiabanian H, et al. Recurrent mutations in epigenetic regulators, RHOA and FYN kinase in peripheral T cell lymphomas. Nat Genet 2014;46(2):166–70.

41. Sakata-Yanagimoto M, Enami T, Yoshida K, et al. Somatic RHOA mutation in angioimmunoblastic T cell lymphoma. Nat Genet 2014;46(2):171–5.

42. Yoo HY, Sung MK, Lee SH, et al. A recurrent inactivating mutation in RHOA GTPase in angioimmunoblastic T cell lymphoma. Nat Genet 2014;46(4):371–5.

43. Zang S, Li J, Yang H, et al. Mutations in 5-methylcytosine oxidase TET2 and RhoA cooperatively disrupt T cell homeostasis. J Clin Invest 2017;127(8):2998–3012.

44. Cortes JR, Ambesi-Impiombato A, Couronne L, et al. RHOA G17V induces T follicular helper cell specification and promotes lymphomagenesis. Cancer Cell 2018;33(2):259–73.e7.

45. Ng SY, Brown L, Stevenson K, et al. RhoA G17V is sufficient to induce autoimmunity and promotes T-cell lymphomagenesis in mice. Blood 2018;132(9):935–47.

46. Waldmann TA, Chen J. Disorders of the JAK/STAT pathway in T cell lymphoma pathogenesis: implications for immunotherapy. Annu Rev Immunol 2017;35: 533–50.

47. Degryse S, de Bock CE, Cox L, et al. JAK3 mutants transform hematopoietic cells through JAK1 activation, causing T-cell acute lymphoblastic leukemia in a mouse model. Blood 2014;124(20):3092–100.

48. Kelly JA, Spolski R, Kovanen PE, et al. Stat5 synergizes with T cell receptor/antigen stimulation in the development of lymphoblastic lymphoma. J Exp Med 2003; 198(1):79–89.

49. Heinrich T, Rengstl B, Muik A, et al. Mature T-cell lymphomagenesis induced by retroviral insertional activation of Janus kinase 1. Mol Ther 2013;21(6):1160–8.

50. Chiarle R, Simmons WJ, Cai H, et al. Stat3 is required for ALK-mediated lymphomagenesis and provides a possible therapeutic target. Nat Med 2005;11(6): 623–9.

51. Wu X, Zhang Y. TET-mediated active DNA demethylation: mechanism, function and beyond. Nat Rev Genet 2017;18(9):517–34.

52. Yang L, Rau R, Goodell MA. DNMT3A in haematological malignancies. Nat Rev Cancer 2015;15(3):152–65.

53. Cortes JR, Palomero T. The curious origins of angioimmunoblastic T-cell lymphoma. Curr Opin Hematol 2016;23(4):434–43.

54. Pan F, Wingo TS, Zhao Z, et al. Tet2 loss leads to hypermutagenicity in haematopoietic stem/progenitor cells. Nat Commun 2017;8:15102.

55. Muto H, Sakata-Yanagimoto M, Nagae G, et al. Reduced TET2 function leads to T-cell lymphoma with follicular helper T-cell-like features in mice. Blood Cancer J 2014;4:e264.

56. Scourzic L, Couronne L, Pedersen MT, et al. DNMT3A(R882H) mutant and Tet2 inactivation cooperate in the deregulation of DNA methylation control to induce lymphoid malignancies in mice. Leukemia 2016;30(6):1388–98.

57. Advani R, Horwitz S, Zelenetz A, et al. Angioimmunoblastic T cell lymphoma: treatment experience with cyclosporine. Leuk Lymphoma 2007;48(3):521–5.

58. Alcazar I, Marques M, Kumar A, et al. Phosphoinositide 3-kinase gamma participates in T cell receptor-induced T cell activation. J Exp Med 2007;204(12): 2977–87.

59. Horwitz SM, Koch R, Porcu P, et al. Activity of the PI3K-delta,gamma inhibitor duvelisib in a phase 1 trial and preclinical models of T-cell lymphoma. Blood 2018; 131(8):888–98.

60. Horwitz SM, Moskowitz AJ, Jacobsen ED, et al. The combination of duvelisib, a PI3K-δ,γ inhibitor, and romidepsin is highly active in relapsed/refractory peripheral T-cell lymphoma with low rates of transaminitis: results of parallel multicenter, phase 1 combination studies with expansion cohorts. Blood 2018; 132(Suppl 1):683.

61. Pilati C, Amessou M, Bihl MP, et al. Somatic mutations activating STAT3 in human inflammatory hepatocellular adenomas. J Exp Med 2011;208(7):1359–66.

62. Koskela HL, Eldfors S, Ellonen P, et al. Somatic STAT3 mutations in large granular lymphocytic leukemia. N Engl J Med 2012;366(20):1905–13.

63. Bilori B, Thota S, Clemente MJ, et al. Tofacitinib as a novel salvage therapy for refractory T-cell large granular lymphocytic leukemia. Leukemia 2015;29(12): 2427–9.

64. Horwitz SM, Feldman TA, Hess BT, et al. The novel SYK/JAK inhibitor cerdulatinib demonstrates good tolerability and clinical response in a phase 2a study in relapsed/refractory peripheral T-Cell lymphoma and cutaneous T-cell lymphoma. Blood 2018;132(Suppl 1):1001.

65. Bejar R, Lord A, Stevenson K, et al. TET2 mutations predict response to hypomethylating agents in myelodysplastic syndrome patients. Blood 2014;124(17): 2705–12.

66. Lemonnier F, Dupuis J, Sujobert P, et al. Treatment with 5-azacytidine induces a sustained response in patients with angioimmunoblastic T-cell lymphoma. Blood 2018;132(21):2305–9.
67. Falchi L, Lue JK, Montanari F, et al. Combined hypomethylating agents (HMA) and histone deacetylase inhibitors (HDACi) exhibit compelling activity in patients with peripheral T-cell lymphoma (PTCL) with high complete response rates in angioimmunoblastic T-cell lymphoma (AITL). Blood 2018;132(Suppl 1):1002.
68. June CH, O'Connor RS, Kawalekar OU, et al. CAR T cell immunotherapy for human cancer. Science 2018;359(6382):1361–5.
69. Ribas A, Wolchok JD. Cancer immunotherapy using checkpoint blockade. Science 2018;359(6382):1350–5.
70. Ramos CA, Ballard B, Zhang H, et al. Clinical and immunological responses after CD30-specific chimeric antigen receptor-redirected lymphocytes. J Clin Invest 2017;127(9):3462–71.
71. Poggio T, Duyster J, Illert AL. Current immunotherapeutic approaches in T cell non-Hodgkin lymphomas. Cancers (Basel) 2018;10(9).
72. Maciocia PM, Wawrzyniecka PA, Philip B, et al. Targeting the T cell receptor beta-chain constant region for immunotherapy of T cell malignancies. Nat Med 2017; 23(12):1416–23.
73. Gomes-Silva D, Srinivasan M, Sharma S, et al. CD7-edited T cells expressing a CD7-specific CAR for the therapy of T-cell malignancies. Blood 2017;130(3): 285–96.
74. Lesokhin AM, Ansell SM, Armand P, et al. Nivolumab in patients with relapsed or refractory hematologic malignancy: preliminary results of a phase Ib study. J Clin Oncol 2016;34(23):2698–704.
75. Latchman Y, Wood CR, Chernova T, et al. PD-L2 is a second ligand for PD-1 and inhibits T cell activation. Nat Immunol 2001;2(3):261–8.
76. Wartewig T, Kurgyis Z, Keppler S, et al. PD-1 is a haploinsufficient suppressor of T cell lymphomagenesis. Nature 2017;552(7683):121–5.
77. Palmer AC, Sorger PK. Combination cancer therapy can confer benefit via patient-to-patient variability without drug additivity or synergy. Cell 2017;171(7): 1678–91.e13.

Overview of Cutaneous T-Cell Lymphomas

Cecilia A. Larocca, MD, Nicole R. LeBoeuf, MD, MPH*

KEYWORDS

- Mycosis fungoides • Sézary syndrome • Cutaneous T-cell lymphoma • Review
- Diagnosis • Histology • Genetics • Therapy

KEY POINTS

- Mycosis fungoides and Sézary syndrome are the most common non-Hodgkin lymphomas to arise from skin-tropic clonal T lymphocytes.
- Significant advances have been made in understanding the genetic and epigenetic aberrations in cutaneous T-cell lymphoma (CTCL).
- Diagnosis of CTCL subtypes requires a combination of clinical, pathologic, and molecular features.
- Several prognostic factors identify patients with poor prognosis.
- Treatment is aimed to minimize morbidity and limit disease progression, as cure is rarely achieved.

INTRODUCTION

Non-Hodgkin lymphoma (NHL) includes a diverse collection of systemic and primary cutaneous lymphomas. Overall cutaneous T-cell lymphomas (CTCLs) represent about 13% of all NHLs, which are further subdivided into a heterogeneous group of lymphomas with vastly different presentations and histologic features.[1] The overall incidence of CTCL is 10.2 per million persons.[2] Although largely indolent, CTCLs can be aggressive in advanced stages, depending on the histologic subtype. Diagnosis requires integration of clinical, pathologic, and molecular features. Among CTCLs, mycosis fungoides (MF) and Sézary Syndrome (SS) are the most prevalent malignancies. Given the rarity of other subtypes, advances in treatment and identification of prognostic factors have been limited to MF and SS. Strides made in characterizing the genomic aberrations in CTCL have focused on SS and to some extent, MF. Treatment is aimed at limiting morbidity and halting disease progression. Hematopoietic stem cell transplantation is the only therapy with curative intent, with well-known significant morbidity and mortality risks.

Department of Dermatology, Center for Cutaneous Oncology, Brigham and Women's Hospital, Dana-Farber Cancer Institute, Harvard Medical School, 450 Brookline Avenue, Boston, MA 02215, USA
* Corresponding author.
E-mail address: nleboeuf@bwh.harvard.edu

Hematol Oncol Clin N Am 33 (2019) 669–686
https://doi.org/10.1016/j.hoc.2019.04.004
0889-8588/19/© 2019 Elsevier Inc. All rights reserved.

CUTANEOUS T-CELL LYMPHOMA CLASSIFICATION

In 2005 the World Health Organization (WHO) and the European Organization for Research and Treatment of Cancer (EORTC) established a consensus classification of primary cutaneous lymphomas.[3] The 2008 WHO/EORTC classification recognized the following as definitive entities: MF and MF variants; SS; primary cutaneous CD30+ lymphoproliferative diseases; subcutaneous panniculitis-like T-cell lymphoma; extranodal natural killer (NK)/T-cell lymphoma, nasal type; and primary peripheral T-cell lymphoma, not otherwise specified. Provisional entities included cutaneous gamma-delta T-cell lymphoma (CGDTCL) and primary cutaneous aggressive epidermotropic cytotoxic CD8+ T-cell lymphoma. These provisional entities have been further defined with the advent of molecular markers, and additional entities were added under the revised fourth edition of the WHO classification in 2016.[4] In this article, the authors review the cutaneous T-cell lymphomas included in the latest WHO classification (**Box 1**). Systemic T-cell lymphomas with frequent skin involvement (eg, adult T-cell leukemia/lymphoma, angioimmunoblastic T-cell lymphoma, systemic EBV+ T-cell lymphoma of childhood) are beyond the scope of this review.

MYCOSIS FUNGOIDES/SÉZARY SYNDROME

Classically, MF and SS arise from skin-tropic memory CD4+ T cells. Although MF and SS have overlapping clinical and histologic presentations and are not distinguished in

---

Box 1
Revised fourth edition (2016) of WHO classification of primary cutaneous T-cell lymphoproliferative disorders

Definitive Entities

Mycosis fungoides and variants

Sézary syndrome

CD30+ lymphoproliferative disorders

Subcutaneous panniculitis-like T-cell lymphoma

Primary cutaneous gamma-delta T-cell lymphoma[a]

Primary cutaneous peripheral T-cell lymphoma, not otherwise specified

Extranodal NK/T-cell lymphomas, nasal type

Provisional Entities

Primary cutaneous aggressive epidermotropic CD8+ cytotoxic T-cell lymphoma

Primary cutaneous acral CD8+ T-cell lymphoma[b]

Primary cutaneous CD4+ small-medium T-cell lymphoproliferative disorder[c]

Hydroa vacciniforme-like lymphoproliferative disorder[c]

Breast implant-associated anaplastic large cell lymphoma[b]

[a] Previously considered provisional entities in 2008 WHO classification

[b] New provisional entities

[c] Renamed from lymphoma to a lymphoproliferative disorder

From Sundram U. Cutaneous Lymphoproliferative Disorders: What's New in the Revised 4th Edition of the World Health Organization (WHO) Classification of Lymphoid Neoplasms. Adv Anat Pathol 2019;26(2):93-113; with permission.

the WHO/EORTC staging criteria, they are considered separate entities.[3] The WHO/ EORTC and the International Society for Cutaneous Lymphoma (ISCL) considers SS to be a clinical syndrome presenting with erythroderma—more than 80% of body surface area (BSA) with diffuse erythema—and leukemic disease.[5] The National Comprehensive Cancer Network (NCCN) considers anyone with a high burden of leukemic disease (B2 in the tumor-node-metastasis-blood [TNMB] staging criteria) to have SS. Evaluation of T-cell surface phenotypes and molecular profiles show distinct patterns between patients with MF versus patients with SS, supporting that these are indeed distinct entities. It is thought that these malignancies arise from different memory T-cell subsets: the skin resident memory T cell in MF and the skin tropic central memory T cell in SS.[6–8]

Diagnosis

The diagnosis of MF/SS is challenging, especially in the early stages.[9] MF and SS have overlapping clinical and histologic features with benign inflammatory dermatoses. Furthermore, molecular studies using traditional polymerase chain reaction (PCR) of the T-cell receptor (TCR) to detect the presence of a T-cell clone in clinical samples has a significant false-negative rate.[6] An algorithm and pathologic criteria have been developed to assist with diagnosis, especially in early stages; however, they have not been formally validated and universally adopted.[10,11] A major advancement in the diagnosis of CTCL, especially in the early stages, is the use of high throughput sequencing (HTS) of the TCRβ and TCRγ gene, which identifies the presence of a T-cell clone with superior sensitivity compared with traditional TCRγ PCR.[12]

The clinical presentation of MF in the early stages resembles persistent eczematous atrophic oval to annular patches or plaques classically distributed in the buttock and hip area (**Fig. 1**A). MF plaques are erythematous oval to annular, indurated or elevated skin lesions with variable amounts of scale (**Fig. 1**B).[5] Advanced disease is characterized by tumors, which must have a diameter of at least 1.0 cm and exhibit a vertical

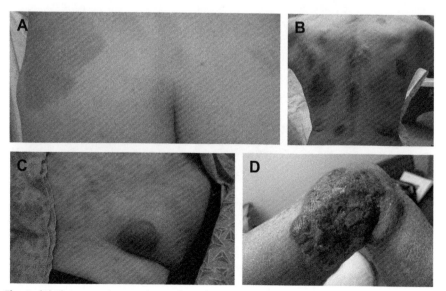

Fig. 1. (*A*) Flat, sometimes scaly patches of mycosis fungoides. (*B*) Plaques of MF. (*C, D*) Tumor stage MF.

phase growth (**Fig. 1**C, D).[5] These lesions may often become ulcerated. Patients with SS often present with erythroderma (**Fig. 2**). Identification and quantification of these clinical lesions (patch, plaque, tumor, and erythroderma) determines the T stage in the WHO/EORTC/ISCL TNMB staging system, adopted by the NCCN.[5]

There are 3 recognized variants of MF: folliculotropic MF (FMF), granulomatous slack skin, and pagetoid reticulosis.[3] FMF often presents in the head and neck region with acneiform papules, comedones, and alopecia nodules (**Fig. 3**).[3] Granulomatous slack skin presents with lax pendulous skin in intertriginous sites.[3] Pagetoid reticulosis presents as a solitary hyperkeratotic plaque on the extremity or acral skin.[3] Granulomatous slack skin and pagetoid reticulosis have indolent behaviors.[3] Overall FMF has a worse prognosis than classic MF, but a subgroup of patients experience indolent disease.[13] Although not considered distinct variants of MF, several unique clinical, histologic, and immunophenotypic subtypes have been described.[14,15]

Early lesions of MF have a superficial atypical lymphoid infiltrate with epidermal tagging (epidermotropism) and variable lymphocytic exocytosis into the epidermis without spongiosis.[3] Pautrier microabscess, clusters of atypical lymphocytes in the epidermis, pathognomonic for MF, may not be present in early stages.[10] Other features include chicken wire–like papillary dermal fibrosis. Atypical lymphocytes are often small to medium in size and have nuclei with cerebriform contours.[3] Advanced lesions, such as tumors, often lack epidermotropism.[10] The immunophenotype of MF/SS is characterized by decreased expression of CD5, CD7, or epidermal/dermal discordance of CD2, CD3, CD5, or CD7.[10] To date there are no clinically used diagnostic molecular markers that can reliably identify malignant T cells from benign T cells. In SS, spongiosis is common.[3] In FMF, there is an atypical lymphocytic

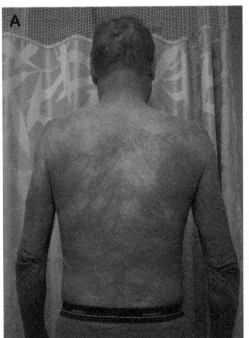
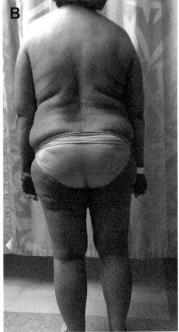

Fig. 2. (*A, B*) Blanching wide-spread erythema over greater than 80% body surface area (erythroderma) characterizes the clinical presentation of SS.

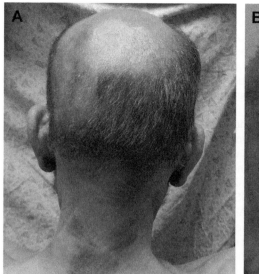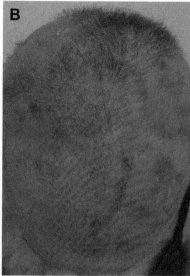

Fig. 3. (*A, B*) Folliculotropic MF with prominence at follicles often leading to alopecia.

folliculotropic infiltrate with variable amounts of follicular mucinosis, periadnexal inflammation, and no epidermotropism.[3] Pagetoid reticulosis can be a CD4+ or CD8+ T-cell infiltrate with marked pagetoid-like atypical lymphocytes, acanthosis, and a mixed reactive infiltrate in the dermis.[3] Granulomatous slack skin has dense granulomatous dermal infiltrates of atypical lymphocytes, macrophages, and many multinucleated giant cells with destruction of the elastic tissue.[3]

Staging of MF/SS revised by the EORTC and ISCL in 2007 and validated in a single-center cohort of 1502 patients was adapted by the NCCN.[5] Staging of MF involves assessment of the burden of disease in the skin (T stage), lymph nodes (N stage), viscera (M stage), and blood (B stage).

Newly diagnosed patients, based on supportive clinical presentation, skin pathology, and TCR PCR detection of clonality in the skin, should undergo evaluation with whole-body imaging (recommended only for patients with BSA greater than 10% or any BSA with high-risk pathologic features) and evaluation of blood for leukemic disease by flow cytometry. Molecular assessment of T-cell clonality by PCR in the blood should be pursued in patients with suspected leukemic disease. Bone marrow biopsies are not routinely pursued unless there is an unexplained hematologic abnormality. Systemic involvement is evaluated by computed tomographic (CT) imaging with contrast or PET/CT. It is recommended that suspicious lymph nodes (>1.5 cm in the long axis on CT imaging) be pathologically evaluated for systemic involvement. Lymph node excision of an accessible suspicious peripheral lymph node is preferred for adequate assessment. In patients with a high burden of skin disease, PET/CT is favored, as it can be used to distinguish dermatopathic (reactive) lymphadenopathy (LN0-2) from that of clinically significant lymphomatous involvement (LN3).[16] On PET/CT imaging, lymph nodes with a standardized uptake value (SUV) of less than or equal to 4.0 can be used as a marker of dermatopathic nodes.[16] Excisional lymph node biopsies should be pursued in cases with an SUV greater than 4.0.

Clinical stage is an important determinant of the risk of disease progression (RDP) and overall survival (OS). Patients with stage IA have a median survival of 35.5 years and a disease-specific survival (DSS) of 90% at 20 years, which is comparable to patients without MF.[17,18] Although these patients have an indolent disease course, there is an 18% RDP at 20 years.[17] Patients with early stage CTCL (Stage IA–IIA) have a median survival of 15.8 to 35.5 years.[17] Patients with advanced disease (Stage IIB–Stage IV) have a poor survival with a median survival of 2.1 to 4.7 years and DSS of 18% to 56% at 5 years.[17] Prognostic factors associated with a higher RDP, poorer OS, and worse DSS include male gender, advanced age, T stage, the presence of a clone in the blood in patients with B0 disease, FMF, large cell transformation, and elevated lactate dehydrogenase.[17] These prognostic factors gave rise to the prognostic index score, developed by the Cutaneous Lymphoma International Consortium, for patients with advanced MF/SS.[19,20] In patients with early stage disease, the burden of malignant T-cell clone (tumor clone frequency [TCF]) in lesional skin predicted RDP and OS.[12] A TCF greater than or equal to 25% was significantly associated with worse progression-free survival (PFS) and OS.[12] This measure was superior to predicting the PFS compared with stage (IB vs IA), presence of plaques, elevated lactate dehydrogenase, age, and the presence of large cell transformation.[12]

Treatment of MF/SS often requires a multidisciplinary approach with involvement of dermatology, medical oncology, and radiation oncology. There are several skin-directed and systemic therapies for the treatment of MF/SS (**Box 2**). Unfortunately, current systemic therapies uncommonly provide durable responses.[21] Increasingly, nonmyeloablative allogeneic stem cell transplantation, the only potential cure for CTCL, is being pursued for advanced stage disease.[22] Given the limited efficacy of existing therapies, all patients are encouraged to participate in clinical trials.

In the last 5 years there have been more than 10 major publications on the genomic landscape of CTCL. A meta-analysis of the 220 genetically profiled patients, largely composed of SS, identified 55 driver mutations and implicated 14 biologically relevant pathways.[23] Striking findings include the high incidence of C-T translocations, a high number of chromosomal abnormalities with copy number variants preferred over single nucleotide variants, and a high number of complex chromosomal structural rearrangements (eg, chromothripsis).[23] Affected pathways broadly include those involved in T-cell activation, function, migration, and differentiation; chromatin modification; cell cycle, survival, and proliferation; and DNA damage response.[23] Present analyses have only rarely yielded readily actionable targets. One such example is the identification of a recurrent novel CTLA-4-CD28 fusion protein, which was successfully targeted by anti-CTLA4 inhibitor ipilimumab in one patient.[24] However, an increasing number of clinical trials are evaluating drugs that target aberrant pathways and surface molecules identified by genomic and transcriptomic analyses in malignant cells such as PI3K, JAK, PD-1, CD47, and microRNA-155 inhibitors.

PRIMARY CUTANEOUS CD30+ LYMPHOPROLIFERATIVE DISORDERS

Primary cutaneous CD30+ lymphoproliferative disorders consist of lymphomatoid papulosis (LyP), primary cutaneous anaplastic large cell lymphoma (PCALCL), and intermediate cases.[3] LyP and PCALCL are believed to exist on a clinical spectrum, where intermediate cases may exhibit features of either.[25,26] Although LyP is not a malignancy, because of its favorable prognosis and self-limiting behavior, patients are at risk for the development of PCALCL.[26,27]

Clinically, LyP presents with recurring crops of small self-healing papulonecrotic lesions (**Fig. 4**).[25] These lesions most often resolve in 2 to 8 weeks but have been reported to take up to 4 months to resolve. This condition may last for months to decades.[28] Although self-limited, a positive T-cell clone may be found in these lesions;

Box 2
Therapies commonly used for treatment of mycosis fungoides/Sézary syndrome

Skin-Directed Therapies

Topical chemotherapy (nitrogen mustard, mechlorethamine)

Topical corticosteroids

Topical immunotherapy (imiquimod)

Topical retinoids (bexarotene; tazarotene)

Phototherapy (nbUVB; PUVA)

Radiation therapy (local external electron beam; brachytherapy; total skin electron beam therapy)

Preferred Systemic Therapies

Alemtuzumab (low dose)[a]

Bexarotene

Brentuximab vedotin

Extracorporeal photopheresis[a]

HDAC-inhibitors (vorinostat, romidepsin)

Interferons (IFNα, IFNγ)

Methotrexate (low dose)

Mogamulizumab

Multiagent chemotherapy[b]

Single-agent chemotherapy (pralatrexate [low or standard dose], gemcitabine, liposomal doxorubicin)

Useful under certain circumstances

Retinoids (acitretin, isotretinoin)

Pembrolizumab

Bortezomib

Chlorambucil

[a] Mainly effective for patients with leukemic disease, as monotherapy for SS or in combination for leukemic MF.

[b] Consider in cases of refractory aggressive disease; extracutaneous disease; PTCL-NOS.

Data from Wilcox RA. Cutaneous T-cell lymphoma: 2017 update on diagnosis, risk-stratification, and management. Am J Hematol 2017;92(10):1085-1102.

---

this has not shown to predict the development of PCALCL.[29] LyP carries an increased risk of developing a secondary hematologic malignancy with a reported prevalence of 9.5% to 61%.[29] The most common secondary malignancies are MF, PCALCL, systemic ALCL, and Hodgkin lymphoma.[27,29] In MF, the presence of LyP lesions is associated with a more favorable prognosis.[17] Patients with LyP have a 10-year DSS of 100%.[26,27] Treatment of LyP depends on symptoms and clinical severity.[25] Close observation may be appropriate in cases of limited disease or those with minimal impact on quality of life.[25] Treatment has not been reported to lower the risk of developing a secondary malignancy.[29]

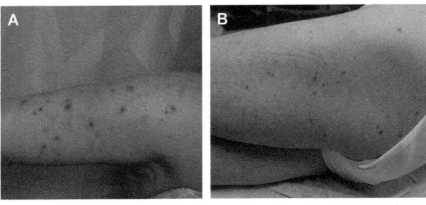

Fig. 4. (*A, B*) Lymphomatoid papulosis with crops of papules and nodules that self-resolve leaving hyperpigmented scars.

Histologically, there are more than 7 subtypes of LyP, which may be indistinguishable from other cutaneous lymphomas (**Table 1**).[26] Patients may have LyP lesions with multiple histologic subtypes.[29] Histologic subtype is not linked to prognosis or clinical morphology.[26] Appreciation of the clinical presentation is crucial to help distinguish LyP from other subtypes of CTCL as well as other CD30 + diseases such as ATLL and nodular reactive lymphoid hyperplasia due to arthropod bite, drug reaction, or infection.[28]

PCALCL classically presents as a large solitary nodule or tumor or group of nodules that typically does not self-resolve; multifocal lesions may also be observed in 22% of cases (**Fig. 5**).[30] Spontaneous regression, partial or total, has been reported to occur in 0% to 44% of cases.[31] The most important diagnostic consideration is systemic

Table 1		
Lymphomatoid papulosis histologic variants		
LyP Type	**Histology**	**CTCL Histologic Mimic**
A	Wedge-shaped infiltrate with a mixed infiltrate consisting of CD30+ atypical large cells, small lymphocytes, multinucleated cells, eosinophils, neutrophils, and histiocytes; variable amounts of epidermotropism	Transformed MF
B	Bandlike and perivascular dermal infiltrate with epidermotropism of small to medium lymphocytes, rare large CD30+ cells	Plaque-stage MF
C	CD30+ diffuse sheet of monotonous population of large atypical lymphocytes, few other admixed inflammatory cells	PCALCL
D	Epidermotropism, dermal, and subcutaneous CD8+	AETCL CGDTCL
E	Angioinvasion, CD8+	NKTCL GDTCL
F	Folliculotropism	FMF
Other	Granulomatous	

Adapted from Kempf W. A new era for cutaneous CD30-positive T-cell lymphoproliferative disorders. Semin Diagn Pathol 2017;34(1):26; with permission.

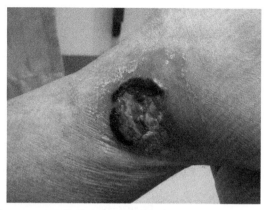

Fig. 5. Primary cutaneous anaplastic large cell lymphoma.

ALCL with secondary cutaneous involvement. Therefore, patients with PCALCL must undergo systemic imaging and flow cytometry blood analysis. PCALCL, as LyP, has a favorable prognosis with 85% to 95% survival at 5 and 10 years.[27,30] However, around 10% of patients develop systemic disease, most often to the draining lymph node basin.[27,30] Survival decreases to 76% to 96% at 5 years with involvement in greater than one nodal basin.[28] PCALCL has been reported to spread to extracutaneous site in 0% to 24% of cases.[28]

Histopathology of PCALCL demonstrates a dense dermal nodular infiltrate with sheets of atypical large anaplastic lymphocytes. By definition, at least 75% of the tumor cells must express CD30.[26] In PCALCL, anaplastic lymphoma kinase (ALK) is almost always negative.[26] Importantly, in systemic ALCL, ALK is positive in only 50% of cases, and therefore, ALK negativity does not rule out systemic ALCL.[26]

LyP and PCALCL often respond to skin-directed therapies (**Table 2**). Systemic therapy is used for refractory or extensive cases of LyP and multifocal PCALCL (see **Table 2**). Numerous topical and systemic therapies have been reported to be efficacious in LyP/PCALCL (see **Table 2**).[25]

SUBCUTANEOUS PANNICULITIS-LIKE T-CELL LYMPHOMA

Subcutaneous panniculitis-like T-cell lymphoma (SPTL) is a rare lymphoma of α/β T-cell phenotype with a favorable prognosis.[3,32] However, these patients are at risk for developing hemophagocytic syndrome (HPS), which heralds an aggressive clinical course and poor prognosis.[32] γ/δ T-cell phenotype, which also involves the subcutaneous tissue, is considered a distinct entity. Clinically, patients present with solitary or diffuse nodules or deeply indurated plaques typically affecting the trunk and extremities.[32] Areas of infiltration may be accompanied with adjacent lipoatrophy and, uncommonly, with ulceration.[32]

On histology there is an atypical lymphoid infiltrate rimming adipocytes resembling a lobular panniculitis.[3] The atypical infiltrate uncommonly extends into the reticular dermis and occasionally infiltrates adnexa.[3] SPTL typically has a CD4−, CD8+, and CD56− phenotype with expression of cytotoxic proteins (granzyme B, TIA-1, perforin) and variable loss of CD2, CD5, and/or CD7.[32] According to case series the 5-year OS and DSS are 82% and 85%, respectively.[32] Patients without HPS have a 5-year OS of 91%, compared with 46% in patients with HPS.[32] Patients are traditionally treated with CHOP-based therapies with sustained clinical remission in up to 64% of patients in case series.[32] Other therapeutic regimens have been used and associated with a

Table 2
Treatments used for the treatment of CD30+ lymphoproliferative diseases

LyP		PCALCL	
First-line Therapy	**Refractory**	**Solitary**	**Multifocal or Refractory Cases**
Observation	Methotrexate	Radiation	Methotrexate
Topical steroids	Brentuximab	Excision	Brentuximab
Phototherapy (nbUVB, PUVA)		Observation (for cases of spontaneous resolution)	Pralatrexate
			Single or multiagent chemotherapy[a]
		Used in isolated case series	
		Intralesional steroid	Isotretinoin
		Intralesional Methotrexate	Interferon
			Oral steroids
		Excimer laser	Thalidomide
		Imiquimod	
		Cryosurgery	

[a] Used in cases with extracutaneous disease.
Modified from Kempf W, Pfaltz K, Vermeer MH, et al. EORTC, ISCL, and USCLC consensus recommendations for the treatment of primary cutaneous CD30-positive lymphoproliferative disorders: lymphomatoid papulosis and primary cutaneous anaplastic large-cell lymphoma. Blood 2011;118(15):4029.

similarly favorable response, suggesting that doxorubicin-based chemotherapy regimens may not be necessary.[32] Solitary lesions have been treated successfully with surgical excision and/or radiation therapy.

CUTANEOUS GAMMA-DELTA T-CELL LYMPHOMA

CGDTCL is a rare and aggressive lymphoma of an activated cytotoxic T-cell phenotype.[3] Three clinical presentations have been observed: extensive panniculitis-like plaques, ulceronecrotic nodules or tumors (**Fig. 6**); solitary or multiple lesions confined to a single anatomic location; or those with MF-like patches.[33] In the latter group, patients typically have a favorable prognosis, but progression to a more aggressive disease with extensive skin ulceration and tumor formation can be observed.[34] In the

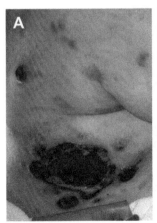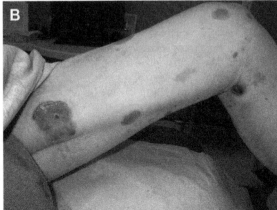

Fig. 6. (*A, B*) Gamma-delta T-cell lymphoma presenting with extensive ulceronecrotic plaques, nodules, and tumors.

largest case series, the 5-year OS rate was 19.9%.[33] Given aggressive disease, patients are most often treated with systemic chemotherapy, but with limited success. Several other therapies have been tried with variable success, including brentuximab.[33,35] Allogeneic stem cell transplantation has lead to cure in isolated cases.[36]

Histologically, there are variable presentations with atypical infiltrates in the epidermis, dermis, and/or subcutis.[4] The immunophenotype is most often CD3+/CD4−/CD8−/CD2+/beta F1−/TIA-1+/granzyme B+/CD7+.[3] CD8+ malignant T cells and rarely CD4+ T cells have been reported.[4] Most often, patients will have dense dermal infiltrates with extension into the subcutaneous tissue and less often into the epidermis.[33] Extensive necrosis and angioinvasion can be observed on pathology with a propensity for ulceration and eschars on examination.[33] Patients with patch-phase CGDTCL primarily exhibit epidermotropism.[33] However, unlike MF patches, there is a pagetoid pattern, scattered necrotic keratinocytes, and a lack of Pautrier microabscesses.[33] It is unclear whether cases with a predominately epidermotropic γδ T-cell phenotype with indolent behavior are best characterized as a variant of MF or CGDTCL.[37] Classic MF lesions have been observed to evolve from a TCR αβ to TCR γδ phenotype.[4]

PRIMARY CUTANEOUS PERIPHERAL T-CELL LYMPHOMA, NOT OTHERWISE SPECIFIED

Primary cutaneous peripheral T-cell lymphoma (PTCL), not otherwise specified (NOS) is assigned to cases of TCL that lack the clinical, histologic, and molecular features to allow further classification within accepted and provisional categories.[3,4] Median survival from small case series is 5.6 years.[38] Patients present with patches, plaques, or tumors.[38] The atypical infiltrate is often dermal but can involve the subcutis.[38] However, as a wastebasket category the features reported earlier will continue to evolve as novel molecular markers, and clinical patterns are identified to help further define entities within this group.

PRIMARY CUTANEOUS AGGRESSIVE EPIDERMOTROPIC CD8+ T-CELL LYMPHOMA

Primary cutaneous aggressive epidermotropic CD8+ T-cell lymphoma is a rare and aggressive lymphoma often characterized by necrotic annular plaques and tumors with frequent mucosal involvement (**Fig. 7**).[3] Patients who progress to systemic involvement often have sites other than lymph nodes involved, such as central nervous system, testis, adrenals, and lung.[4,39,40] Mean survival is 32 months, and at 5 years average survival is 18%.[39] Treatment is difficult, but responses have been documented to total skin irradiation combined with bexarotene and combination chemotherapy with the goal of permitting allogeneic stem cell transplantation.[39,40]

Histologically, there is often a dense pagetoid infiltrate that can completely efface the epidermis with extension into the dermis.[4,39] The epidermis may be hyperplastic with necrotic keratinocytes and with overlying hyperkeratosis or parakeratosis.[39] The subcutis is uncommonly involved and no angioinvasion with destruction is observed.[39] The immunophenotype is of CD3+/CD8+/αβ T cells (rarely CD8− or TCRβ negative) with an activated cytotoxic phenotype expressing TIA-1, granzyme B, and perforin.[39] CD56 may be positive.[4] CD30 is typically negative.[4]

PRIMARY CUTANEOUS ACRAL CD8+ T-CELL LYMPHOMA

This is a new provisional entity in the 2016 WHO classification.[4] It is an indolent lymphoma with a favorable prognosis characterized by involvement of facial and/or acral sites.[41–43] Lesions are often solitary with a predilection for the ear.[4] They respond to

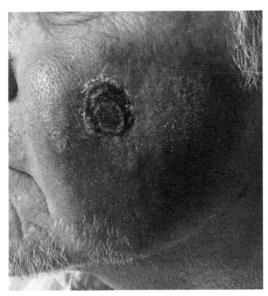

Fig. 7. Aggressive epidermotropic cutaneous T-cell lymphoma.

local treatment, such as intralesional steroids, excision, or radiation.[41–45] Recurrence is rare and no documented cases of progressive disease have been documented. In the past it has been considered a phenotypic variant of CD4+ small/medium T-cell lymphoproliferative disorder (SMTCL).[43]

Histologically, the CD8+ infiltrate is located in the dermis with a grenz zone and lacks significant cytologic atypia compared with aggressive epidermotropic cytotoxic CD8+ T-cell lymphoma.[4,42–44] It may express cytotoxic marker T1A-1 and to lesser degree granzyme B and perforin.[4] There may be loss of CD2, CD5, and CD7. Unlike SMTCL there is no expression of PD-1 and CXCL13. CD30 is negative.[4] TCR gene rearrangement studies are often positive.[4] Systemic leukemia with secondary involvement of the skin must be excluded.

PRIMARY CUTANEOUS CD4+ SMALL/MEDIUM T-CELL LYMPHOPROLIFERATIVE DISORDER

Primary cutaneous CD4+ small/medium T-cell lymphoproliferative disorder (SMTCL) is an indolent lymphoproliferative disorder presenting with solitary or few lesions on the head and neck area (**Fig. 8**).[3] Treatment with local therapy such as excision, intralesional steroids, and radiation can be curative.[4] Cutaneous relapses at distinct sites can be observed and treated likewise. Across several retrospective large case series there are isolated cases of SMTCL with fatal systemic involvement, which raises questions regarding the diagnosis of SMTCL. In other fatal cases, the presence of tumors, multifocal lesions, and a high proliferation index (Ki-67 >50%) were noted and could exclude the diagnosis of SMTCL in favor of PTCL, NOS.[46] A systemic workup is recommended in all suspected cases of SMTCL and those with systemic involvement at staging are best categorized as PTCL, NOS.

As acral CD8+ TCL, SMTCL has a grenz zone and a dermal infiltrate with small and occasionally large lymphocytes mixed with plasma cells and histiocytes, which can have a granulomatous pattern.[4,46] The immunophenotype is of CD4+, $\alpha\beta$T-cells with no expression of cytotoxic markers.[4,46] Mild perifollicular and periadnexal

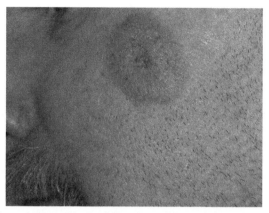

Fig. 8. Small-medium pleomorphic T-cell lymphoproliferative disorder.

involvement may be present. CD20+ B cells may be scattered to numerous.[4,43,46] Markers of follicular helper T cells (PD-1, CXCL13, CD10, BCL6, ICOS) have been reported.[4,43,46] Clonal T cells are often present and occasionally concurrent clonal immunoglobulin H rearrangements have been identified.[43] SMTCL may be difficult to distinguish from cutaneous lymphoid hyperplasia.[4]

BREAST IMPLANT–ASSOCIATED ANAPLASTIC T-CELL LYMPHOMA

Breast implant–associated anaplastic T-cell lymphoma (BI-ALCL), the most recently described T-cell lymphoma, was first recognized in the 2016 WHO classification.[4] It has been reported most often in patients with a history of textured silicone breast implants following medical or cosmetic surgery.[47] Clinically it usually presents as a delayed seroma (more than 1 year from implantation) adjacent to the implant, characterized by breast swelling, asymmetry, or tenderness.[47] In more advanced disease, patients may present with cutaneous lesions, capsular contracture, a breast mass, or with regional lymphadenopathy.[47]

Patients should be evaluated with an ultrasound or breast MRI.[48] The seroma should be sampled via fine-needle aspiration (at least 10 mL but ideal >50 mL) for cytology, flow cytometry, and T-cell clonality.[47,48] A clone may not always be identified.[47] Atypical lymphocytes are large and pleomorphic and may resemble high-grade breast carcinoma.[48] Therefore, immunophenotyping is essential, evaluating for T-cell markers and CD30.[48] PET/CT should be obtained in all patients to evaluate for capsular and extracapsular disease before surgical intervention.[48] There is a validated staging system for BI-ALCL supported by the NCCN.[48] BI-ALCL in the early stages is a localized disease with good prognosis; OS is 100% at 3 years.[47] Complete surgical removal of the implant, capsule, and any chest wall masses is essential.[48] Incomplete resection should be considered for surgical reexcision, adjuvant radiation, and/or systemic therapy.[48] Patients with lymph node involvement have a 5-year OS of 75%.[47] There is no standard systemic therapy in patients with advanced, relapsed, or disseminated disease.[48] CHOP-based chemotherapy regimens are usually given with curative intent.[47] Brentuximab vedotin has been used as a second-line agent.[47]

EXTRANODAL NATURAL KILLER/T-CELL LYMPHOMA, NASAL TYPE

Extranodal NK/T-cell lymphoma, nasal type is an Epstein–bar virus (EBV)-associated lymphoma with an aggressive behavior and poor prognosis.[4] Patients are predominately from Asia or South America.[49] It classically presents in the nasal cavity, nasopharynx, or oropharynx with frequent metastasis to the skin, salivary gland, testis, and gastrointestinal tract.[49] In the United States and Europe, the presenting feature is nasal obstruction or a bleeding mass in the nasal cavity or upper aerodigestive tract (nasopharynx, paranasal sinuses, tonsils, hypopharynx, and larynx).[50] Nasal involvement may not be clinically apparent at diagnosis, emphasizing the importance of PET/CT imaging to evaluate for occult nasal primaries. It is recommended that suspected cases of nonnasal NK/T-cell lymphomas be confirmed by PET/CT and nasal panendoscopy performed irrespective of initial site of presentation.[50] The median survival is 20 months.[51] Three-year OS is 47%.[51]

Most of the cases are of NK-cell origin (CD2+, CD56+, surface CD3−, germline TCR), but rare cases are of T-cell lineage (CD3+, CD56−, granzyme B+, expressing a clonal TCRαβ or rarely TCRγδ).[49] Histologically, there are small to medium lymphoid cells mixed with small lymphocytes, plasma cells, eosinophils, and histiocytes. The atypical infiltrate is often angiocentric and angiodestructive.[49]

Anthracycline-based chemotherapy regimens are largely ineffective.[50,52] Current treatment strategies, even in local, early stage disease use concurrent chemoradiation or sandwich strategies with an L-asparaginase-based regimen, such as SMILE (dexamethasone, methotrexate, ifosfamide, L-asparaginase, and etoposide) combined with radiation at doses of greater than or equal to 50 Gy.[50] Serial plasma cell-free EBV DNA monitoring can be a useful predictor of disease burden and activity.[50] Whole blood is less useful, as it contains EBV-infected memory B cells.[50] Immunotherapy has been successfully used in refractory cases.[53] Patients with advanced or relapsed lymphoma that achieve complete remission may be considered for allogeneic hematopoietic stem cell transplantation.[50,52]

HYDROA VACCINIFORME-LIKE LYMPHOPROLIFERATIVE DISORDER

Hydroa vacciniforme-like lymphoproliferative disorder (HVLPD) is an EBV-associated T-cell or NK-cell lymphoproliferative disorder. In 2016 it was renamed as a "lymphoproliferative disorder," previously characterized as a "lymphoma" in 2008, given its unpredictable prognosis.[4] It exists on the spectrum of hydroa vacciniforme, a rare benign photosensitive eruption characterized by scarring vesicles and edematous plaques on sun-exposed sites but may evolve into an aggressive systemic EBV-associated T-cell lymphoma (EBV+ TCL).[4] It is most often reported in children but does rarely occur in adults primarily from Asia or indigenous populations of Mexico, Central America, or South America.[4,54] Patients with HVLPD often present with pruritic erythematous vesicles and edematous plaques, usually on sun exposed sites.[4] Lesions are larger and more indurated compared with hydroa vacciniforme and may become necrotic with overlying eschars (**Fig. 9**).[4] Lesions may be chronic and may be reported to occur at sites of insect bites.[55] In adults, lesions are often limited to the face and extremities.[55] Progression to systemic involvement represents evolution into an EBV+ TCL.[4,54] Prognosis is difficult to assess, given the presence of few case series in the literature.[55] Adult onset portends a worse prognosis.[55]

On histology, hydroa vacciniforme-like lymphoma has a superficial and deep atypical infiltrate of small to medium lymphocytes with a perivascular and periadnexal distribution.[4,55] Epidermotropism, intraepidermal vesicles, and epidermal necrosis may be seen.[4] Extension of the infiltrate into the subcutis is often associated with angiocentricity and vascular destruction.[4,54,55] There is an admixed inflammatory infiltrate with neutrophils, eosinophils, small lymphocytes, plasma cells, and mast cells.[4,54,55] The origin may be of T cells (CD3+, CD4+, CD8+, or double negative with expression

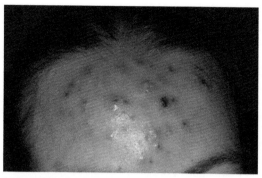

Fig. 9. Hydroa vacciniforme-like lymphoproliferative disorder.

of TCRαβ or TCRγδ), NK cells (CD56+), or both.[4] Cytotoxic markers, namely T1A-1, are commonly positive. Epstein–Barr encoding region in situ hybridization expression is mandatory.[4] NK-cell phenotype and CD30 expression may carry a better prognosis.[4] Adult onset, T-cell phenotype, and mast cell infiltration are associated with a worse prognosis.[55]

SUMMARY

Cutaneous oncology has experienced several advancements in the lymphoma realm, thanks to novel molecular and genomic studies. The advent of HTS for TCR has enhanced our ability to diagnose MF/SS earlier and to predict which patients are at risk for disease progression. Major insights into disease biology have been made through genomic studies of MF/SS. There is increasing recognition of unique CTCL subtypes with distinct clinicopathologic features and prognosis. However, many cases remain a diagnostic challenge. Although there are increasing numbers of clinical trials for novel therapies for MF/SS, treatment of aggressive and rare CTCL subtypes has seen little advancement.

REFERENCES

1. Bradford PT, Devesa SS, Anderson WF, et al. Cutaneous lymphoma incidence patterns in the United States: a population-based study of 3884 cases. Blood 2009;113(21):5064–73.
2. Korgavkar K, Xiong M, Weinstock M. Changing incidence trends of cutaneous T-cell lymphoma. JAMA Dermatol 2013;149(11):1295–9.
3. Willemze R, Jaffe ES, Burg G, et al. WHO-EORTC classification for cutaneous lymphomas. Blood 2005;105(10):3768–85.
4. Sundram U. Cutaneous lymphoproliferative disorders: what's new in the revised 4th edition of the World Health Organization (WHO) classification of lymphoid neoplasms. Adv Anat Pathol 2018;26(2):93–113.
5. Olsen E, Vonderheid E, Pimpinelli N, et al. Revisions to the staging and classification of mycosis fungoides and Sezary syndrome: a proposal of the International Society for Cutaneous Lymphomas (ISCL) and the cutaneous lymphoma task force of the European Organization of Research and Treatment of Cancer (EORTC). Blood 2007;110(6):1713–22.
6. Kirsch IR, Watanabe R, O'Malley JT, et al. TCR sequencing facilitates diagnosis and identifies mature T cells as the cell of origin in CTCL. Sci Transl Med 2015; 7(308):308ra158.

7. Watanabe R, Gehad A, Yang C, et al. Human skin is protected by four functionally and phenotypically discrete populations of resident and recirculating memory T cells. Sci Transl Med 2015;7(279):279ra239.

8. Campbell JJ, Clark RA, Watanabe R, et al. Sezary syndrome and mycosis fungoides arise from distinct T-cell subsets: a biologic rationale for their distinct clinical behaviors. Blood 2010;116(5):767–71.

9. Scarisbrick JJ, Quaglino P, Prince HM, et al. The PROCLIPI international registry of early stage Mycosis Fungoides identifies substantial diagnostic delay in most patients. Br J Dermatol 2018. [Epub ahead of print].

10. Guitart J, Kennedy J, Ronan S, et al. Histologic criteria for the diagnosis of mycosis fungoides: proposal for a grading system to standardize pathology reporting. J Cutan Pathol 2001;28(4):174–83.

11. Pimpinelli N, Olsen EA, Santucci M, et al. Defining early mycosis fungoides. J Am Acad Dermatol 2005;53(6):1053–63.

12. de Masson A, O'Malley JT, Elco CP, et al. High-throughput sequencing of the T cell receptor beta gene identifies aggressive early-stage mycosis fungoides. Sci Transl Med 2018;10(440) [pii:eaar5894].

13. van Santen S, Roach RE, van Doorn R, et al. Clinical staging and prognostic factors in folliculotropic mycosis fungoides. JAMA Dermatol 2016;152(9):992–1000.

14. Ahn CS, ALSayyah A, Sangüeza OP. Mycosis fungoides: an updated review of clinicopathologic variants. Am J Dermatopathol 2014;36(12):933–48 [quiz: 949–51].

15. Virmani P, Myskowski PL, Pulitzer M. Unusual variants of mycosis fungoides. Diagn Histopathol (Oxf) 2016;22(4):142–51.

16. Tsai EY, Taur A, Espinosa L, et al. Staging accuracy in mycosis fungoides and sezary syndrome using integrated positron emission tomography and computed tomography. Arch Dermatol 2006;142(5):577–84.

17. Agar NS, Wedgeworth E, Crichton S, et al. Survival outcomes and prognostic factors in mycosis fungoides/Sezary syndrome: validation of the revised International Society for Cutaneous Lymphomas/European Organisation for Research and Treatment of Cancer staging proposal. J Clin Oncol 2010;28(31):4730–9.

18. Kim YH, Liu HL, Mraz-Gernhard S, et al. Long-term outcome of 525 patients with mycosis fungoides and Sezary syndrome: clinical prognostic factors and risk for disease progression. Arch Dermatol 2003;139(7):857–66.

19. Scarisbrick JJ, Kim YH, Whittaker SJ, et al. Prognostic factors, prognostic indices and staging in mycosis fungoides and Sezary syndrome: where are we now? Br J Dermatol 2014;170(6):1226–36.

20. Scarisbrick JJ, Prince HM, Vermeer MH, et al. Cutaneous lymphoma international consortium study of outcome in advanced stages of mycosis fungoides and sezary syndrome: effect of specific prognostic markers on survival and development of a prognostic model. J Clin Oncol 2015;33(32):3766–73.

21. Wilcox RA. Cutaneous T-cell lymphoma: 2017 update on diagnosis, risk-stratification, and management. Am J Hematol 2017;92(10):1085–102.

22. Kharfan-Dabaja MA, Kumar A, Ayala E, et al. Clinical practice recommendations on indication and timing of hematopoietic cell transplantation in mature T Cell and NK/T cell lymphomas: an international collaborative effort on behalf of the guidelines committee of the American Society for Blood and Marrow Transplantation. Biol Blood Marrow Transplant 2017;23(11):1826–38.

23. Park J, Yang J, Wenzel AT, et al. Genomic analysis of 220 CTCLs identifies a novel recurrent gain-of-function alteration in RLTPR (p.Q575E). Blood 2017;130(12):1430–40.

24. Sekulic A, Liang WS, Tembe W, et al. Personalized treatment of Sezary syndrome by targeting a novel CTLA4:CD28 fusion. Mol Genet Genomic Med 2015;3(2): 130–6.

25. Kempf W, Pfaltz K, Vermeer MH, et al. EORTC, ISCL, and USCLC consensus recommendations for the treatment of primary cutaneous CD30-positive lymphoproliferative disorders: lymphomatoid papulosis and primary cutaneous anaplastic large-cell lymphoma. Blood 2011;118(15):4024–35.

26. Kempf W. A new era for cutaneous CD30-positive T-cell lymphoproliferative disorders. Semin Diagn Pathol 2017;34(1):22–35.

27. Liu HL, Hoppe RT, Kohler S, et al. CD30+ cutaneous lymphoproliferative disorders: the Stanford experience in lymphomatoid papulosis and primary cutaneous anaplastic large cell lymphoma. J Am Acad Dermatol 2003;49(6):1049–58.

28. Sauder MB, O'Malley JT, LeBoeuf NR. CD30(+) lymphoproliferative disorders of the skin. Hematol Oncol Clin North Am 2017;31(2):317–34.

29. Wieser I, Oh CW, Talpur R, et al. Lymphomatoid papulosis: treatment response and associated lymphomas in a study of 180 patients. J Am Acad Dermatol 2016;74(1):59–67.

30. Bekkenk MW, Geelen FA, van Voorst Vader PC, et al. Primary and secondary cutaneous CD30(+) lymphoproliferative disorders: a report from the Dutch Cutaneous Lymphoma Group on the long-term follow-up data of 219 patients and guidelines for diagnosis and treatment. Blood 2000;95(12):3653–61.

31. Greisser J, Palmedo G, Sander C, et al. Detection of clonal rearrangement of T-cell receptor genes in the diagnosis of primary cutaneous CD30 lymphoproliferative disorders. J Cutan Pathol 2006;33(11):711–5.

32. Willemze R, Jansen PM, Cerroni L, et al. Subcutaneous panniculitis-like T-cell lymphoma: definition, classification, and prognostic factors: an EORTC Cutaneous Lymphoma Group Study of 83 cases. Blood 2008;111(2):838–45.

33. Guitart J, Weisenburger DD, Subtil A, et al. Cutaneous gammadelta T-cell lymphomas: a spectrum of presentations with overlap with other cytotoxic lymphomas. Am J Surg Pathol 2012;36(11):1656–65.

34. da Silva Almeida AC, Abate F, Khiabanian H, et al. The mutational landscape of cutaneous T cell lymphoma and Sezary syndrome. Nat Genet 2015;47(12): 1465–70.

35. Rubio-Gonzalez B, Zain J, Garcia L, et al. Cutaneous gamma-delta T-cell lymphoma successfully treated with brentuximab vedotin. JAMA Dermatol 2016; 152(12):1388–90.

36. Gibson JF, Alpdogan O, Subtil A, et al. Hematopoietic stem cell transplantation for primary cutaneous gammadelta T-cell lymphoma and refractory subcutaneous panniculitis-like T-cell lymphoma. J Am Acad Dermatol 2015;72(6): 1010–5.e5.

37. Merrill ED, Agbay R, Miranda RN, et al. Primary cutaneous T-Cell lymphomas showing gamma-delta (gammadelta) phenotype and predominantly epidermotropic pattern are clinicopathologically distinct from classic primary cutaneous gammadelta T-cell lymphomas. Am J Surg Pathol 2017;41(2):204–15.

38. Tolkachjov SN, Weenig RH, Comfere NI. Cutaneous peripheral T-cell lymphoma, not otherwise specified: a single-center prognostic analysis. J Am Acad Dermatol 2016;75(5):992–9.

39. Berti E, Tomasini D, Vermeer MH, et al. Primary cutaneous CD8-positive epidermotropic cytotoxic T cell lymphomas. A distinct clinicopathological entity with an aggressive clinical behavior. Am J Pathol 1999;155(2):483–92.

40. Gormley RH, Hess SD, Anand D, et al. Primary cutaneous aggressive epidermotropic CD8+ T-cell lymphoma. J Am Acad Dermatol 2010;62(2):300–7.
41. Goodlad JR. Indolent CD8-positive lymphoid proliferation of acral sites: identifying the sheep in wolf's clothing. Br J Dermatol 2015;172(6):1480–1.
42. Kluk J, Kai A, Koch D, et al. Indolent CD8-positive lymphoid proliferation of acral sites: three further cases of a rare entity and an update on a unique patient. J Cutan Pathol 2016;43(2):125–36.
43. Virmani P, Jawed S, Myskowski PL, et al. Long-term follow-up and management of small and medium-sized CD4(+) T cell lymphoma and CD8(+) lymphoid proliferations of acral sites: a multicenter experience. Int J Dermatol 2016;55(11): 1248–54.
44. Greenblatt D, Ally M, Child F, et al. Indolent CD8(+) lymphoid proliferation of acral sites: a clinicopathologic study of six patients with some atypical features. J Cutan Pathol 2013;40(2):248–58.
45. Hathuc VM, Hristov AC, Smith LB. Primary cutaneous acral CD8(+) T-cell lymphoma. Arch Pathol Lab Med 2017;141(11):1469–75.
46. James E, Sokhn JG, Gibson JF, et al. CD4 + primary cutaneous small/medium-sized pleomorphic T-cell lymphoma: a retrospective case series and review of literature. Leuk Lymphoma 2015;56(4):951–7.
47. Mehta-Shah N, Clemens MW, Horwitz SM. How I treat breast implant-associated anaplastic large cell lymphoma. Blood 2018;132(18):1889–98.
48. Clemens MW, Horwitz SM. NCCN consensus guidelines for the diagnosis and management of breast implant-associated anaplastic large cell lymphoma. Aesthet Surg J 2017;37(3):285–9.
49. Tse E, Kwong YL. Diagnosis and management of extranodal NK/T cell lymphoma nasal type. Expert Rev Hematol 2016;9(9):861–71.
50. Tse E, Kwong YL. How I treat NK/T-cell lymphomas. Blood 2013;121(25): 4997–5005.
51. Kommalapati A, Tella SH, Ganti AK, et al. Natural killer/T-cell neoplasms: analysis of incidence, patient characteristics, and survival outcomes in the United States. Clin Lymphoma Myeloma Leuk 2018;18(7):475–9.
52. Tse E, Kwong YL. Management of advanced NK/T-cell lymphoma. Curr Hematol Malig Rep 2014;9(3):233–42.
53. Kwong YL, Chan TSY, Tan D, et al. PD1 blockade with pembrolizumab is highly effective in relapsed or refractory NK/T-cell lymphoma failing l-asparaginase. Blood 2017;129(17):2437–42.
54. Quintanilla-Martinez L, Ridaura C, Nagl F, et al. Hydroa vacciniforme-like lymphoma: a chronic EBV+ lymphoproliferative disorder with risk to develop a systemic lymphoma. Blood 2013;122(18):3101–10.
55. Wen PF, Zhang M, Wang TT, et al. Comparative study of the clinical pathology, immunophenotype, epstein-barr virus infection status, and gene rearrangements in adult and children patients with hydroa vacciniforme-like lymphoproliferative disorder. Am J Dermatopathol 2019;41(1):7–15.

Allogeneic Stem Cell Transplantation and Chimeric Antigen Receptor (CAR) T-Cell Therapy for the Treatment of Non-Hodgkin Lymphoma

Bradley D. Hunter, MD, MPH[a,b,]*, Yi-Bin Chen, MD[b],
Caron A. Jacobson, MD, MMSc[a]

KEYWORDS

- Non-Hodgkin lymphoma • B-cell lymphoma • T-cell lymphoma
- Chimeric antigen receptor T-cell therapy • Allogeneic stem cell transplant

KEY POINTS

- There remains widely variable practice in the treatment of relapsed or refractory non-Hodgkin lymphomas.
- Allogeneic stem cell transplant and CAR T-cell therapies are curative intent modalities for appropriately selected patients.
- Outcomes for patients with non-Hodgkin lymphoma who undergo allogeneic stem cell are generally favorable.
- CAR T-cell therapy should be considered before allogeneic stem cell transplant for patients with aggressive B-cell lymphomas.

INTRODUCTION

Lymphoma represents approximately 5% of all cancers diagnosed in the United States, with an estimated incidence in 2018 of 83,180 cases (National Cancer Institute SEER Program, https://seer.cancer.gov/statfacts/). For most B- and T-cell lymphomas, chemoimmunotherapy (with the possible addition of radiotherapy in limited-stage disease) is the standard of care for front-line therapy with curative intent

Relevant Disclosures: B.D. Hunter has nothing to disclose. Y-.B. Chen has consulted for Takeda, Magenta, Incyte, Kiadis. C.A. Jacobson has consulted for Kite, Novartis, Precision Biosciences, Celgene, Pfizer, and Bayer.
[a] Dana Farber Cancer Institute, 450 Brookline Avenue, Boston, MA 02215, USA;
[b] Massachusetts General Hospital, 0 Emerson Place, Suite 118, Boston, MA 02114, USA
* Corresponding author. Dana Farber Cancer Institute, Smith 353, 450 Brookline Avenue, Boston, MA 02215.
E-mail address: bdhunter@mgh.harvard.edu

Hematol Oncol Clin N Am 33 (2019) 687–705
https://doi.org/10.1016/j.hoc.2019.03.005
0889-8588/19/© 2019 Elsevier Inc. All rights reserved.

for aggressive lymphomas or a prolonged disease-free interval for patients with indolent disease. There are numerous chemotherapeutic, targeted, and immunotherapy options that exist for patients who relapse or have refractory disease; however, despite the myriad of available treatments, there remains a substantial subset of patients who are not able to achieve a prolonged disease-free interval with conventional chemotherapy or targeted agents. For these patients, hematopoietic stem cell transplantation (HCT), either autologous or allogeneic, remains an option for consolidative or curative treatment. Additionally, chimeric antigen receptor (CAR) T-cell therapy has emerged as a treatment option for patients with relapsed/refractory B-cell lymphomas, with two agents receiving Food and Drug Administration (FDA) approval in 2017 (axicabtagene ciloleucel [axi-cel] and tisagenlecleucel). Even within the realm of stem cell transplant and other cellular therapies, there is a great degree of nuance associated with treatment planning beyond the choice of therapy itself, including donor selection, conditioning regimen, and prophylaxis of infectious and immune complications. Published studies to date vary widely in their selected approach to transplant and cellular therapies. This review summarizes available data related to allogeneic HCT and CAR T-cell therapy for the treatment of lymphoma, providing clinicians with tools to aid in the selection of appropriate therapy and determining when to refer to a transplant specialist in the management of patients with T- and B-cell lymphomas.

T-CELL LYMPHOMAS

T-cell lymphomas make up approximately 10% of all lymphomas in the United States and up to 20% in Asia.[1] All the currently available data for T-cell lymphomas come from nonrandomized, retrospective studies (**Table 1**). In general, T-cell lymphomas are thought to be more sensitive to an immunologic graft-versus-lymphoma effect compared with their B-cell counterparts. However, few studies have compared outcomes of allogeneic HCT with chemotherapy alone approaches. When compared in retrospective studies, the outcomes for HCT seem to be superior.[2] The caveat remains that these data are subject to inherent selection bias for patients who remain in remission and are healthy enough to undergo allogeneic transplant. In general, patients with T-cell lymphomas who experience relapse do so within the first year (90% in large series)[3] after allogeneic HCT with rare relapses after 2 years. For those who do relapse, many respond to post-transplant therapies with reported remission rates in the post-transplant setting ranging from 30% to 67% in some series.[4,5]

For patients with peripheral T-cell lymphoma not otherwise specified, the most common histology of T-cell non-Hodgkin lymphomas, long-term survival with allogeneic HCT tends to be between 40% and 50%, whereas for patients who do not undergo HCT, 5-year overall survival (OS) is 10%.[6] Reported outcomes seem similar for patients receiving HCT in first remission compared with those that undergo transplant for relapsed/refractory disease; however, definitive prospective data are clearly lacking. One retrospective trial compared autologous transplant with allogeneic transplant and did not find significant survival differences based on the type of transplant.[7] Although refractory disease at the time of HCT has been shown to be predictive of inferior survival, one study of 284 patients reported that approximately 50% of patients who received allogeneic transplant in the setting of progressive disease were still alive at 2 years post-transplant.[3]

A few specific histologies where allogeneic HCT in CR1 may be considered standard of care merit individual mention. In the two studies involving patients with

Table 1
Allogeneic transplantation for T-cell lymphoma

Author, Year	Patients, n	Disease	Timing	Transplant[a]	NRM/Relapse (y)	Survival (y)
Dodero et al,[4] 2012	52	PTCL NOS, 23 ALCL, 11 AITL, 9 Others, 9	All patients with relapsed/refractory disease 52% with prior autoSCT 75% with chemosensitive disease at time of transplant	RIC MRD (63%) MUD (25%) Haplo (12%)	NRM 12% (5) Relapse 49% (5)	PFS 50% (5) OS 40% (5)
Smith et al,[36] 2013	126	PTCL-NOS, 63 AITL, 12 ALCL, 51	30% in CR (14% in CR1)	MAC 59% RIC 36% MRD 60% MUD 16% Mismatch-unrel 24%	NRM 27%–32% (3) Relapse 32%–40% (3)	PFS 33%–36% (3) OS 39%–52% (3)
Corradini et al,[2] 2014	61 ITT 38 transplant	PTCL-NOS, AITL, ALK-negative ALCL, EATL	Patients transplanted in first remission All patients received alemtuzumab before transplant	MAC MRD 57% MUD 43%	NRM 13% (4) Relapse 17% (4)	ITT-PFS 44% (4) 4-y PFS 69% (allo pts) ITT OS 49% (4) OS 69% (4) (allo pts)
Schmitz et al,[7] 2015	ITT 58 24 transplant	PTCL NOS	Patients transplanted in first remission	Auto vs Allo RIC	NR	ITT EFS 41% (1) ITT OS 69% (1)
Jacobsen et al,[37] 2011	52	PTCL, 20 CTCL, 8 ALCL, 6 AITL, 5 ENKL, 4 HSTL, 4 NKTCL, 5 ATLL, 1	44% in CR (19% in CR1) 31% in PR	MAC 60% RIC 40% MRD 46% MUD 37% Mismatch-rel 4% Mismatch-unrel 13%	NRM 27% (3) Relapse 43% (3)	PFS 30% (3) OS 41% (3)

(continued on next page)

Table 1
(continued)

Author, Year	Patients, n	Disease	Timing	Transplant[a]	NRM/Relapse (y)	Survival (y)
Mehta-Shah et al,[10] 2017	284	NOS, 78; AITL, 50; ALCL, 31; ATLL, 15; HSTL, 25; ENKL, 34; EATL, 4; CTCL, 21; SPTL, 9; GDTL, 3; BPDCN, 4	60.5% in CR; 33.1% in PR; 21% transplanted in first remission, rest beyond first line	MAC 46%; RIC 52%; MRD 40%; MUD 37%; Mismatch; Haplo 8%; UCB 9%	NRM 13.2% (1); Relapse 31% (4)	PFS 48% (2); OS 60% (2); PTCL NOS PFS 56% (2); AITL PFS 62% (2); ALK neg ALCL PFS 30% (2)
Mamez et al,[3] 2018 (SFGM-TC)	284	PTCL NOS, 111; AITL, 82; ALCL, 43; Others, 48	62% in CR; 27% in PR; 28% as part of frontline treatment; 36% after 2 lines; 25% after 3 or more lines	MAC 38%; RIC 62%; MRD 45%; MUD 36%; Mismatch 5%; UCB 12%; Haplo 2%	NRM 24% (2); Relapse 22% (2)	OS 64% (2)
Kanate et al,[8] 2018 (CIBMTR)	82	ENKL	12% with chemorefractory disease; 38% with previous ʟ-asparaginase; 30% treated with allo as part of frontline therapy	MAC 38%; RIC 59%; MRD 61%; MUD 28%; UCB 6%; Haplo 4%	NRM 30% (3); Relapse 42% (3)	PFS 28% (3); OS 34% (3)
Tse et al,[9] 2014 (Asia Lymphoma Study Group)	18	ENKL	50% in CR1, 39% in CR2	MAC 78%; RIC 22%; MRD 67%; MUD 33%	NRM 33% (2); Relapse 28% (2)	PFS 51% (5); OS 57% (5)

Tanase et al,[11] 2015 (EBMT)	18 Allo 7 Auto	HSTL	39% in CR 44% in PR Median time from diagnosis to transplant = 5 mo Patients had received between 1–7 prior lines of treatment		NRM 40% (3) Relapse 12% (3)	PFS 48% (3) OS 54% (3)
Hishizawa et al,[12] 2010	386	ATLL	32% in CR Most patients transplanted within 6 mo of diagnosis	MAC 67% RIC 33% MRD 56% MUD 33% Mismatch 6% UCB 6%	TRM 37% (3) Relapse 35% (3)	OS 33% (3)
Bazarbachi et al,[13] 2014	17	ATLL Acute, 7 Lymphoma, 10	54% in CR1 23% in PR	MAC 24% RIC 76% MRD 35% MUD 41% Haplo 18%	NRM 17% (3) Relapse 48% (3)	EFS 26% (3) OS 34% (3)
Fujiwara et al,[14] 2017 (TRUMP)	131	ATLL Acute, 62 Lymphoma, 46 Chronic, 2 Missing, 21	82% in first relapse, 18% 2nd relapse No patients were in remission 42% performed before 2007	MAC 47% RIC 47% MRD 29% MUD 42% UCB 23% Mismatch-rel 6%	NRM 37% (3) Relapse 51% (3)	OS 13% (3)
Duarte et al,[15] 2014 (EBMT)	60	CTCL MF, 36 SS, 24	67% had advanced stage disease at time of transplantation; 53% with chemosensitive disease, 47% with chemorefractory disease; 42% received T-cell depletion therapy	MAC 27% RIC 73% MRD 75% MUD 25%	NRM 22% (7) Relapse 45% (7)	PFS 32% (5) PFS 30% (7) OS 46% (5) OS 44% (7)

(continued on next page)

Table 1
(continued)

Author, Year	Patients, n	Disease	Timing	Transplant[a]	NRM/Relapse (y)	Survival (y)
Lechowicz et al,[38] 2014 (CIBMTR)	129	CTCL MF/SS	6% of patients in CR at time of transplant, 34% of patients had never achieved CR	MAC 46% RIC 64% MRD 50% MUD 43% Mismatch-rel 7%	NRM 22% (5) Relapse 61% (5)	PFS 17% (5) OS 32% (5)
Hosing et al,[5] 2015	47	CTCL	89% received total body electron beam radiation before transplant 15% in CR 60% in PR	MRD 45% MUD 51% Mismatch 4%	NRM 17% (2) Relapse 50% (4)	PFS 26% (4) OS 51% (4)

Abbreviations: AITL, angioimmunoblastic T-cell lymphoma; ALCL, anaplastic large cell lymphoma; ATLL, adult T-cell leukemia/lymphoma; BPDCN, blastic plasmacytoid dendritic cell neoplasm; CR, complete response; CTCL, cutaneous T-cell lymphoma; EATL, enteropathy-associated T-cell lymphoma; ENKL, extranodal natural killer T-cell lymphoma; GDTL, gamma-delta T-cell lymphoma; HSTL, hepatosplenic T-cell lymphoma; ITT, intention to treat; MAC, myeloablative conditioning; MF, mycosis fungoides; MRD, matched related donor; MUD, matched unrelated donor; NKTCL, natural killer T-cell lymphoma; NR, not reported; NRM, nonrelapse mortality; OS, overall survival; PFS, progression-free survival; PR, partial response; PTCL-NOS, peripheral T-cell lymphoma, not otherwise specified; RIC, reduced-intensity conditioning; SPTL, subcutaneous panniculiits-like T-cell lymphoma; SS, Sézary syndrome; UCB, umbilical cord blood donor.

[a] Not all columns sum to 100% because of missing data from the published studies.

extranodal natural killer cell lymphoma, long-term progression-free survival (PFS) and OS were 28% to 51% and 51% to 57%, respectively.[8,9] In both studies, there was no difference in outcome for patients transplanted in CR1 versus delayed transplant. Conditioning regimen choice or intensity did not seem to affect outcomes, although patient numbers were small.

For hepatosplenic T-cell lymphoma, outcomes seem to be favorable with reported 5-year PFS and OS of 48% and 54%, respectively. A large retrospective experience of 284 patients with T-cell lymphomas (which included 25 patients with hepatosplenic T-cell lymphoma) was recently reported at the 2017 American Society of Hematology meeting, with a 2-year PFS of 48% and OS of 60%; specific survival estimates for hepatosplenic T-cell lymphoma patients were not delineated because there were not significant survival differences based on tumor histology.[10] Additionally, patients who have refractory disease at the time of transplant have been shown to have reasonable outcomes, with PFS of 50% at 3 years in one series.[11]

For patients with adult T-cell leukemia/lymphoma, outcomes with transplant tend to be poor with rapid relapse, occurring in one study at a median of 2.5 months after allogeneic HCT.[12] Autologous HCT does not seem to be an effective treatment, with early relapse and mortality in limited reporting.[13] The largest series to date comes from the Japanese experience with reported 3-year OS of 33%.[12] Notable risk factors associated with inferior OS include remission status other than complete response, age, performance status, and stem cell transplant before 2007. Among these, achieving remission before transplant seems to be particularly important; one study that included only patients who were not in remission at the time of transplant reported dismal outcomes, with a 3-year OS of 13%.[14]

Finally, patients with relapsed/refractory cutaneous T-cell lymphomas who undergo allogeneic transplant have reported 5-year OS of 30% to 50%. Relapse is common with most studies reporting PFS of less than 30% at 4 years. There is a discrepancy between PFS and OS, which demonstrates that many patients may survive long after they relapse, likely caused by disease biology and alternative treatment options. Indeed, one study reported that 8/27 patients who relapsed after HCT were still alive with a median follow-up of 8 years (Duarte).[15]

INDOLENT B-CELL LYMPHOMAS

In the modern era, outcomes for patients with indolent B-cell lymphomas who undergo allogeneic HCT are favorable (**Table 2**). Long-term OS has ranged between 45% and 85%, with most studies reporting survival of greater than 60%. Among indolent disease, follicular lymphoma (FL) and chronic lymphocytic leukemia (CLL) are the most common subtypes. Survival for FL in large series seems to be superior to that of CLL (66% and 45%, respectively).[16,17] However, a recent update to the largest reported series of patients with CLL receiving allogeneic HCT reported that factors associated with poor outcome include age, performance status, remission status before HCT, unrelated donor type, and unfavorable sex-mismatch (notably, 17p deletion did not affect survival).[18] For well-selected patients, 2-year nonrelapse mortality (NRM) was 11% and 5-year Event-free survival (EFS) was approximately 60%.[18]

Indolent B-cell lymphomas tend to be slow growing, and although incurable, are treatable with a multitude of good treatment options, and most patients survive for two decades or more. Given that the average age at diagnosis is 60+ years, many patients will not need a transplant and will die with, rather than of, these lymphomas. In regards to allogeneic HCT for indolent B-cell lymphomas in general, NRM in the modern era mostly ranges between 10% and 25%, with rates of relapse ranging for the

Table 2
Allogeneic transplantation for indolent B-cell lymphoma

Author, Year	Patients, n	Donor Type	Conditioning	NRM (y)	Relapse	PFS	OS
Hosing et al,[39] 2003	44	MRD (89%) MUD (4%) Mismatch-related (7%)	MAC	NR	NR	49% (4)	45% (4)
Corradini et al,[40] 2007	63	MRD (95%) Mismatch-related (5%)	RIC	14% (3)	29% (3)	57% (3)	69% (3)
Rezvani et al,[41] 2008	46	MRD (53%) MUD (27%) Mismatch-related (2%) Mismatch-unrelated (18%)	RIC	42% (3)	14% (3)	43% (3)	52% (3)
Hari et al,[19] 2008 (CIBMTR)	208 Stratified by conditioning	MRD	MAC (58%) RIC (42%)	25% (3) 28% (3)	8% (3)[a] 17% (3)	67% (3) 55% (3)	71% (3) 62% (3)
Kuruvilla et al,[42] 2008	39	MRD (82%) MUD (5%) Mismatch-related (13%)	MAC (95%) RIC (5%)	18% (5)	3% (5)	76% (5)	79% (5)
Pinana et al,[43] 2010	37	MRD	RIC	37% (4)	8% (4)	57% (4)	57% (4)
Thomson et al,[44] 2010	82	MRD (48%) MUD (40%) Mismatch-unrelated (12%)	RIC (inc. anti-CD52)	15% (4)	26% (4)	76% (4)	76% (4)
Shea et al,[45] 2011	44	MRD	RIC	9% (3)	NR	75% (3)	81% (3)
Khouri et al,[46] 2012	47	MRD (96%) MUD (4%)	RIC	15% (9)	6% (9)	78% (11)	72% (11)
Tada et al,[47] 2012	46	MRD (50%) MUD (50%)	MAC (15%) RIC (85%)	16% (5)	15% (5)	70% (5)	77% (5)
Evens et al,[48] 2013	49	MRD (63%) MUD (37%)	NR	24% (3)	16% (3)	NR	61% (3)
Robinson et al,[49] 2013	149	MRD (80%) MUD (20%)	RIC	22% (3)	20% (5)	57% (5)	67% (5)

Study	N	Donor Type	Conditioning				
McClune et al,[50] 2014 (CIBMTR)	580	NR	NR	24% (1)	26% (3)	42% (3)	52% (3)
Klyuchnikov et al,[16] 2015 (CIBMTR)	268 (all FL)	MRD (53%) MUD (38%) Mismatch (8%)	RIC	26% (5)	20% (5)	68% (5)	66% (5)
Yano et al,[51] 2015	46	NR	RIC	23% (5)	15% (5)	75% (5)	81% (5)
Cassaday et al,[52] 2015	89	MRD (53%) MUD (47%)	RIC	NR	NR	46% (3)	63% (3)
Laport et al,[53] 2016 (BMT CTN)	62	MRD (53%) MUD (47%)	RIC	13% (3)	16% (3)	71% (3)	82% (3)
Armand et al,[54] 2016	59	MRD (40%) MUD (60%)	RIC	NR	NR	53%–71% (2)	63%–82% (2)
Picleanu & Novelli,[55] 2017	77	NR	MAC (17%) RIC (83%)	7% (6 mo)	NR	51% (5)	58% (5)
Dodero et al,[56] 2017	57	NR	RIC	16% (1)	17% (3)	60%–70% (3)	66%–76% (3)
Van Gelder et al,[17] 2017 (EBMT)	2589 (all CLL)	MRD (51%) Other (49%)	MAC (23%) RIC (77%)	36% (5)	29% (5)	35% (5)	45% (5)
Warlick et al,[57] 2018	23	NR	RIC	17% (2)	0% (5)	NR	78% (5)

Abbreviations: CIBMTR, Center for International Blood and Marrow Transplant Research; CLL, chronic lymphocytic leukemia; EBMT, European Society for Blood and Marrow Transplantation; FL, follicular lymphoma; MAC, myeloablative conditioning; MRD, matched related donor; MUD, matched unrelated donor; NR, not reported; NRM, nonrelapse mortality; RIC, reduced-intensity conditioning.
a P<.05.

most part between 15% and 25%. Studies reporting allogeneic transplants for the treatment of indolent B-cell lymphomas have largely used reduced-intensity conditioning (RIC). One large study using data from the Center for International Blood and Marrow Research (CIBMTR) compared regimen intensity and reported an increased risk of relapse in patients who received RIC regimens, but no significant differences were seen in PFS or OS.[19] In the largest published series to date of patients with indolent B-cell lymphomas, which included 580 patients in the CIBMTR database, 3-year PFS was 42%. Other CIBMTR analyses that have only included patients with FL have reported long-term PFS has been more than 65%.[16,19] Because of these impressive survival rates for FL, others have suggested that allogeneic transplantation be a preferred treatment to autologous transplant for patients with relapsed or refractory disease.[20] Although cure rates seem high for allogeneic HCT in CLL and FL, most patients never undergo such therapy because of improved alternative therapies and advanced age at diagnosis followed by even more advanced age at a time when allogeneic transplant would be considered. However, for younger patients with either multiply relapsed/refractory disease or those with clearly identified high-risk biology, allogeneic HCT is likely the treatment choice that will maximize survival.

AGGRESSIVE B-CELL LYMPHOMAS

Allogeneic HCT remains an effective therapeutic option for patients with relapsed diffuse large B-cell lymphoma (DLBCL) (**Table 3**). As opposed to conditioning therapy for indolent B-cell lymphomas, conditioning regimens for aggressive B-cell lymphomas tend to be more mixed; however, RIC conditioning still tends to predominate. Analyses of large cohorts using CIBMTR data reported higher relapse rates, lower NRM, and in some series, superior OS with RIC conditioning.[21-23] In one series the survival benefit of RIC lost statistical significance after controlling for chemoresistant disease.[22] Given the retrospective nature of the studies, and the heterogeneity of included patients, it is difficult to make meaningful comparisons among published series. As expected given retrospective data, outcomes vary widely, with rates of relapse and NRM ranging between 26% and 50% and 9% and 56%, respectively. Long-term survival ranges between 18% and 77%. Long-term OS in large series ranges between 18% and 54% with better outcomes reported in series that included only patients with prior autologous stem cell transplant[22,24,25] (selecting out patients with primary refractory disease) and series with high proportions of patients with grade 3 FL.[26] Recent studies have looked for potential differences in outcomes based on double-expressor lymphoma or double-hit lymphoma status and did not find a significant difference in survival outcomes for those with double-expressor lymphoma or those with double hit lymphoma.[27,28] Although allogeneic stem cell transplant remains a reasonable treatment option for patients with aggressive B-cell lymphomas, the advent of CAR T-cell therapy and its ability to produce durable remissions calls into question if allogeneic HCT should be reserved for patients who fail CAR T-cell therapy.

CHIMERIC ANTIGEN RECEPTOR T-CELL THERAPIES FOR NON-HODGKIN LYMPHOMAS

CAR T-cell therapy represents one of the most exciting new modalities for the treatment of lymphoma. Despite 5-year survival rates of 60% to 70%, approximately 50% of patients with advanced DLBCL relapse or develop refractory disease. Before the advent of CAR T-cell therapy, outcomes for patients with primary refractory DLBCL or disease that relapsed within 1 year after autologous stem cell transplant was dismal, with a median OS of 6.3 months and less than 10% of patients being

Table 3
Allogeneic transplantation for aggressive B-cell lymphoma

Author, Year	Patients, n	Prior Auto-HCT	Donor	Conditioning Regimen	NRM (y)	Relapse (y)	PFS (y)	OS (y)
Thomson et al,[58] 2009	48 62% DLBCL 38% tFL	69%		RIC (100%)	32% (4)	33% (4)	47% (4)	48% (4)
Sirvent et al,[59] 2010	68 100% DLBCL	79%	MRD (82%) MUD (12%) Mismatch-unrel (6%)	RIC (100%)	23% (1)	41% (2)	44% (2)	49% (2)
Lazarus, et al,[60] 2010 (CIBMTR)	79 100% DLBCL	0%	MRD	MAC (100%)	43% (3)	33% (3)	24% (3)	26% (3)
Van Kampen et al,[24] 2011 (EBMT)	101 100% DLBCL	100%	MRD (71%) MUD (29%)	MAC (37%) RIC (63%)	28% (3)	30% (3)	42% (3)	54% (3)
Rigacci et al,[25] 2012 (GITMO)	165 100% DLBCL Stratified by donor type	100%	MRD (65%) MUD (35%)	MAC (30%) RIC (70%)	19% (2)[a] 32% (2)	NR	32% (2)	39% (2)
Bacher et al,[21] 2012 (CIBMTR)	396 100% DLBCL Stratified by conditioning	32%	MRD (33%) MUD (42%) Mismatch-unrel (25%)	MAC (42%) RIC (58%)	56% (5)[b] 36% (5)	26% (5)[b] 38% (5)	18% (5) 23% (5)	18% (5) 20% (5)
Hamadani et al,[23] 2013 (CIBMTR)	533 90% DLBCL 10% G3FL Stratified by conditioning	25%	MRD (66%) MUD (23%) Mismatch-unrel (11%)	MAC (58%) RIC (42%)	53% (3)[b] 42% (3)	28% (3)[b] 35% (3)	19% (3) 23% (3)	19% (3)[b] 28% (3)

(continued on next page)

Table 3
(continued)

Author, Year	Patients, n	Prior Auto-HCT	Donor	Conditioning Regimen	NRM (y)	Relapse (y)	PFS (y)	OS (y)
Fenske et al,[22] 2016 (CIBMTR)	503 / 100% DLBCL / Stratified by conditioning	100%	MRD (50%) / MUD (23%) / Mismatch-unrel (26%)	MAC (25%) / RIC (75%)	31% (5)	40% (5)	27% (5) / 30% (5)	28% (5)[a] / 37% (5)
Klyuchnikov et al,[26] 2016 (CIBMTR)	70 / 100% G3FL	0%	MRD (59%) / MUD (38%) / Mismatch-unrel (3%)	RIC	27% (5)	20% (5)	51% (5)	54% (5)
Kawashima et al,[27] 2018	37 (DEL) / 23 (w/o DEL) / Stratified by histology	32%	MRD (32%) / MUD (16%) / Mismatch (19%) / Haplo (5%) / UCB (27%)	MAC (7%) / RIC (93%)	22% (2) / 9% (2)	NR	20% (2)[b] / 78% (2)	46% (2)[b] / 77% (2)
Herrera et al,[28] 2018	31 (w/o DEL or DHL) / 37 (DEL) / 10 (DHL) / Stratified by histology	58%	MRD (36%) / MUD (42%) / Mismatch-unrel (10%) / Haplo (4%) / UCB (8%)	MAC (23%) / RIC (77%)	23% (4) / 20% (4) / 20% (4)	38% (4) / 50% (4) / 40% (4)	39% (4) / 30% (4) / 40% (4)	49% (5) / 31% (5) / 50% (4)

Abbreviations: DEL, double-expressor lymphoma; DHL, double-hit lymphoma; DLBCL, diffuse large B-cell lymphoma; G3FL, grade 3 follicular lymphoma; MAC, myeloablative conditioning; MRD, matched related donor; MUD, matched unrelated donor; NR, not reported; tFL, transformed follicular lymphoma; UCB, umbilical cord blood donor.

[a] $P = .055$.

[b] $P < .05$ P value is less than 0.05.

able to achieve a complete response to subsequent therapy.[29] Two CD19 CAR T-cell therapies have been FDA approved (axicabtagene ciloleucel, tisagenlecleucel) for the treatment of relapsed/refractory DLBCL, primary mediastinal B-cell lymphoma, and transformed FL after 2 prior lines of chemotherapy. To date, studies using CD19 CAR T cells have demonstrated response rates of 70% to 80% with durable responses of greater than 40% in patients with aggressive B-cell lymphomas and up to 70% for patients with indolent lymphomas (**Table 4**).[30,31] The most common complications associated with CAR T-cell therapy are the cytokine release syndrome and neurotoxicity (NT). In reported studies to date, 13% to 22% of patients have experienced grade 3 + cytokine release syndrome, and 12% to 28% have experienced grade 3 + NT. Both cytokine release syndrome and NT tend to be fully reversible, although rarely patients have experienced incomplete resolution of NT. The most feared complication of NT is fatal cerebral edema, which has not been reported in either of the studies that led to FDA approval for CAR T-cell products in B-cell lymphomas.[30,31] Deaths directly attributable to CAR T-cell therapy were reported at 0% to 2%.[30,31] Because CD19 is a pan B-cell marker, one frequent long-term toxicity is prolonged B-cell aplasia. B-cell aplasia increases the risk of infection but can often be effectively managed with infectious disease prophylaxis and replacement of intravenous immunoglobulin. Therapies that target pan T-cell markers run the risk of prolonged T-cell aplasia, which is far more immunosuppressive than B-cell aplasia. As CD5 CAR T-cell trials are currently underway, toxicity data will be important in

Table 4
CAR T-cell therapies for non-Hodgkin lymphoma

Author, Year	Patients, n	CAR T-cell Product	3 + CRS	3 + NT	ORR	PFS (y)	OS (y)
Kochenderfer et al,[61] 2015	4 DLBCL 4 PMBCL 4 CLL 1 tCLL 1 SMZL	CD19/CD28	NR	NR	80%	NR	NR
Turtle et al,[62] 2016	11 DLBCL 11 tIndolent 4 MCL 6 FL	CD19/4-1BB (delivered in a fixed 1:1 CD4/CD8 ratio)	13%	28%	72%	NR	NR
Neelapu et al,[31] 2017	77 DLBCL 8 PMBCL 16 tFL (should probably report response rates and survival stats based separated by histology)	CD19/CD28 (axicabtagene ciloleucel)	13%	28%	82%	44% (1)	59% (1)
Schuster et al,[63] 2017	14 DLBCL 14 FL	CD19/4-1BB (CTL019)	18%	11%	64%	43% (2) 71% (2)	NR
Schuster et al,[30] 2018	88 DLBCL 21 tFL	CD19/4-1BB (CTL019, tisagenlecleucel)	22%	12%	52%	NR	49% (1)

Abbreviations: CRS, cytokine release syndrome; MCL, mantle cell lymphoma; NT, neurotoxicity; PMBCL, primary mediastinal B-cell lymphoma; NR, not reported; ORR, overall response rate; SMZL, splenic marginal zone lymphoma; tCLL, transformed CLL (Richter transformation); tIndolent, transformed indolent B-cell lymphoma.

determining if meaningful survival can still be achieved in this setting. For T-cell lymphomas that express markers that are not universally expressed on normal T-cells (ie, CD30), there is the promise of more effective selection of tumor cells and reduced toxicity. As previous studies have demonstrated that CD19 low-expressing or negative cells are still able to be eliminated with CD19 CAR T-cell therapy,[30] it follows that either only low levels of antigen density may be required to activate a CAR T-cell response, or other tumor-specific antigens are ultimately recognized when the immune system is activated by CD19 CAR T-cells. The latter offers some hope that CAR T-cell therapies for T-cell lymphomas may not need a pan T-cell target to be effective. Currently, there are many other CAR T-cell targets in clinical trials, including new targets (CD5, CD7, TRBC1, CD20, CD22, CD30); dual target CARs (CD30/CCR4, CD19/CD22, CD19/CD20); CARs with multiple costimulatory domains (CD19 CAR with CD28 and 4-1BB costimulatory domains); CARs that express unique markers or cytokines (ie, CD19 with expression of intrerleukin-15 and HER1t, other examples include CD40L and 4IBBL); and CD19 CARs with concurrent administration of immunomodulatory antibodies, such as PD-1/PD-L1 checkpoint blockade, 41BB agonist antibodies, and so forth. Additionally, Boolean or logic-gated CARs are under development, which can require dual engagement of separate receptors[32] (can also be inhibited in the presence of dual engagement)[33] to activate with the hope of improving specificity and thereby reducing off-target effects. Beyond the use of CAR T-cells, the development of chimeric T-cell antigen couplers, which co-opt the T-cell receptor, offer the potential for improved cytotoxic efficiency and less toxicity.[34] At a minimum, they offer an alternative cellular therapy approach to currently approved CD19 CAR T cells. At this point, CAR T-cell therapy is standard of care for patients with refractory or multiply relapsed (after autologous stem cell transplant) aggressive B-cell lymphomas and should be considered before allogeneic transplant. In addition to their clinical effectiveness, further study is needed to explore the cost-effectiveness of CAR T-cell therapy. A recent analysis of cost-effectiveness for pediatric patients treated with CAR T-cell therapy for acute lymphoblastic leukemia concluded that at current pricing (infusion cost of $475,000 for tisagenlecleucel), long-term survival of 40% was needed for the therapy to be cost-effective.[35] The current high cost of CAR T-cell therapy underscores the potential advantage that an effective, off-the-shelf, allogeneic product could have in reducing the cost of treatment and making such therapies available to a larger population of patients.

SUMMARY

The studies presented in this review indicate that allogeneic HCT remains an effective therapy for select patients with lymphoma, although much depends on histology, disease biology, clinical behavior, and alternative options. For patients with peripheral T-cell lymphomas, reported outcomes in retrospective studies comparing autologous versus allogeneic stem cell transplant as consolidation therapy have shown similar survival, and many opt for autologous approaches in this setting given the lower risk of NRM; however, for the more aggressive T-cell lymphomas and for relapsed/refractory disease, allogeneic stem cell transplant should be considered standard of care. In general, the outcomes for patients with relapsed/refractory aggressive B-cell lymphomas are poorer than those with other lymphomas. The long-term survival rate is at best comparable with the rate of durable response seen with CAR T-cell therapy, and many of the included studies in this review report survival that is inferior to that reported in CAR T-cell trials. Given the low rates of NRM reported to date for CAR T-cell therapy, there is a strong argument for preferentially selecting CAR

T-cell therapy for patients with relapsed or refractory aggressive B-cell lymphomas and reserving allogeneic HCT for patients who relapse after or are refractory to CAR T-cell therapy. For indolent B-cell lymphomas, outcomes after allogeneic HCT are favorable for the right patient, and it is not yet clear if CAR T-cell therapy will result in superior outcomes. CAR T-cell therapy for T-cell lymphomas remains in early stages of development. If effective therapies are developed, the management of T-cell aplasia will be a larger barrier to implementation than that of B-cell aplasia. Areas of focus for future study include strategies to decrease NRM for allogeneic stem cell transplants, and the development of safer, less expensive, and more effective CAR T-cell products, especially those that can safely eradicate T-cell lymphomas.

REFERENCES

1. Schmitz N, Lenz G, Stelljes M. Allogeneic hematopoietic stem cell transplantation for T-cell lymphomas. Blood 2018;132(3):245–53.
2. Corradini P, Vitolo U, Rambaldi A, et al. Intensified chemo-immunotherapy with or without stem cell transplantation in newly diagnosed patients with peripheral T-cell lymphoma. Leukemia 2014;28(9):1885–91.
3. Mamez A, Dupont A, Blaise D, et al. Allogeneic stem cell transplantation for peripheral T-cell lymphomas: a study of 284 patients from the Societe Francophone de Greffe de Moelle et de Therapie Cellulaire. 44th Annual Meeting of the EBMT. Lisbon, March 18-21, 2018.
4. Dodero A, Spina F, Narni F, et al. Allogeneic transplantation following a reduced-intensity conditioning regimen in relapsed/refractory peripheral T-cell lymphomas: long-term remissions and response to donor lymphocyte infusions support the role of a graft-versus-lymphoma effect. Leukemia 2012;26(3):520–6.
5. Hosing C, Bassett R, Dabaja B, et al. Allogeneic stem-cell transplantation in patients with cutaneous lymphoma: updated results from a single institution. Ann Oncol 2015;26(12):2490–5.
6. Chihara D, Fanale MA, Miranda RN, et al. The survival outcome of patients with relapsed/refractory peripheral T-cell lymphoma-not otherwise specified and angioimmunoblastic T-cell lymphoma. Br J Haematol 2017;176(5):750–8.
7. Schmitz N, Nickelsen M, Altmann B, et al. Allogeneic or autologous transplantation as first-line therapy for younger patients with peripheral T-cell lymphoma: results of the interim analysis of the AATT trial. J Clin Oncol 2015;33(15):8507.
8. Kanate AS, DiGilio A, Ahn KW, et al. Allogeneic haematopoietic cell transplantation for extranodal natural killer/T-cell lymphoma, nasal type: a CIBMTR analysis. Br J Haematol 2018;182(6):916–20.
9. Tse E, Chan TS, Koh LP, et al. Allogeneic haematopoietic SCT for natural killer/T-cell lymphoma: a multicentre analysis from the Asia Lymphoma Study Group. Bone Marrow Transplant 2014;49(7):902–6.
10. Mehta-Shah N, Teja S, Tao Y, et al. Successful treatment of mature T-cell lymphoma with allogeneic stem cell transplantation: the largest multicenter retrospective analysis. Blood 2017;130:4597.
11. Tanase A, Schmitz N, Stein H, et al. Allogeneic and autologous stem cell transplantation for hepatosplenic T-cell lymphoma: a retrospective study of the EBMT Lymphoma Working Party. Leukemia 2015;29(3):686–8.
12. Hishizawa M, Kanda J, Utsunomiya A, et al. Transplantation of allogeneic hematopoietic stem cells for adult T-cell leukemia: a nationwide retrospective study. Blood 2010;116(8):1369–76.

13. Bazarbachi A, Cwynarski K, Boumendil A, et al. Outcome of patients with HTLV-1-associated adult T-cell leukemia/lymphoma after SCT: a retrospective study by the EBMT LWP. Bone Marrow Transplant 2014;49(10):1266–8.

14. Fujiwara H, Fuji S, Wake A, et al. Dismal outcome of allogeneic hematopoietic stem cell transplantation for relapsed adult T-cell leukemia/lymphoma, a Japanese nation-wide study. Bone Marrow Transplant 2017;52(3):484–8.

15. Duarte RF, Boumendil A, Onida F, et al. Long-term outcome of allogeneic hematopoietic cell transplantation for patients with mycosis fungoides and Sezary syndrome: a European society for blood and marrow transplantation lymphoma working party extended analysis. J Clin Oncol 2014;32(29):3347–8.

16. Klyuchnikov E, Bacher U, Kroger NM, et al. Reduced-intensity allografting as first transplantation approach in relapsed/refractory grades one and two follicular lymphoma provides improved outcomes in long-term survivors. Biol Blood Marrow Transplant 2015;21(12):2091–9.

17. van Gelder M, de Wreede LC, Bornhauser M, et al. Long-term survival of patients with CLL after allogeneic transplantation: a report from the European Society for Blood and Marrow Transplantation. Bone Marrow Transplant 2017;52(3):372–80.

18. Schetelig J, de Wreede LC, van Gelder M, et al. Risk factors for treatment failure after allogeneic transplantation of patients with CLL: a report from the European Society for Blood and Marrow Transplantation. Bone Marrow Transplant 2017; 52(4):552–60.

19. Hari P, Carreras J, Zhang MJ, et al. Allogeneic transplants in follicular lymphoma: higher risk of disease progression after reduced-intensity compared to myeloablative conditioning. Biol Blood Marrow Transplant 2008;14(2):236–45.

20. Epperla N, Hamadani M. Hematopoietic cell transplantation for diffuse large B-cell and follicular lymphoma: current controversies and advances. Hematol Oncol Stem Cell Ther 2017;10(4):277–84.

21. Bacher U, Klyuchnikov E, Le-Rademacher J, et al. Conditioning regimens for allotransplants for diffuse large B-cell lymphoma: myeloablative or reduced intensity? Blood 2012;120(20):4256–62.

22. Fenske TS, Ahn KW, Graff TM, et al. Allogeneic transplantation provides durable remission in a subset of DLBCL patients relapsing after autologous transplantation. Br J Haematol 2016;174(2):235–48.

23. Hamadani M, Saber W, Ahn KW, et al. Impact of pretransplantation conditioning regimens on outcomes of allogeneic transplantation for chemotherapy-unresponsive diffuse large B cell lymphoma and grade III follicular lymphoma. Biol Blood Marrow Transplant 2013;19(5):746–53.

24. van Kampen RJ, Canals C, Schouten HC, et al. Allogeneic stem-cell transplantation as salvage therapy for patients with diffuse large B-cell non-Hodgkin's lymphoma relapsing after an autologous stem-cell transplantation: an analysis of the European Group for Blood and Marrow Transplantation Registry. J Clin Oncol 2011;29(10):1342–8.

25. Rigacci L, Puccini B, Dodero A, et al. Allogeneic hematopoietic stem cell transplantation in patients with diffuse large B cell lymphoma relapsed after autologous stem cell transplantation: a GITMO study. Ann Hematol 2012;91(6):931–9.

26. Klyuchnikov E, Bacher U, Woo Ahn K, et al. Long-term survival outcomes of reduced-intensity allogeneic or autologous transplantation in relapsed grade 3 follicular lymphoma. Bone Marrow Transplant 2016;51(1):58–66.

27. Kawashima I, Inamoto Y, Maeshima AM, et al. Double-expressor lymphoma is associated with poor outcomes after allogeneic hematopoietic cell transplantation. Biol Blood Marrow Transplant 2018;24(2):294–300.

28. Herrera AF, Rodig SJ, Song JY, et al. Outcomes after allogeneic stem cell transplantation in patients with double-hit and double-expressor lymphoma. Biol Blood Marrow Transplant 2018;24(3):514–20.

29. Crump M, Neelapu SS, Farooq U, et al. Outcomes in refractory diffuse large B-cell lymphoma: results from the international SCHOLAR-1 study. Blood 2017; 130(16):1800–8.

30. Schuster SJ, Bishop MR, Tam CS, et al. Tisagenlecleucel in adult relapsed or refractory diffuse large B-cell lymphoma. N Engl J Med 2018;380(1):45–56.

31. Neelapu SS, Locke FL, Bartlett NL, et al. Axicabtagene ciloleucel CAR T-cell therapy in refractory large B-cell lymphoma. N Engl J Med 2017;377(26):2531–44.

32. Kloss CC, Condomines M, Cartellieri M, et al. Combinatorial antigen recognition with balanced signaling promotes selective tumor eradication by engineered T cells. Nat Biotechnol 2013;31(1):71–5.

33. Fedorov VD, Themeli M, Sadelain M. PD-1- and CTLA-4-based inhibitory chimeric antigen receptors (iCARs) divert off-target immunotherapy responses. Sci Transl Med 2013;5(215):215ra172.

34. Helsen CW, Hammill JA, Lau VWC, et al. The chimeric TAC receptor co-opts the T cell receptor yielding robust anti-tumor activity without toxicity. Nat Commun 2018;9(1):3049.

35. Lin JK, Lerman BJ, Barnes JI, et al. Cost effectiveness of chimeric antigen receptor T-cell therapy in relapsed or refractory pediatric B-cell acute lymphoblastic leukemia. J Clin Oncol 2018. https://doi.org/10.1200/JCO.2018.79.0642.

36. Smith SM, Burns LJ, van Besien K, et al. Hematopoietic cell transplantation for systemic mature T-cell non-Hodgkin lymphoma. J Clin Oncol 2013;31(25): 3100–9.

37. Jacobsen ED, Kim HT, Ho VT, et al. A large single-center experience with allogeneic stem-cell transplantation for peripheral T-cell non-Hodgkin lymphoma and advanced mycosis fungoides/Sezary syndrome. Ann Oncol 2011;22(7):1608–13.

38. Lechowicz MJ, Lazarus HM, Carreras J, et al. Allogeneic hematopoietic cell transplantation for mycosis fungoides and Sezary syndrome. Bone Marrow Transplant 2014;49(11):1360–5.

39. Hosing C, Saliba RM, McLaughlin P, et al. Long-term results favor allogeneic over autologous hematopoietic stem cell transplantation in patients with refractory or recurrent indolent non-Hodgkin's lymphoma. Ann Oncol 2003;14(5):737–44.

40. Corradini P, Dodero A, Farina L, et al. Allogeneic stem cell transplantation following reduced-intensity conditioning can induce durable clinical and molecular remissions in relapsed lymphomas: pre-transplant disease status and histotype heavily influence outcome. Leukemia 2007;21(11):2316–23.

41. Rezvani AR, Norasetthada L, Gooley T, et al. Non-myeloablative allogeneic haematopoietic cell transplantation for relapsed diffuse large B-cell lymphoma: a multicentre experience. Br J Haematol 2008;143(3):395–403.

42. Kuruvilla J, Pond G, Tsang R, et al. Favorable overall survival with fully myeloablative allogeneic stem cell transplantation for follicular lymphoma. Biol Blood Marrow Transplant 2008;14(7):775–82.

43. Pinana JL, Martino R, Gayoso J, et al. Reduced intensity conditioning HLA identical sibling donor allogeneic stem cell transplantation for patients with follicular lymphoma: long-term follow-up from two prospective multicenter trials. Haematologica 2010;95(7):1176–82.

44. Thomson KJ, Morris EC, Milligan D, et al. T-cell-depleted reduced-intensity transplantation followed by donor leukocyte infusions to promote graft-versus-

lymphoma activity results in excellent long-term survival in patients with multiply relapsed follicular lymphoma. J Clin Oncol 2010;28(23):3695–700.

45. Shea T, Johnson J, Westervelt P, et al. Reduced-intensity allogeneic transplantation provides high event-free and overall survival in patients with advanced indolent B cell malignancies: CALGB 109901. Biol Blood Marrow Transplant 2011; 17(9):1395–403.

46. Khouri IF, Saliba RM, Erwin WD, et al. Nonmyeloablative allogeneic transplantation with or without 90yttrium ibritumomab tiuxetan is potentially curative for relapsed follicular lymphoma: 12-year results. Blood 2012;119(26):6373–8.

47. Tada K, Kim SW, Asakura Y, et al. Comparison of outcomes after allogeneic hematopoietic stem cell transplantation in patients with follicular lymphoma, diffuse large B-cell lymphoma associated with follicular lymphoma, or de novo diffuse large B-cell lymphoma. Am J Hematol 2012;87(8):770–5.

48. Evens AM, Vanderplas A, LaCasce AS, et al. Stem cell transplantation for follicular lymphoma relapsed/refractory after prior rituximab: a comprehensive analysis from the NCCN lymphoma outcomes project. Cancer 2013;119(20):3662–71.

49. Robinson SP, Canals C, Luang JJ, et al. The outcome of reduced intensity allogeneic stem cell transplantation and autologous stem cell transplantation when performed as a first transplant strategy in relapsed follicular lymphoma: an analysis from the Lymphoma Working Party of the EBMT. Bone Marrow Transplant 2013; 48(11):1409–14.

50. McClune BL, Ahn KW, Wang HL, et al. Allotransplantation for patients age >/=40 years with non-Hodgkin lymphoma: encouraging progression-free survival. Biol Blood Marrow Transplant 2014;20(7):960–8.

51. Yano S, Mori T, Kanda Y, et al. Favorable survival after allogeneic stem cell transplantation with reduced-intensity conditioning regimens for relapsed/refractory follicular lymphoma. Bone Marrow Transplant 2015;50(10):1299–305.

52. Cassaday RD, Storer BE, Sorror ML, et al. Long-term outcomes of patients with persistent indolent B cell malignances undergoing nonmyeloablative allogeneic transplantation. Biol Blood Marrow Transplant 2015;21(2):281–7.

53. Laport GG, Wu J, Logan B, et al. Reduced-intensity conditioning with fludarabine, cyclophosphamide, and high-dose rituximab for allogeneic hematopoietic cell transplantation for follicular lymphoma: a phase two multicenter trial from the blood and marrow transplant clinical trials network. Biol Blood Marrow Transplant 2016;22(8):1440–8.

54. Armand P, Kim HT, Sainvil MM, et al. The addition of sirolimus to the graft-versus-host disease prophylaxis regimen in reduced intensity allogeneic stem cell transplantation for lymphoma: a multicentre randomized trial. Br J Haematol 2016; 173(1):96–104.

55. Picleanu AM, Novelli S. Allogeneic hematopoietic stem cell transplantation for non-Hodgkin's lymphomas: a retrospective analysis of 77 cases. Ann Hematol 2017;96(5):787–96.

56. Dodero A, Patriarca F, Milone G, et al. Allogeneic stem cell transplantation for relapsed/refractory B cell lymphomas: results of a multicenter phase II prospective trial including rituximab in the reduced-intensity conditioning regimen. Biol Blood Marrow Transplant 2017;23(7):1102–9.

57. Warlick ED, DeFor TE, Bejanyan N, et al. Reduced-intensity conditioning followed by related and unrelated allografts for hematologic malignancies: expanded analysis and long-term follow-up. Biol Blood Marrow Transplant 2018;25(1): 56–62.

58. Thomson KJ, Morris EC, Bloor A, et al. Favorable long-term survival after reduced-intensity allogeneic transplantation for multiple-relapse aggressive non-Hodgkin's lymphoma. Journal of clinical oncology: official journal of the American Society of Clinical Oncology 2009;27(3):426–32.
59. Sirvent A, Dhedin N, Michallet M, et al. Low nonrelapse mortality and prolonged long-term survival after reduced-intensity allogeneic stem cell transplantation for relapsed or refractory diffuse large B cell lymphoma: report of the Societe Francaise de Greffe de Moelle et de Therapie Cellulaire. Biol Blood Marrow Transplant 2010;16(1):78–85.
60. Lazarus HM, Zhang MJ, Carreras J, et al. A comparison of HLA-identical sibling allogeneic versus autologous transplantation for diffuse large B cell lymphoma: a report from the CIBMTR. Biol Blood Marrow Transplant 2010;16(1):35–45.
61. Kochenderfer JN, Dudley ME, Kassim SH, et al. Chemotherapy-refractory diffuse large B-cell lymphoma and indolent B-cell malignancies can be effectively treated with autologous T cells expressing an anti-CD19 chimeric antigen receptor. J Clin Oncol 2015;33(6):540–9.
62. Turtle CJ, Hanafi LA, Berger C, et al. Immunotherapy of non-Hodgkin's lymphoma with a defined ratio of CD8+ and CD4+ CD19-specific chimeric antigen receptor-modified T cells. Sci Transl Med 2016;8(355):355ra116.
63. Schuster SJ, Svoboda J, Chong EA, et al. Chimeric antigen receptor T cells in refractory B-cell lymphomas. N Engl J Med 2017;377(26):2545–54.

Noncellular Immune Therapies for Non-Hodgkin Lymphoma

Alex F. Herrera, MD

KEYWORDS

- Immunotherapy • Non-Hodgkin lymphoma • Checkpoint blockade • PD-1 • CD47
- Bispecific antibody • Antibody drug conjugate

KEY POINTS

- Several novel noncellular immunotherapies are demonstrated to be safe and effective in the treatment of non-Hodgkin lymphoma (NHL).
- Blockade of immune checkpoints, such as PD-1 or CD47, has resulted in antitumor activity in NHL.
- Antibody drug conjugates deliver a potent chemotherapy directly to tumor cells that harbor a specific target of interest.
- Bispecific antibodies are molecules with dual specificity that bring immune cells in proximity to tumor cells to trigger an antitumor immune response.

INTRODUCTION

Non-Hodgkin lymphomas (NHLs) are a diverse group of diseases, encompassing mature B-cell, T-cell, and natural killer (NK) cell malignancies and ranging in behavior from indolent to highly aggressive. For many years, the traditional treatment of NHL centered on chemotherapy. However, the introduction of rituximab, a monoclonal antibody directed against CD20, ushered in the era of immunotherapy for NHLs. Since the introduction of rituximab, there has been a tremendous proliferation of noncellular immune therapies for NHL, ranging from additional naked monoclonal antibodies to antibody-drug conjugates to bispecific T-cell engaging antibodies to antibodies targeting immune checkpoints. In this article, novel immune therapies that

Disclosure Statement: The author has the following disclosures: BMS—research funding, consultancy; Genentech—research funding, consultancy; Merck—research funding, consultancy; Seattle Genetics—research funding, consultancy; Pharmacyclics—research funding; Immune Design—research funding; Kite Pharma—research funding, consultancy; Gilead Sciences—research funding; Adaptive Biotechnologies—consultancy.
Department of Hematology and Hematopoietic Cell Transplantation, City of Hope National Medical Center, 1500 East Duarte Road, Duarte, CA 91010, USA
E-mail address: aherrera@coh.org

Hematol Oncol Clin N Am 33 (2019) 707–725
https://doi.org/10.1016/j.hoc.2019.03.007
0889-8588/19/© 2019 Elsevier Inc. All rights reserved.
hemonc.theclinics.com

have been used for the treatment of NHL are reviewed. The data supporting the use of rituximab have been reviewed extensively; this article focuses on novel immune therapies other than rituximab that remain in use or are actively being studied in clinical trials.

MONOCLONAL ANTIBODIES
Obinutuzumab

Obinutuzumab is a glycoengineered type II monoclonal antibody directed against CD20 with greater antibody-dependent cellular cytotoxicity, direct cell death, and phagocytic properties as compared with rituximab. These enhancements to anti-CD20 therapy have resulted in demonstrated efficacy of obinutuzumab in patients with indolent B-cell lymphoma who are refractory to rituximab and improved efficacy compared with rituximab as front-line therapy for follicular lymphoma (FL). The randomized phase III GADOLIN trial demonstrated prolonged median progression-free survival (PFS) and overall survival (OS) in patients with rituximab-refractory indolent B-cell NHL who received obinutuzumab added to bendamustine, which led to the Food and Drug Administration (FDA) approval of obinutuzumab in patients with rituximab-refractory FL.[1] Similarly, the randomized phase III GALLIUM study evaluated obinutuzumab-based chemoimmunotherapy as compared with rituximab-based chemoimmunotherapy followed by maintenance of the anti-CD20 mAb. Obinutuzumab prolonged 3-year PFS (80% vs 73.3%), but a higher rate of severe adverse events (AE) and grade 3 to 5 AEs was observed in the obinutuzumab arm.[2] Based on these data, obinutuzumab was approved by the FDA in combination with chemotherapy in patients with previously untreated FL. Although obinutuzumab improved outcomes in FL, no improvement in outcome was observed when obinutuzumab was used as part of frontline chemoimmunotherapy in patients with newly diagnosed diffuse large B-cell lymphoma (DLBCL).[3]

Mogamulizumab

Mogamulizumab is a first-in-class defucosylated anti-CCR4 antibody with enhanced antibody-dependent cellular toxicity that has been evaluated in T-cell lymphomas. CCR4 is a chemokine that is commonly expressed on tumor cells in T-cell lymphomas, including peripheral T-cell lymphomas (PTCL), adult T-cell leukemia-lymphoma (ATLL), and cutaneous T-cell lymphomas (CTCL) including mycosis fungoides (MF) and Sezary syndrome (SS). Mogamulizumab has been studied in Japan for the treatment of PTCL or CTCL (35% overall response rate [ORR], median PFS 3 months), as well as ATLL (ORR 50%, median PFS 5.2 months), and is approved by Japanese authorities for CCR4+ ATLL and CTCL.[4,5] The international randomized phase III MAVORIC trial compared mogamulizumab with vorinostat in 372 patients with relaxed/refractory (R/R) CTCL who had received a median of 3 prior lines of therapy. Mogamulizumab treatment was tolerable, with the most common AEs being infusion-related reactions, rash, diarrhea, and fatigue. Mogamulizumab produced higher overall global (35%) and skin (44%) responses compared with vorinostat (global 6% and skin 22%) and the investigator-assessed median PFS was 7.7 months in the mogamulizumab arm compared with 3.1 months in the vorinostat arm. The mediation duration of response to mogamulizumab by compartment was 25.5 months in blood, 20.6 months in skin, and 15.5 months in lymph nodes.[6] Based on these data, mogamulizumab was approved by the FDA for use in patients with R/R MF or SS after failure of one line of treatment.

Hu5F9-G4

Hu5F9-G4 (5F9) is a first-in-class monoclonal antibody that targets CD47, which has demonstrated promising safety and activity in patients with B-cell NHL. CD47 is expressed on the surface of tumor cells and acts as a "don't eat me" signal, allowing the tumor to avoid phagocytosis by macrophages and resulting in cytotoxic adaptive immune responses. 5F9 blocks the "don't eat me" signal and stimulates an antitumor immune response. In a phase Ib/II study, 22 patients with R/R DLBCL (n = 15) or FL (n = 7) were treated with 5F9 in combination with rituximab. Therapy was well tolerated with 41% of patients having chills, 36% having headache, and 27% of patients having fever; nearly all AEs were grade 1 to 2. The ORR was 50%, including 40% ORR and 27% complete response (CR) rate in patients with DLBCL and a 71% ORR and 43% CR rate in patients with FL. At the time of presentation, 90% of patients were in ongoing response (median follow-up of 4.4 months), with one patient in a response for 13 plus months.[7] The phase II portion of the study is ongoing (NCT02953509).

ANTIBODY DRUG CONJUGATES

Antibody drug conjugates (ADCs) are compound molecules that allow the delivery of potent chemotherapy into a cell that expresses a target of interest. Cytotoxic agents are covalently linked to monoclonal antibodies directed against cellular targets that are usually ubiquitously present on a particular malignant cell. Brentuximab vedotin (BV), an ADC with an auristatin payload directed against CD30, was the initial ADC developed for the treatment of hematologic malignancies, in particular, classic Hodgkin lymphoma (HL). Since the development and subsequent FDA approval of BV for the treatment of HL and anaplastic large cell lymphoma (ALCL), multiple other ADCs have been developed for the treatment of NHLs (**Table 1**).

Polatuzumab Vedotin

Polatuzumab vedotin (PoV) is an ADC with a monomethyl auristatin E (MMAE) payload directed against CD79b, a part of the B-cell receptor complex that is ubiquitously expressed on B cells. PoV has been studied in B-cell NHL (B-NHL) and CLL as a single agent and in multiple PoV-based combination studies in patients with B-NHL. After initial efficacy and tolerability was observed in B-NHL, subsequent phase II studies evaluated PoV with rituximab or with obinutuzumab in patients with R/R FL or DLBCL: PoV plus rituximab resulted in an ORR of 56% with a CR rate of 15% in R/R DLBCL, whereas patients with R/R FL had an ORR of 70% and a CR rate of 40% and PoV plus obinutuzumab yielded a best ORR of 52% and CR rate of 29% in R/R DLBCL and patients with R/R FL had an ORR of 78% and CR rate of 30%.[8] In a separate phase II study, PoV was combined with 6 cycles of bendamustine and either rituximab or obinutuzumab in patients with R/R DLBCL or FL in a study that included a randomized cohort of rituximab-bendamustine, BR versus PoV plus rituximab-bendamustine. In patients with R/R DLBCL randomized to PoV + BR (n = 40), the best ORR and CR rate were 70% and 57.5%, respectively as compared with 32.5% and 20%, respectively, in patients who received BR (n = 40). PFS and OS were significantly longer in patients who received PoV-BR (median OS 12.4 months vs 4.7 months), with a higher frequency of peripheral neuropathy and cytopenias in the PoV-BR group. In patients with R/R FL, the CR rate at the end of 6 cycles of PoV + BR (n = 39, 69%) was similar to BR (n = 41, 63%) and PFS was also similar (17 vs 17.3 months).[9] Based on these findings, the FDA and European Medicines Agency granted PoV breakthrough therapy and PRIME designation, respectively, for the treatment of R/R DLBCL. PoV has also

Table 1
Clinical trials evaluating antibody-drug conjugates in non-Hodgkin lymphoma

Target	Drug/Regimen[a]	Phase	N[b]	Population	Response Data	DOR/PFS	Ref
CD19	**Denintuzumab mafodotin** q3w, q6w	1	62 (60)	R/R B-NHL	ORR 33% CR 22%	DOR 40 wk	Moskowitz et al,[21] 2015
	Coltuximab ravtansine q3w x ≤ 6	1	39 (35)	R/R BCL	ORR 17%		Younes et al,[48] 2012
	Coltuximab ravtansine qw (W1-4), then q2w	2	NA (41)	CD19 + R/R DLBCL	ORR 44% CR 12%		Trneny et al,[23] 2014
	Coltuximab ravtansine qw x ≤ 12	1	44 (43)	R/R B-NHL	ORR 30% CR/CRu 15%	DOR 10 wk	Ribrag et al,[22] 2014
	Coltuximab ravtansine qw (W1-4), then q2w (W5-8) + R	2	52 (45)	R/R DLBCL	ORR 31%	PFS 3.9 mo OS 9.0 mo DOR 8.6 mo	Coiffier et al,[24] 2016
	Loncastuximab tesirine q3w	1	138 (68)	R/R B-NHL	B-NHL: ORR 60% CR 35% DLBCL: ORR 55% CR 37%		Herrera et al,[40] 2018
CD22	**Pinatuzumab vedotin** q3w	1	75 (73)	R/R DLBCL, iNHL, or CLL	Refractory DLBCL: ORR 25% iNHL: ORR 42% CLL: ORR 0%	Refractory DLBCL: PFS 4.0 mo iNHL: PFS 7.6 mo	Advani et al,[49] 2017
	Pinatuzumab vedotin q3w + R	2	63 (63)	R/R DLBCL or FL	DLBCL: ORR 57% CR 24% FL: ORR 62% CR 10%	DLBCL PFS 5.2 mo	Morschhauser et al,[8] 2014

Regimen	Phase	N (evaluable)	Population	Response	Outcome	Reference
Inotuzumab ozogamicin q4w × ≤8	2	81 (81)	FL, MZL, or SLL refractory to R, R + CT, or RIT	ORR 67% CR 31%	PFS 13 mo	Ogura et al,[50] 2016
Inotuzumab ozogamicin q4w × ≤8 + R	1	10 (10)	R/R CD22+ B-NHL	ORR 80% CR/CRu 70%	DOR >1 y	Ogura et al,[18] 2012
Inotuzumab ozogamicin q3w ≤6 + R-CVP	1	48 (32)	R/R CD22+ B-NHL	iNHL: ORR 100% CR 24% aNHL: ORR 57%		Ogura et al,[51] 2016
Inotuzumab ozogamicin q3w ≤6 + R-GDP	1	55 (55)	R/R B-NHL	FL: ORR 71% DLBCL: ORR 33% MCL: ORR 62%		Sangha et al,[52] 2017
Inotuzumab ozogamicin q4w × ≤8 + R	1/2	118 (111)	R/R CD20 + CD22+ B-NHL with prior R	FL: ORR 87% DLBCL: ORR 74%	FL: DOR NR DLBCL: DOR 18 mo	Fayad et al,[17] 2013
Inotuzumab ozogamicin q3w ≤6 + R, then ASCT	2	63 (63)	High-risk R/R DLBCL	ORR 29%	2-y PFS 61% in pts undergoing HDT-ASCT	Wagner-Johnston et al,[19] 2015
Arm 1: Inotuzumab ozogamicin q4w + R Arm 2: R + bendamustine or gemcitabine	3	338 (332)	CD22 + R/R a B-NHL not candidates for HDT	Arm 1: ORR 41% CR 18% Arm 2: ORR 44% CR 16%	Arm 1: OS 9.5 mo Arm 2: OS 9.5 mo	Dang et al,[20] 2018

(continued on next page)

Table 1
(continued)

Target	Drug/Regimen[a]	Phase	N[b]	Population	Response Data	DOR/PFS	Ref
CD25	**Camidanlumab tesirine** q3w	1	86 (68)	R/R HL or NHL	B-NHL: ORR 31% CR 19% PTCL: 50% ORR		Horwitz et al,[53] 2017
CD30	**BV** q3w	2	53 (52)	R/R DLBCL w undetectable CD30 expn	ORR 31% CR 12%		Bartlett et al,[54] 2017
	Cohort 1: **BV** q3w Cohort 2: **BV** q3w + R	2	49 (48)	R/R DLBCL w detectable CD30 expn	Cohort 1: ORR 44% CR 17% Cohort 2: ORR 46% CR 15%	Cohort 1: PFS 4.0 mo	Jacobsen et al,[11] 2015
	Part 1: **BV** q3w + RCHOP Part 2: **BV** q3w + RCHP	2	11[c] (10)	1L DLBCL w IPI 1–3 or aaIPI 2–3	Part 1: ORR 91% Part 2: ORR 82%	Part 1: 18-mo PFS CD30 + 79% CD30%–58% 18-mo OS CD30 + 92% CD30%–71%	Budde et al,[15] 2016
	BV Q3W	2	58	R/R ALCL	ORR 86% CR 57%	DOR 12.6 mo PFS 13.3 mo	Pro et al,[12] 2012
	BV Q3W	2	35	R/R PTCL NOS R/R AITL	ORR 34%, CR 14% ORR 54%, CR 38%	DOR 7.6 mo PFS 5.5 mo	Horwitz et al,[13] 2014

Target	Regimen	Phase	N (N)	Indication	Response	Survival	Reference
	BV-CHP Q3Wd	3	226	R/R CD30 + PTCL	CR 68%	PFS 48.2 mo	Horwitz et al,[16] 2019
	BV	3	131	R/R MF, 1° cutaneous ALCL	ORR4 56%	PFS 16.7 mo	Prince et al,[14] 2017
CD79b	PoV q3w	1	7 (7)	R/R B-NHL	ORR 43% CR 29%		Hatake et al,[55] 2016
	PoV or PoV + R q3w	1	95 (95)	R/R B-NHL or CLL	NHL PoV: ORR 55% PoV + R: ORR 78% CLL PoV: ORR 0%	NHL PoV PFS 5.7 mo DOR 6.2 mo PoV + R mPFS 12.5 mo mDOR 12.3 mo	Palanca-Wessels et al,[56] 2015
	PoV q3w + R	2	59 (59)	R/R DLBCL or FL	DLBCL: ORR 56% CR 15% FL: ORR 70% CR 40%		Morschhauser et al,[8] 2014
	PoV q3w x ≤ 8 + R-CHP	1/2	45 (45)	1L DLBCL	ORR 91% CR 78%		Tilly et al,[10] 2017
	PoV q3w x 8 + G	1/2	70 (44)	R/R DLBCL or FL	DLBCL: ORR 52% CR 29% FL: ORR 78% CR 30%		Phillips et al,[57] 2016

(continued on next page)

Table 1
(continued)

Target	Drug/Regimen[a]	Phase	N[b]	Population	Response Data	DOR/PFS	Ref
	PoV q3w x 8 + G-CHP	1/2	21 (19)	1L or R/R DLBCL	ORR 91% CR 81%		Forero-Torres et al,[58] 2017
	PoV q3w + B+ (R or G) vs BR	1/2	65[d] (64)	R/R DLBCL or FL not eligible for HSCT	DLBCL For BR: CR 15% For PoV + BR: CR 40% FL For PoV + BR: ORR 100% CR 67% For PoV + BG: ORR 85% CR 65%	DLBCL BR: OS 4.7 mo PoV + BR: OS 11.8 mo	Matasar et al,[59] 2017

Abbreviations: A, aggressive; aaIPI, age-adjusted international prognostic index; ASCT, autologous stem cell transplant; B, bendamustine; BCL, B-cell lymphoma; B-NHL, B-non-Hodgkin lymphoma; BV, brentuximab vedotin; C, cycle; CLL, chronic lymphocytic leukemia; CR, complete response; CRu, complete response unconfirmed; CT, chemotherapy; DLBCL, diffuse large B-cell lymphoma; DOR, duration of response; expn, expression; FL, follicular lymphoma; G, obinutuzumab; GGT, gamma-glutamyl transferase; HDT, high-dose therapy; HSCT, hematopoietic stem cell transplant; iNHL, indolent NHL; InO, inotuzumab ozogamicin; IPI, international prognostic index; L, line; MZL, marginal zone lymphoma; NHL, non-Hodgkin lymphoma; NOS, not otherwise specified; NR, not reached; ORR, overall response rate; OS, overall survival; PFS, progression-free survival; PoV, polatuzumab vedotin; Pts, patients; q2w, once every 2 weeks; q3w, once every 3 weeks; q4w, once every 4 weeks; qw, once weekly; R, rituximab; R/R, relapsed or refractory; RCHOP, rituximab, cyclophosphamide, doxorubicin, vincristine, and prednisone; R-CHP, rituximab, cyclophosphamide, doxorubicin and prednisone; R-CVP, rituximab, cyclophosphamide, vincristine, and prednisolone; R-GDP, rituximab, gemcitabine, dexamethasone, and cisplatin; RIT, radioimmunotherapy; SLL, small lymphocytic lymphoma; W, week.

[a] All ADCs were administered intravenously.
[b] Safety population (evaluable efficacy population).
[c] Patients in Part 2. Number of patients in Part 1 not specified.
[d] Total population (combined PoV + BR, and PoV + BG) for FL data; for DLBCL data, n = 80.

been evaluated as part of initial therapy (cyclophosphamide, doxorubicin, and predni-sone with either rituximab, R-CHP, or obinutuzumab, G-CHP) in patients with newly diagnosed DLBCL, resulting in an end of treatment ORR and CR rate after R-CHP (n = 45) of 91% and 78%, respectively.[10] There is currently a randomized, double-blinded, placebo-controlled, phase III trial evaluating the addition of PoV to R-CHP compared with R-CHOP as initial therapy for DLBCL (NCT03274492).

Brentuximab Vedotin

In addition to its success in treating HL, BV has been studied in the treatment of B-NHL, PTCL, and CTCL. In a phase II study of BV in patients with R/R B-NHL or PTCL, CD30 expression was an eligibility criterion for enrollment; however, there was wide variability in CD30 expression, and in a subsequent central review some pa-tients were found to be CD30 negative. In patients with DLBCL (n = 48), the ORR was 44% with a CR rate of 17%, and in a separate cohort of DLBCL patients combining BV with rituximab (n = 15) the response rate was 46%. Only 1 of 6 patients enrolled with primary mediastinal large B-cell lymphoma (PMBCL) responded (CR) and the ORR among 6 patients with gray zone lymphoma (features intermediate between DLBCL and HL) was 50% with 1 CR (17%).[11]

Anaplastic large cell lymphoma is a subtype of PTCL with universal CD30 expres-sion, making it a ripe target for CD30-directed therapy. BV was highly effective in a pivotal phase II study in patients with R/R ALCL, demonstrating an ORR of 86% and CR rate of 57% and a duration of response of 12.6 months.[12] Based on these re-sults, BV was approved for use in patients with R/R ALCL. Results with BV were less promising in patients with R/R non-ALCL PTCL (n = 34), with an ORR of 41% and CR rate of 24% but responses varied by PTCL subtype with a 54% ORR and 38% CR rate in patients with angioimmunoblastic T-cell lymphoma (n = 13) as compared with a 33% ORR and 14% CR rate in patients with PTCL, not otherwise specified. The safety profile of BV across these studies was similar to what was observed in studies of BV in HL, with peripheral neuropathy and neutropenia being the main notable AEs.[13] In the randomized phase III ALCANZA study, patients with CD30-positive R/R MF or primary cutaneous ALCL who received BV had a higher rate of objective global response last-ing at least 4 months (56%) and median PFS (16.7 months) as compared with physi-cian's choice therapy (oral methotrexate or oral bexarotene—12.5% and 3.5 months).[14] Based on these findings, the FDA approved BV for use in patients with R/R CTCL who have failed at least one prior therapy.

BV has also been studied as part of frontline therapy in patients with CD30-positive PTCL and B-NHL. In patients with previously untreated DLBCL with an international prognostic index score of 3 or higher (n = 11), 6 cycles of R-CHP plus BV resulted in an ORR of 91% and CR rate of 82% at the end of treatment with a peripheral neu-ropathy rate of 55%.[15] After initial studies demonstrated promise with the addition of BV to CHP as frontline therapy in CD30 + PTCL, the randomized phase III ECHELON-2 study of CHP + BV versus CHOP confirmed that CHP + BV produced a superior median PFS of 48.2 months compared with 20.8 months in patients who received CHOP and led to the FDA approval of BV in the frontline setting for CD30 + PTCL.[16]

ANTI-CD22 ANTIBODY DRUG CONJUGATES

Two anti-CD22 ADCs have been studied in B-NHL—pinatuzumab vedotin (PiV), which has an MMAE payload, and inotuzumab ozogamicin (InO), which has a calicheamicin-based payload. In the phase II ROMULUS study, the ORR to PiV plus rituximab in pa-tients with R/R DLBCL was 57% with a CR rate of 24% and a median duration of response (DOR) of 5.2 months. Similar response rates to PiV plus rituximab were observed in FL (62% ORR, 10% CR). The most common side effects observed with PiV were fatigue, peripheral neuropathy, and neutropenia.[8] Clinical trials of InO have had variable results, with initial studies of InO monotherapy or InO plus rituximab demonstrating promising efficacy but subsequent larger studies yielding lower response rates and a randomized phase III study of InO + R versus either BR or gemcitabine with rituximab showing no difference in ORR, PFS, or OS between the InO + R and chemotherapy arms.[17–20]

ANTI-CD19 ANTIBODY DRUG CONJUGATES

Several anti-CD19 ADCs have been evaluated in B-NHL, including denintuzumab mafodotin, coltuximab ravtansine, and most recently, loncastuximab tesirine (ADCT-402). Although a phase I trial of denintuzumab mafodotin demonstrated reasonable antitumor activity in patients with R/R B-NHL (n = 60, primarily DLBCL) with an ORR of 33% and a CR rate of 22%, 84% of patients experienced superficial keratopathy, usually managed with dose reductions and topical corticosteroids.[21] Initial studies of coltuximab ravtansine also demonstrated moderate activity in B-NHL (ORR 17%–44%), but a subsequent phase II of coltuximab ravtansine plus rituximab in patients with R/R DLBCL did not meet the prespecified efficacy target (ORR $\geq$40%).[22–24] As with denintuzumab mafodotin, coltuximab ravtansine resulted in ocular AEs that were typically mild, as well as cytopenias and peripheral neuropathy. In an initial phase I study of loncastuximab tesirine (ADCT-402), an anti-CD19 ADC with a pyrrolobenzodiazepine (PBD) dimer payload, the observed response rate in B-NHL has been higher than with other anti-CD19 ADCs with impressive efficacy (ORR 55%, 37% CR, DOR 4.9 months) as a single agent in patients with R/R DLBCL who received higher doses ($\geq$120 µg/kg) of the medication. At the time of reporting, the maximum tolerated dose had not been reached, and notable AEs included grade 3 or higher neutropenia (15%) or elevated gamma-glutamyl transferase (GGT) (15%) and rash of any grade observed in 52% of patients.[25]

CAMIDANLUMAB TESIRINE (ADCT-301)

Similar to loncastuximab tesirine (ADCT-402), camidanlumab tesirine (ADCT-301) is an anti-CD25 ADC with a PBD dimer payload. In a phase I study, camidanlumab tesirine produced a 31% ORR and 19% CR rate among 16 patients with B-cell lymphoma treated at higher doses and an ORR of 50% observed among the 10 patients with PTCL. Like with loncastuximab tesirine (ADCT-402), the most common grade $\geq$3 AEs were hematologic (thrombocytopenia, 9%) and elevated GGT (13%). Dose-limiting toxicities were observed at a range of doses of camidanlumab tesirine, including mucositis/enteritis, elevated creatinine, rash/pruritis, and lip ulceration and skin infection.[26] A study of camidanlumab tesirine in R/R PTCL and HL is ongoing (NCT02432235).

BISPECIFIC T-CELL ENGAGER ANTIBODIES

Bispecific T-cell engager (BiTE) antibodies are molecules with dual specificity that target both a tumor antigen and an immune cell, bringing them in close physical proximity in order to trigger an antitumor immune response. Blinatumomab was the initial BiTE antibody directed against CD19 on B-cells and the CD3ε subunit of the T-cell receptor complex and is approved for use in the treatment of acute lymphoblastic leukemia as a continuous infusion with stepwise dosing to reach the target dose. After blinatumomab showed promising efficacy in a phase I study of patients with B-NHL, a phase II study evaluated 25 patients with R/R DLBCL at a target dose of 112 μg/d, producing an ORR of 43% with 19% CR. Despite dexamethasone prophylaxis, neurologic toxicities were notable, including grade ≥3 encephalopathy (9%), aphasia (9%), as well as tremor, speech disorder, dizziness, somnolence, and disorientation (4% each).[27]

Novel T-cell engaging antibodies that target CD20 and CD3 are currently being evaluated in B-NHL. In a multicenter phase I/Ib study, the CD20/CD3 BiTE antibody mosunetuzumab was administered to 98 patients with R/R B-NHL (DLBCL n = 55, FL n = 29, MCL n = 3, other B-NHL n = 11). Mosunetuzumab was well tolerated—cytokine release syndrome was the most common treatment emergent AE (21%, all grade 1–2) and grade ≥3 neutropenia was observed in 13% of patients. Unlike with blinatumomab, neurologic toxicities were uncommon. The ORR among the 66 evaluable patients who received a target dose of at least 1.2 mg was 41%, including 61% (50% CR) in patients with FL and 33% (21% CR) in patients with DLBCL. Notably, responses occurred in patients who had failed prior chimeric antigen receptor-modified T cells and were refractory to prior anti-CD20–directed therapy. At the time of presentation with a median follow-up of 12 months, all patients who achieved a CR remained in remission.[28] Another CD20/CD3 T-cell–engaging antibody with a 2:1 format (each molecule has 2 x CD20 binders and 1 x CD3 binder), CD20-TCB (RG6026), has been evaluated in 64 patients with R/R B-NHL (aggressive B-NHL n = 47, FL n = 17) with a similar safety profile observed. At a target dose of 300 μg or above (n = 29), the ORR and CR rate were 38% and 24%, respectively, including 33% ORR and 21% CR in patients with DLBCL (n = 24).[29]

PD-1 BLOCKADE

The advent of checkpoint blockade has reshaped the therapeutic landscape of oncology, enacting a major paradigm shift in the way we care for many cancers. In a range of solid tumors and in HL, programmed death receptor-1 (PD-1) blockade, in particular, has become a cornerstone of therapy. In patients with NHL, PD-1 blockade has demonstrated antitumor activity, but the efficacy varies considerably by NHL subtype as might be expected because NHL encompasses a broad range of diseases (**Table 2**).

PD-1 is an immune checkpoint that normally serves to dampen immune responses.[30] Tumor cells can co-opt this pathway to evade attack by the host immune system.[30] A wide range of NHLs express PD-1 or PD-L1, and molecular analyses have demonstrated that genetic alterations involving the PD-1 ligands and their overexpression are critical in the pathogenesis of PMBCL and Epstein-Barr virus (EBV)-associated posttransplant lymphoproliferative disorders.[31,32] An early anti-PD-1 antibody, pidilizumab, produced responses as a single agent in patients with R/R FL, CLL, and HL[33] and yielded a 66% ORR when used in combination with rituximab in patients with R/R FL who were still sensitive to rituximab.[34] In a multicenter phase II study of pidilizumab consolidation after autologous stem cell transplant (ASCT) in patients with R/R DLBCL, the PFS at 16 months was 72%, including 70% in patients who were PET + at the time of ASCT.[35]

Since these initial studies, there has been a proliferation of studies evaluating a range of anti-PD-1 (nivolumab, pembrolizumab) or anti-PD-L1 (atezolizumab, durvalumab, avelumab) antibodies as single agents or in combination with other immunotherapies, targeted therapies, or chemotherapy. The adverse effect profile of PD-1 blockade has been summarized extensively elsewhere[36]; in brief, the agents have

Table 2
Clinical trials evaluating PD-1/PD-L1 blockade in non-Hodgkin lymphoma

Agents	Phase	Population	N	ORR	CR	DOR (median)	PFS (median)	Ref
Pidilizumab	2	R/R FL, rituximab sensitive	32	66%	52%	20.2 mo	18.8 mo	Westin et al,[34] 2014
Pidilizumab	2	R/R DLBCL, post-ASCT	68	51% (n = 35)	34% (n = 35)	NA	16m PFS 72% PET + at ASCT: 16m PFS 70%	Armand et al,[35] 2013
Nivolumab	1/2	R/R FL	Ph 1: 10 Ph 2: 92	Ph 1: 40% Ph 2: 4%	Ph 1: 10% Ph 2: 1%	Ph 1: NA Ph 2: 10.9 mo	Ph 1: not reached Ph 2: 2.2 mo	Lesokhin et al,[37] 2016
Pembrolizumab + rituximab	2	R/R FL, rituximab sensitive	25	64%	48%	14.1 mo	11.4 mo	Nastoupil et al,[38] 2017
Atezolizumab + obinutuzumab	1b	R/R FL	26	57%	NA	NA	NA	Palomba et al,[39]
Durvalumab + ibrutinib	1/2	R/R FL	27	26%	4%	11.3 mo	10.2 mo	Herrera et al,[40] 2018
Nivolumab	1/2	R/R DLBCL	Ph 1: 11 Ph 2: 121 total 87 prior ASCT 34 no ASCT	36% 10% 3%	18% 3% 0%	NA 11 mo 8 mo	7 mo 1.9 mo 1.4 mo	Lesokhin et al,[37] 2016; Ansell et al,[41] 2019
Atezolizumab + obinutuzumab	1b	R/R DLBCL	23	16%	NA	NA	NA	Palomba et al,[39]

Durvalumab + ibrutinib	½	R/R DLBCL	GCB: 16 Non-GCB: 16	13% 38%	6% 31%	NA	2.9 mo 4.1 mo	Herrera et al,[40] 2018
Pembrolizumab	1b, 2	R/R PMBCL	Ph 1b: 21 Ph 2: 53	48% 45%	33% 13%	Not reached	10.4 mo 5.5 mo	Armand et al,[42] 2018
Pembrolizumab	2	RT	9	44%	11%	NA	5.4 mo	Ding et al,[43] 2017
Nivolumab + ibrutinib	2	RT	23	43%	35%	9.3 mo	NA	Jain et al,[44] 2018
Nivolumab	1	R/R PTCL	5	40%	0%	NA	14 mo	Lesokhin et al,[37] 2016
Nivolumab	1	R/R MF R/R CTCL	13 3	15% 0%	0% 0%	NA	10 mo 7 mo	Lesokhin et al,[37] 2016
Pembrolizumab	2	R/R MF/SS	24	38%	4%	NA	Not reached	Khodadoust et al,[45] 2016
Pembrolizumab	2	R/R NKTL	7	100%	100%	10 mo	Not reached	Kwong et al,[46] 2017
Pembrolizumab	2	R/R NKTL	7	57%	29%	4.1 mo	4.8 mo	Li et al,[47] 2018

Abbreviations: ASCT, autologous stem cell transplantation; CR, complete response; CTCL, cutaneous T-cell lymphoma; DLBCL, diffuse large B-cell lymphoma; DOR, duration of response; FL, follicular lymphoma; MF, mycosis fungoides; NA, not available; NKTL, NK T-cell lymphoma; ORR, overall response rate; PFS, progression-free survival; PMBCL, primary mediastinal large B-cell lymphoma; R/R, relapsed or refractory; RT, Richter transformation; SS, Sezary syndrome.

been well tolerated in patients with NHL. PD-1 blockade results in unique immune-related toxicities resulting in organ/tissue inflammation, including most commonly endocrinopathy (eg, thyroiditis), dermatitis, pneumonitis, hepatitis, and colitis. The efficacy data on PD-1 blockade are reviewed by NHL subtype in the subsequent sections.

PD-1 Blockade in Follicular Lymphoma

After an initial phase I study of nivolumab in hematologic malignancies demonstrated an ORR of 40% in 10 patients with R/R FL, only 4% of patients had objective responses in a phase II study (NCT02038946).[37] A phase II trial of pembrolizumab plus rituximab enrolled 25 evaluable patients with an ORR of 64% and CR rate of 48%. Sixty percent of patients were in ongoing response at a median follow-up time of 11 months.[38] A phase Ib study of atezolizumab combined with obinutuzumab enrolled 26 patients with R/R FL and demonstrated an ORR of 57%. There was no association between PD-L1 expression by immunohistochemistry and response to atezolizumab/obinutuzumab or to pembrolizumab/rituximab in the previous study.[39] Ibrutinib (560 mg daily) was combined with durvalumab in a phase Ib/II study that enrolled 27 patients with R/R FL. The efficacy seemed similar to ibrutinib monotherapy with an ORR of 26% and CR rate of 4%, a median DOR of 11.3 months and a median PFS of 10.2 months.[40] Interpretation of the data on PD-1 blockade in FL is challenging because of the heterogeneity of the treatment and patient characteristics enrolled (ie, rituximab sensitive vs refractory), but it does seem that the response rates are highest when PD-1 blockade is combined with an anti-CD20 antibody that the patient is still sensitive or naïve to.

PD-1 Blockade in Aggressive B-NHL

Similar to FL, after a 36% ORR was observed in R/R de novo DLBCL patients treated with nivolumab in a phase I study, only 10% of patients had an objective response in the phase II study.[37,41] Likewise, in a phase Ib trial of atezolizumab plus obinutuzumab, the ORR was 16% among 23 patients with R/R DLBCL.[39] A phase Ib/II study of ibrutinib plus durvalumab enrolled 35 patients with R/R de novo DLBCL, including 17 patients with germinal center subtype (GCB) DLBCL and 16 with non-GCB DLBCL assessed by the Hans criteria. The ORR in GCB DLBCL was 13%, whereas the ORR in non-GCB DLBCL was 38% with CR 31%. Five of 7 non-GCB DLBCL patients had a DOR of at least 8 months. The investigators concluded that activity of the combination was not demonstrated beyond what would be expected with single-agent ibrutinib.[40]

Although the results of PD-1 blockade in de novo DLBCL have varied, PD-1 blockade has demonstrated more promise in patients with PMBCL. Armand and colleagues[42] recently presented results of 21 patients with R/R PMBCL patients treated with pembrolizumab as part of a phase I study (ORR 48%, CR 33%), along with phase II results that showed that the ORR was 45% and CR rate 13%. The 1-year PFS was 47% in the phase Ib patients and 38% in the phase II patients. Notably, all patients who had achieved a CR in the phase II study remained in remission at the time of presentation. Based on these results, pembrolizumab was approved by the FDA for use in patients with refractory PMBCL or patients who have relapsed after 2 or more lines of therapy.

Patients with Richter transformation (RT) of CLL represent another subset of aggressive B-NHL that may benefit from PD-1 blockade. A phase II study of pembrolizumab in patients with CLL and RT demonstrated no objective responses in patients with CLL, but there was a 44% ORR (4/9) in patients with RT, including 1 patient with CR, with a median PFS of 5.4 months in RT patients.[43] Jain and colleagues[44] reported the findings of a phase II study of ibrutinib (420 mg daily) combined with nivolumab in

23 patients with RT, including 11 patients who received prior ibrutinib therapy. The ORR was 43% with a CR rate of 35% and a median duration of response of 9.3 months.

PD-1 Blockade in T-cell Lymphomas

In the initial phase I study of nivolumab in hematologic malignancies, the ORR was 15% in patients with MF (n = 13) and 40% in PTCL (n = 5)—all responses were PR. No objective responses were observed in patients with other types of CTCL.[37] A phase II study of pembrolizumab in 24 patients with R/R MF or SS showed a higher ORR of 38%, with one patient achieving a CR and 8 of 9 responses ongoing with a median duration of 32 weeks. Although the safety of pembrolizumab in patients with MF/SS was similar to previous studies in other diseases, 40% of patients with SS developed a skin flare reaction.[45] A subtype of PTCL that may be particularly sensitive to PD-1 blockade is extranodal NK/T-cell lymphomas (NKTLs). NKTL are EBV-associated tumors, and there is evidence that EBV-driven tumors have upregulation of PD-L1.[32] In one small report, 7 patients with R/R NKTL were treated with pembrolizumab and all patients responded, including 2 patients who achieved clinical, radiologic, and molecular (EBV viral load) CR and 3 patients believed to have clinical and radiologic CR. At a median follow-up time of 6 months, all 5 patients remained in sustained CR.[46] In another study, pembrolizumab resulted in an ORR of 57% in 7 patients with R/R NKTL. Notably, 2 out of 7 patients had grade 3 pneumonitis.[47]

SUMMARY

Since the introduction of rituximab, immunotherapy has been central to the treatment of NHL. The armamentarium of novel noncellular immunotherapies continues to expand with the introduction of newer monoclonal antibodies that are engineered to enhance tumor cell killing or that are targeting different cellular antigens, effective new ADCs, and antibodies that block PD-1 or possibly other immune checkpoints in the future. The ongoing development of new and effective immunotherapies presents both important therapeutic opportunities as well as new challenges regarding how to introduce these drugs into the clinic. Many unanswered questions remain, including the practical question of how to sequence these novel immunotherapies or how to sequence them with the effective cellular immunotherapies that are now available. In addition to the sequencing of immunotherapies, an important question will be whether these drugs can be more effective earlier in the course of a patient's therapy. Furthermore, there are a large number of ongoing clinical trials and others in development that are studying immunotherapy combinations in order to improve the efficacy of these drugs, and it is still not clear whether these combinations will increase response rates or response durability or which ones will prove most effective. Finally, the reality is that despite the promising antitumor activity exhibited by many novel immunotherapies, there are many patients who will not respond to these drugs. It will be important to identify predictive biomarkers for immunotherapeutic agents or combinations, because the goal should be to treat the patients most likely to benefit from immunotherapy approaches. With a rapidly expanding range of effective noncellular immunotherapy options for the treatment of NHL, how to optimize immunotherapy for NHL will be a critically important task in the coming years.

REFERENCES

1. Cheson BD, Chua N, Mayer J, et al. Overall survival benefit in patients with rituximab-refractory indolent non-Hodgkin lymphoma who received

obinutuzumab plus bendamustine induction and obinutuzumab maintenance in the GADOLIN study. J Clin Oncol 2018;36(22):2259–66.

2. Marcus R, Davies A, Ando K, et al. Obinutuzumab for the first-line treatment of follicular lymphoma. N Engl J Med 2017;377(14):1331–44.

3. Vitolo U, Trneny M, Belada D, et al. Obinutuzumab or rituximab plus cyclophosphamide, doxorubicin, vincristine, and prednisone in previously untreated diffuse large B-Cell lymphoma. J Clin Oncol 2017;35(31):3529–37.

4. Ogura M, Ishida T, Hatake K, et al. Multicenter phase II study of mogamulizumab (KW-0761), a defucosylated anti-cc chemokine receptor 4 antibody, in patients with relapsed peripheral T-cell lymphoma and cutaneous T-cell lymphoma. J Clin Oncol 2014;32(11):1157–63.

5. Ishida T, Joh T, Uike N, et al. Defucosylated anti-CCR4 monoclonal antibody (KW-0761) for relapsed adult T-cell leukemia-lymphoma: a multicenter phase II study. J Clin Oncol 2012;30(8):837–42.

6. Kim YH, Bagot M, Pinter-Brown L, et al. Mogamulizumab versus vorinostat in previously treated cutaneous T-cell lymphoma (MAVORIC): an international, open-label, randomised, controlled phase 3 trial. Lancet Oncol 2018;19(9):1192–204.

7. Advani R, Flinn I, Popplewell L, et al. CD47 blockade by Hu5F9-G4 and rituximab in non-Hodgkin's lymphoma. N Engl J Med 2018;379(18):1711–21.

8. Morschhauser F, Flinn I, Advani RH, et al. Updated results of a phase II randomized study (ROMULUS) of polatuzumab vedotin or pinatuzumab vedotin plus rituximab in patients with relapsed/refractory non-Hodgkin lymphoma. Blood 2014; 124(21):4457.

9. Sehn LH, Herrera AF, Matasar MJ, et al. Addition of polatuzumab vedotin to bendamustine and rituximab (BR) improves outcomes in transplant-ineligible patients with relapsed/refractory (R/R) diffuse large B-cell lymphoma (DLBCL) versus BR alone: Results from a randomized phase 2 study. Poster presented at: 59th Annual Meeting & Exposition for the American Society of Hematology. Atlanta, GA, December 10, 2017.

10. Tilly H, Sharman J, Bartlett N, et al. Pola-R-CHP: polatuzumab vedotin combined with rituximab, cyclophosphamide, doxorubicin, prednisone for patients with previously untreated diffuse large B-cell lymphoma. Hematol Oncol 2017;35:90–1.

11. Jacobsen ED, Sharman JP, Oki Y, et al. Brentuximab vedotin demonstrates objective responses in a phase 2 study of relapsed/refractory DLBCL with variable CD30 expression. Blood 2015;125(9):1394–402.

12. Pro B, Advani R, Brice P, et al. Brentuximab vedotin (SGN-35) in patients with relapsed or refractory systemic anaplastic large-cell lymphoma: results of a phase II study. J Clin Oncol 2012;30(18):2190–6.

13. Horwitz SM, Advani RH, Bartlett NL, et al. Objective responses in relapsed T-cell lymphomas with single-agent brentuximab vedotin. Blood 2014;123(20): 3095–100.

14. Prince HM, Kim YH, Horwitz SM, et al. Brentuximab vedotin or physician's choice in CD30-positive cutaneous T-cell lymphoma (ALCANZA): an international, open-label, randomised, phase 3, multicentre trial. Lancet 2017;390(10094):555–66.

15. Budde LE, Halwani A, Yasenchak CA, et al. Results of an ongoing phase 2 study of brentuximab vedotin with rchp as frontline therapy in patients with high-intermediate/high-risk diffuse large B cell lymphoma (DLBCL). Blood 2016; 128(22):104.

16. Horwitz S, O'Connor OA, Pro B, et al. Brentuximab vedotin with chemotherapy for CD30-positive peripheral T-cell lymphoma (ECHELON-2): a global, double-blind, randomised, phase 3 trial. Lancet 2019;393(10168):229–40.

17. Fayad L, Offner F, Smith MR, et al. Safety and clinical activity of a combination therapy comprising two antibody-based targeting agents for the treatment of non-Hodgkin lymphoma: results of a phase I/II study evaluating the immunoconjugate inotuzumab ozogamicin with rituximab. J Clin Oncol 2013;31(5):573–83.

18. Ogura M, Hatake K, Ando K, et al. Phase I study of anti-CD22 immunoconjugate inotuzumab ozogamicin plus rituximab in relapsed/refractory B-cell non-Hodgkin lymphoma. Cancer Sci 2012;103(5):933–8.

19. Wagner-Johnston ND, Goy A, Rodriguez MA, et al. A phase 2 study of inotuzumab ozogamicin and rituximab, followed by autologous stem cell transplant in patients with relapsed/refractory diffuse large B-cell lymphoma. Leuk Lymphoma 2015;56(10):2863–9.

20. Dang NH, Ogura M, Castaigne S, et al. Randomized, phase 3 trial of inotuzumab ozogamicin plus rituximab versus chemotherapy plus rituximab for relapsed/refractory aggressive B-cell non-Hodgkin lymphoma. Br J Haematol 2018;182(4): 583–6.

21. Moskowitz CH, Fanale MA, Shah BD, et al. A phase 1 study of denintuzumab mafodotin (SGN-CD19A) in relapsed/refactory B-lineage non-Hodgkin lymphoma. Blood 2015;126(23):182.

22. Ribrag V, Dupuis J, Tilly H, et al. A dose-escalation study of SAR3419, an anti-CD19 antibody maytansinoid conjugate, administered by intravenous infusion once weekly in patients with relapsed/refractory B-cell non-Hodgkin lymphoma. Clin Cancer Res 2014;20(1):213–20.

23. Trneny M, Verhoef G, Dyer MJ, et al. Starlyte phase II study of coltuximab ravtansine (CoR, SAR3419) single agent: clinical activity and safety in patients (pts) with relapsed/refractory (R/R) diffuse large B-cell lymphoma (DLBCL; NCT01472887). J Clin Oncol 2014;32(15_suppl):8506.

24. Coiffier B, Thieblemont C, de Guibert S, et al. A phase II, single-arm, multicentre study of coltuximab ravtansine (SAR3419) and rituximab in patients with relapsed or refractory diffuse large B-cell lymphoma. Br J Haematol 2016;173(5):722–30.

25. Kahl BS, Hamadani M, Caimi P, et al. Encouraging early results from the first in-human clinical trial of Adct-402 (Loncastuximab Tesirine), a novel pyrrolobenzodiazepine-based antibody drug conjugate, in relapsed/refractory B-Cell Lineage Non-Hodgkin Lymphoma. Poster presented at: 59th Annual Meeting & Exposition for the American Society of Hematology. Atlanta, GA, December 9, 2017.

26. Collins G, Horwitz SM, Davies A, et al. Adct-301 (camidanlumab tesirine), a novel pyrrolobenzodiazepine-based CD25-targeting antibody drug conjugate, in a phase 1 study of relapsed/refractory non-Hodgkin lymphoma shows activity in T-cell lymphoma. Blood 2018;132:1658.

27. Viardot A, Goebeler ME, Hess G, et al. Phase 2 study of the bispecific T-cell engager (BiTE) antibody blinatumomab in relapsed/refractory diffuse large B-cell lymphoma. Blood 2016;127(11):1410–6.

28. Budde LE, Sehn LH, Assouline S, et al. Mosunetuzumab, a full-length bispecific CD20/CD3 antibody, displays clinical activity in relapsed/refractory B-cell non-Hodgkin lymphoma (NHL): interim safety and efficacy results from a phase 1 study. Blood 2018;132:399.

29. Hutchings M, Iacoboni G, Morschhauser F, et al. CD20-Tcb (RG6026), a novel "2:1" format T-cell-engaging bispecific antibody, induces complete remissions in relapsed/refractory B-cell non-Hodgkin's lymphoma: preliminary results from a phase I first in human trial. Blood 2018;132:226.

30. Pardoll DM. The blockade of immune checkpoints in cancer immunotherapy. Nat Rev Cancer 2012;12(4):252–64.

31. Green MR, Monti S, Rodig SJ, et al. Integrative analysis reveals selective 9p24.1 amplification, increased PD-1 ligand expression, and further induction via JAK2 in nodular sclerosing Hodgkin lymphoma and primary mediastinal large B-cell lymphoma. Blood 2010;116(17):3268–77.

32. Green MR, Rodig S, Juszczynski P, et al. Constitutive AP-1 activity and EBV infection induce PD-L1 in Hodgkin lymphomas and posttransplant lymphoproliferative disorders: implications for targeted therapy. Clin Cancer Res 2012;18(6):1611–8.

33. Berger R, Rotem-Yehudar R, Slama G, et al. Phase I safety and pharmacokinetic study of CT-011, a humanized antibody interacting with PD-1, in patients with advanced hematologic malignancies. Clin Cancer Res 2008;14(10):3044–51.

34. Westin JR, Chu F, Zhang M, et al. Safety and activity of PD1 blockade by pidilizumab in combination with rituximab in patients with relapsed follicular lymphoma: a single group, open-label, phase 2 trial. Lancet Oncol 2014;15(1):69–77.

35. Armand P, Nagler A, Weller EA, et al. Disabling immune tolerance by programmed death-1 blockade with pidilizumab after autologous hematopoietic stem-cell transplantation for diffuse large B-cell lymphoma: results of an international phase II trial. J Clin Oncol 2013;31(33):4199–206.

36. Brahmer JR, Lacchetti C, Schneider BJ, et al. Management of immune-related adverse events in patients treated with immune checkpoint inhibitor therapy: American society of clinical oncology clinical practice guideline. J Clin Oncol 2018;36(17):1714–68.

37. Lesokhin AM, Ansell SM, Armand P, et al. Nivolumab in patients with relapsed or refractory hematologic malignancy: preliminary results of a phase Ib study. J Clin Oncol 2016;34(23):2698–704.

38. Nastoupil N, Westin JR, Fowler NH, et al. High complete response rates with pembrolizumab in combination with rituximab in patients with relapsed follicular lymphoma: results of an open-label, phase II study. Blood 2017;130:414.

39. Palomba L, Till BG, Park SI, et al. A phase Ib study evaluating the safety and clinical activity of atezolizumab combined with obinutuzumab in patients with relapsed or refractory non-hodgkin lymphoma (NHL). Hematol Oncol 2017;35: 137–8.

40. Herrera AF, Goy A, Mehta A, et al. Activity and safety of ibrutinib and durvalumab in patients with relapsed or refractory follicular lymphoma (FL) or diffuse large B-cell lymphoma (DLBCL). 30th EORTC-NCI-AACR Symposium on molecular targets and Cancer therapeutics. Dublin (Ireland), November 13, 2018; [abstract: 7].

41. Ansell SM, Minnema MC, Johnson P, et al. Nivolumab for relapsed/refractory diffuse large B-cell lymphoma in patients ineligible for or having failed autologous transplantation: a single-arm, phase II study. J Clin Oncol 2019;37(6):481–9.

42. Armand P, Rodig SJ, Melnichenko V, et al. Pembrolizumab in patients with relapsed or refractory primary mediastinal large B-cell lymphoma (PMBCL): data from the keynote-013 and keynote-170 studies. Blood 2018;132:228.

43. Ding W, LaPlant BR, Call TG, et al. Pembrolizumab in patients with CLL and Richter transformation or with relapsed CLL. Blood 2017;129(26):3419–27.

44. Jain N, Ferrajoli A, Basu S, et al. A phase II trial of nivolumab combined with ibrutinib for patients with richter transformation. Blood 2018;132:296.

45. Khodadoust M, Rook AH, Porcu P, et al. Pembrolizumab for treatment of relapsed/refractory mycosis fungoides and sezary syndrome: clinical efficacy in a citn multicenter phase 2 study. Blood 2016;128:181.

46. Kwong YL, Chan TSY, Tan D, et al. PD1 blockade with pembrolizumab is highly effective in relapsed or refractory NK/T-cell lymphoma failing l-asparaginase. Blood 2017;129(17):2437–42.

47. Li X, Cheng Y, Zhang M, et al. Activity of pembrolizumab in relapsed/refractory NK/T-cell lymphoma. J Hematol Oncol 2018;11(1):15.

48. Younes A, Kim S, Romaguera J, et al. Phase I multidose-escalation study of the anti-CD19 maytansinoid immunoconjugate SAR3419 administered by intravenous infusion every 3 weeks to patients with relapsed/refractory B-cell lymphoma. J Clin Oncol 2012;30(22):2776–82.

49. Advani RH, Lebovic D, Chen A, et al. Phase I study of the anti-CD22 antibody-drug conjugate pinatuzumab vedotin with/without rituximab in patients with relapsed/refractory B-cell non-Hodgkin lymphoma. Clin Cancer Res 2017;23(5): 1167–76.

50. Goy A, Forero A, Wagner-Johnston N, et al. A phase 2 study of inotuzumab ozogamicin in patients with indolent B-cell non-Hodgkin lymphoma refractory to rituximab alone, rituximab and chemotherapy, or radioimmunotherapy. Br J Haematol 2016;174(4):571–81.

51. Ogura M, Tobinai K, Hatake K, et al. Phase I study of inotuzumab ozogamicin combined with R-CVP for relapsed/refractory CD22+ B-cell non-Hodgkin lymphoma. Clin Cancer Res 2016;22(19):4807–16.

52. Sangha R, Davies A, Dang NH, et al. Phase 1 study of inotuzumab ozogamicin combined with R-GDP for the treatment of patients with relapsed/refractory CD22+ B-cell non-Hodgkin lymphoma. J Drug Assess 2017;6(1):10–7.

53. Horwitz SM, Fanale MA, Spira AI, et al. Interim data from the first clinical study of ADCT-301, a novel pyrrolobenzodiazapine-based antibody drug conjugate, in relapsed/refractory hodgkin/non-Hodgkin lymphoma. Hematol Oncol 2017;35: 270–1.

54. Bartlett NL, Smith MR, Siddiqi T, et al. Brentuximab vedotin activity in diffuse large B-cell lymphoma with CD30 undetectable by visual assessment of conventional immunohistochemistry. Leuk Lymphoma 2017;58(7):1607–16.

55. Hatake K, Kinoshita T, Terui Y, et al. A phase I pharmacokinetic and safety study of polatuzumab vedotin in Japanese patients with relapsed/refractory b-cell non-Hodgkin lymphoma: A comparison with non-Japanese DCS4968g study. J Clin Oncol 2016;34(15_suppl):e19070.

56. Palanca-Wessels MC, Czuczman M, Salles G, et al. Safety and activity of the anti-CD79B antibody-drug conjugate polatuzumab vedotin in relapsed or refractory B-cell non-Hodgkin lymphoma and chronic lymphocytic leukaemia: a phase 1 study. Lancet Oncol 2015;16(6):704–15.

57. Phillips T, Brunvand M, Chen A, et al. Polatuzumab vedotin combined with obinutuzumab for patients with relapsed or refractory non-Hodgkin lymphoma: preliminary safety and clinical activity of a phase Ib/II study. Blood 2016;128(22):622.

58. Forero-Torres A, Kolibaba KS, Tilly H, et al. Polatuzumab vedotin combined with obinutuzumab, cyclophosphamide, doxorubicin, and prednisone (G-CHP) for patients with previously untreated diffuse large B-cell lymphoma (DLBCL): updated results of a phase Ib/II study. Blood 2017;130(Suppl 1):4120.

59. Matasar M, Herrera AF, Kamdar M, et al. Polatuzumab vedotin plus bendamustine and rituximab or obinutuzumab in relapsed/refractory fl or dlbcl: updated results of a phase 1B/2 study. Hematol Oncol 2017;35:271–2.

Targeting Biology in Non-Hodgkin Lymphoma

Mayur Narkhede, MD, Maryam Sarraf Yazdy, MD, Bruce D. Cheson, MD*

KEYWORDS

- Non-Hodgkin lymphoma • Intracellular oncogenic pathways • Targeted agents
- Monoclonal antibodies

KEY POINTS

- Increased understanding of the biology of NHL has led to the development of drugs that target specific abnormalities of B-cell function and the tumor microenvironment.
- Targeted agents that show promise as single agents are being combined with other targeted agents to develop efficacious regimens.
- Carefully conducted clinical trials are essential before exposing patients to untested doublets or triplets.

INTRODUCTION

The birth of chemotherapy occurred during World War I when mustard gas was dumped on Allied soldiers, leading to skin ulcerations, blindness, and secondary malignancies, among other untoward effects. However, it also resulted in lymphopenia and atrophic lymph nodes. Subsequently a derivative, nitrogen mustard, was administered to patients with lymphoma, resulting in impressive, albeit transient, responses. This class of drugs, alkylating agents, has formed the foundation of almost all of our current lymphoma chemotherapy regimens, including drugs such as cyclophosphamide and bendamustine. Unfortunately, decades of clinical research focused on mixing and matching various chemotherapy agents with no improvement in outcome.

Disclosure Statement: M. Narkhede: Nothing to disclose. M.S. Yazdy: Received honoraria from Bayer as a speaker and holds a consultancy role for Abbvie. Research funding (to institution) – Roche-Genentech. B. Cheson: Consulting/Advisory Boards – Abbvie, Astra Zeneca, TG Therapeutics, Celgene, Roche-Genentech, Bayer, Epizyme, Gilead, Pharmacyclics, Karyopharm, Morphosys, Astellas. Research funding (to institution) – Abbvie, Roche-Genentech, TG Therapeutics, AstraZeneca, Epizyme, Trillium, Pharmacyclics, Gilead. Speaker – Bayer.
Lombardi Comprehensive Cancer Center, Medstar Georgetown University Hospital, Lombardi Comprehensive Cancer Center Podium A, 3800 Reservoir Road Northwest, Washington, DC 20007, USA
* Corresponding author.
E-mail address: bdc4@georgetown.edu

Hematol Oncol Clin N Am 33 (2019) 727–738
https://doi.org/10.1016/j.hoc.2019.03.006
0889-8588/19/© 2019 Elsevier Inc. All rights reserved.

THE ERA OF TARGETED AGENTS

The history of targeted therapies dates back more than a century, to Professor Paul Ehrlich, who conceptualized the "magic bullet," that would specifically target organisms or tumor cells, sparing the remainder of the body substances. The sketches in his monograph were quite similar to our current concept of the structure of monoclonal antibodies.[1]

It was not until an appropriate tumor target could be identified (eg, CD20), as well as the capacity to manufacture sufficient quantities of therapeutic antibodies, that the age of targeted therapies began.[2,3] The initial result was the chimeric monoclonal antibody rituximab, which first demonstrated single-agent activity in the relapsed setting and, subsequently, as a front-line therapy for patients with follicular lymphoma (FL).[4,5] When subsequently combined with chemotherapy, rituximab was the first agent to prolong the survival of patients with FL or diffuse large B-cell lymphoma (DLBCL).[6,7] Nonetheless, the cure rate for FL remains disappointingly low, and there is considerable room for improvement in other lymphoma histologies.

In 2004, given the encouraging results with a single antibody, investigators from the Cancer and Leukemia Group B were the first to test combinations of biological agents, starting with doublets of monoclonal antibodies,[8,9] demonstrating a high level of efficacy in previously untreated patients with FL. They next piloted the combination of rituximab with the immunomodulatory agent lenalidomide (R^2).[10,11] Not only was R^2 active in the relapsed setting, but, as initial therapy, produced overall response rates (ORRs) of 85% to 95% with 5-year progression-free survival (PFS) of 70% and overall survival (OS) of 100% after a median follow-up of 5 years.[10,11] These results are consistent with those achievable with multiagent chemoimmunotherapy. These observations led to the phase 3 RELEVANCE trial, in which 1030 previously untreated patients with FL were randomized to either R^2 or chemoimmunotherapy with either rituximab (R)-cyclophosphamide, vincristine, and prednisone (R-CVP), R-cyclophosphamide, adriamycin, vincristine, and prednisone (R-CHOP), or R-bendamustiune. The co-primary endpoints of complete response (CR) at 30 months and PFS were similar between the arms. Thus, the nonchemotherapy approach with R^2 was as effective as chemoimmunotherapy, but with fewer side effects, except for rash, and can be considered as a standard treatment option.[12] Similarly, in an another phase 3 trial, the R^2 regimen in comparison with rituximab alone in relapsed or refractory (R/R) FL or marginal zone lymphoma achieved a prolonged PFS, with an OS benefit in the FL subset, providing another efficacious nonchemotherapeutic option in indolent non-Hodgkin lymphoma (NHL).[13]

The increasing number of novel targeted agents that target the cell surface, including monoclonal antibody-based therapies, those that interfere with intracellular pathways, and others that are directed at the microenvironment, has further stimulated interest in clinical research (**Fig. 1**).

TARGETING THE CELL SURFACE

Following the success of rituximab, a myriad of anti-CD20s were developed. The most promising has been obinutuzumab, which, when combined with chemotherapy as initial therapy for patients with FL and chronic lymphocytic leukemia/small lymphocytic lymphoma (CLL/SLL), was superior to R-based chemoimmunotherapy, prolonging only PFS in FL but both PFS and OS in CLL.[14,15] In addition, obinutuzumab plus bendamustine followed by obinutuzumab maintenance prolonged PFS and OS over bendamustine monotherapy in rituximab-refractory patients with indolent NHL.[16,17] Unfortunately, obinutuzumab has shown less promise against DLBCL.[18] Other

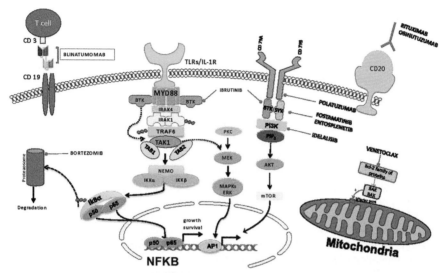

Fig. 1. Summary of mechanism of action of targeted agents. BTK, Bruton's tyrosine kinase; PI3K, phosphoinositide 3-kinase; SYK, spleen tyrosine kinase; TLR, Toll-like receptors. (*Data from* Yang G, Zhou Y, Liu X, et al. A mutation in MYD88 (L265P) supports the survival of lymphoplasmacytic cells by activation of Bruton tyrosine kinase in Waldenström macroglobulinemia. Blood 2013;122(7):1222–32.)

unconjugated monoclonal antibodies in development include MOR-208 (anti-CD-19), which, when combined with lenalidomide in R/R DLBCL, achieved an ORR of 58% with 33% CRs and a median PFS of 16.2 months, superior to most other regimens in this setting, and has been granted U.S. Food and Drug Administration (FDA) Breakthrough Designation.[19] Further studies in FL and CLL are warranted.

Attempts to improve on the monoclonal antibody include antibody-drug conjugates (ADC). The first to demonstrate activity was brentuxmab vedotin (BV), which involves an anti-CD30 monoclonal antibody bound to auristatin, a tubulin toxin. Excellent response rates have been reported in patients with Hodgkin lymphoma (HL) either in the R/R setting or combined with chemotherapy in the front line.[20,21] Impressive activity has been reported in anaplastic large-cell NHL as well.[22] In the recently published ECHELON-2 trial, CHP + BV prolonged survival compared with CHOP in the initial treatment of peripheral T-cell lymphoma, setting a new standard.[23]

Polatuzumab vedotin (pola) joins an anti-CD79b antibody to the same linker and toxin as BV. When combined with rituximab, it has demonstrated impressive response rates and PFS in FL and DLBCL.[24] In a randomized study, the addition of pola to bendamustine and rituximab (BR) resulted in a longer median OS of 11.8 months and a longer median PFS of 6.7 months compared with 4.7 and 2 months, respectively, for BR in relapsed DLBCL, although this benefit was not observed in FL.[25] This combination has received Breakthrough Designation from the FDA. Other ADCs are also in development.

Bispecific T-cell engagers (BiTEs) are constructs that bind to the lymphoma cell and help to approximate the effector cells. Blinatumomab has impressive activity in acute lymphoblastic leukemia and some B-NHLs, but is associated with potentially serious neurotoxicity.[26] Other BiTEs are being developed that target different antigens and effectors for their treatment in NHL; however, toxicity remains a concern (NCT03192202, NCT02290951). Chimeric antigen receptor T cells targeting CD19 have impressive activity in DLBCL with durable responses in heavily pretreated patients.[27] Different chimeric antigen receptor constructs targeting other B- and T-cell antigens are in development.

INTRACELLULAR PATHWAYS
Bruton's Tyrosine Kinase

Stimulating the B-cell receptor activates many intracellular pathways, prolonging cellular survival. Some of the most relevant of these include Bruton's tyrosine kinase (BTK). The first inhibitor of BTK was ibrutinib, which, in R/R CLL/SLL, achieved a response rate of 89%, and 87% in treatment-naive patients, with PFS superior to standard biological and chemoimmunotherapeutic regimens, including bendamustine-rituximab and fludarabine-cyclophosphamide-rituximab.[28,29] Problematic toxicities include atrial fibrillation in 6% and spontaneous bleeding in about 40% of patients, which is serious in 4% to 10%.[30] A second-generation BTK inhibitor, acalabrutinib, seems to have comparable activity, perhaps with less toxicity.[31]

Approximately 90% of patients with Waldenström macroglobulinemia (WM) have mutations of the myeloid differentiation response protein 88 (MYD88).[32] MYD88[MUT] leads to activation of BTK, and, subsequently, constitutive activation of nuclear factor κB and STAT3 signaling, leading to cellular proliferation. Ibrutinib and acalabrutinib achieve response rates of 90% or greater in R/R WM or in the front-line setting and have become a standard treatment of R/R and treatment-naive patients.[33,34]

Ibrutinib is also extremely effective in mantle cell lymphoma, with responses in 68% of patients with R/R disease, and a median PFS of 13.9 months.[35] Activity has been demonstrated in marginal zone lymphomas, with an ORR of 48% and a median PFS of 14.2 months.[36] Surprisingly, recent data showed only a 20.9% response rate in FL and 31% in activated a B-cell subtype of DLBCL; thus, its role in these histologies is questionable.[37,38]

Phosphoinositol 3-Kinase

The phosphatidylinositol 3-kinase (PI3K) pathway is an essential cell signaling pathway that converts external growth stimuli into intracellular processes leading to proliferation and differentiation of cells. The PI3K pathway is dysregulated in FL, mantle cell lymphoma, and DLBCL, leading to activation of downstream effectors, such as protein kinase B (AKT)/mammalian target of rapamycin (mTOR) pathway, in turn leading to growth, proliferation, and chemoresistance.[39–41] Several inhibitors of the PI3K pathway are commercially available or in development. Idelalisib is a Δ-isoform-specific inhibitor approved with an ORR of 58%, a CR of 6%, and a median PFS of 11.2 months in third-line or greater.[42] Unfortunately, up to 54% of patients experienced a grade 3 or higher adverse event, with discontinuation of idelalisib in 20% of the patients. Some of the most frequently reported adverse events limiting its use include diarrhea, colitis, pneumonitis, transaminitis, and dermatitis (**Table 1**).[42,43]

Copanlisib is a pan-class I PI3K inhibitor with predominant activity against the α- and δ-isoforms that is approved by the FDA for the treatment of R/R FL in the third-line setting as it resulted in an ORR of 59% and CR of 14%, and a median PFS of 11.2 months. Notable toxicities with copanlisib are transient hypertension and hyperglycemia that need to be monitored and managed closely before, during, and after the infusions[44,45] (see **Table 1**; **Table 2**).

Duvelisib is the most recently FDA-approved PI3K inhibitor in patients with CLL/SLL and FL who have received at least 2 previous therapies.[46] In the DUO trial, patients achieved an ORR of 74% and partial remission of 73%; however, the toxicity profile specifically diarrhea (15%), colitis (12%), and pneumonia (18%) were concerning

Table 1
Approved and emerging PI3K inhibitors

	Copanlisib	Idelalisib	Duvelisib	Umbralisib (TGR1202)
Current indication(s)	3rd-line FL	3rd-line FL; 3rd-line SLL; 2nd-line CLL	3rd-line FL; 3rd-line SLL; 2nd-line CLL	N/A
Mechanism of action	PI3Ki (α,δ)	PI3Ki (δ)	PI3Ki (δ,γ)	PI3Ki (δ), cMyc
Administration	IV	Oral	Oral	Oral
Dosing schedule	60 mg day 1, 8, 15 (28-d cycle)	150 mg, twice daily	25 mg, twice daily	Once daily
Study population	≥3rd line (FL, n = 104)	≥3rd line (FL, n = 72)	≥3rd line (FL, n = 83)	≥2nd line (FL, n = 12)
ORR (FL), %	59	54	41	53
PFS (FL), mo	11.2	11	8.3	16
CR (FL), %	14	8	1.2	12

Modified from Cheson BD, O'Brien S, Ewer MS, et al. Optimal management of adverse events from copanlisib in the treatment of patients with non-hodgkin lymphomas. Clin Lymphoma Myeloma Leuk 2019;19(3):137; with permission.

(see **Tables 1** and **2**). Umbralisib (previously TGR-1202) is being investigated in indolent NHL and CLL/SLL and seems to have a more favorable toxicity profile than other PI3Ks (NCT03269669, NCT03178201, NCT01882803).[47]

Bcl-2 Inhibition

Venetoclax is a specific Bcl-2 inhibitor with activity in a variety of B-NHL. Alone and in combination with rituximab, it has shown impressive activity in CLL/SLL, with a substantial proportion of patients experiencing eradication of minimal residual disease, generally not achieved with other kinase inhibitors.[48,49] The MURANO trial combined venetoclax and rituximab and compared it with BR for its use in the R/R setting.[49] Venetoclax plus rituximab was superior to BR with a longer PFS (84% vs 36% at 2 years) and higher ORR (92.3% vs 72.3%) and CR (26.8% vs 8.2%). This PFS advantage was also seen in patients with deletion 17p. More patients became minimal residual disease-negative compared with BR (84% vs 23%). Venetoclax has been found to be active in R/R mantle cell lymphoma with an ORR of 75%, CR rate of 21%, and a median PFS of 14 months.[50] Surprisingly, venetoclax has shown limited single-agent activity in FL, a disease thought to be Bcl-2 driven.[50]

Other Pathways and Targets

Drugs that target other pathways, such as spleen tyrosine kinase (entospletinib, fostamatinib), janus-2 kinase, or mTOR (eg, everolimus, temsirolomus), have only modest activity, and the rationale for further development in NHL is questionable.[43,51,52]

Enhancer of zeste homolog 2 (EZH2) is an epigenetic regulator of gene expression and plays a critical role in many forms of cancer. Activating mutations of EZH2 occur in 20% of patients with lymphoma and can function as oncogenic drivers, especially in FL and GCB DLBCL. Tazemetostat is an oral, first-in-class, selective, reversible, inhibitor of mutated and wild-type EZH2. Although activity in DLBCL has been disappointing, in FL, the ORR in mutated and unmutated patients is 71% and 33%, respectively.[53]

Table 2
PI3K inhibitor adverse event

	Copanlisib	Idelalisib	Duvelisib	Umbralisib (TGR1202)[4]
Black box warning	None	Fatal and/or serious toxicities: • Hepatotoxicity (11%–18%) • Severe diarrhea or colitis (14%–19%) • Pneumonitis (4%) • Infections (21%–36%) • Intestinal perforation	Fatal and/or serious toxicities: • Cutaneous reactions (5%) • Severe diarrhea or colitis (18%) • Pneumonitis (5%) • Infections (31%)	N/A
Grade ≥3 AEs				
Hyperglycemia	41% (infusion-related)	N/A	N/A	N/A
Hypertension	26% (infusion-related)	N/A	N/A	N/A
Pneumonitis, % Lung infection, %	1 16	16	14	<1.5[a] 5[e]
Diarrhea, % Colitis, %	5 1[c]	14	15 12	3 <1.5[a]
Alanine aminotransferase increased, %	1.4	18	3	3
Aspartate aminotransferase increased, %	1.4	12	3	3

[a] All grades.
[c] Patient had medical history of diverticulosis.
[e] Pneumonia only.
Adapted from Cheson BD, O'Brien S, Ewer MS, et al. Optimal management of adverse events from copanlisib in the treatment of patients with Non-Hodgkin Lymphomas. Clin Lymphoma Myeloma Leuk 2019;19(3):137; with permission.

Exportin 1 (XPO1) is the major nuclear export protein for tumor suppressor proteins and oncoprotein mRNAs. Selinexor is an oral, selective XPO1 inhibitor that reactivates multiple tumor suppressor proteins relevant to NHL and reduces levels of c-Myc, Bcl-2, and Bcl-6. Responses can be achieved in about 30% of select patients who did not progress during a prolonged wash-out period. The most troublesome adverse effects include fatigue, a wasting syndrome with nausea and anorexia, vomiting and diarrhea, as well as myelosuppression. Although PFS data are not available, the median duration of response is 23 months in DLBCL.[54]

TARGETING THE TUMOR MICROENVIRONMENT

Most cells in a lymphoma-involved node are other than lymphoma but are, in contrast, effector and inflammatory cells that have been rendered ineffective in tumor killing. Drugs that target the microenvironment include lenalidomide (vide supra).[12]

Checkpoint inhibitors, which activate dormant effector cells, are extremely active in HL, in contrast to NHL. Nivolumab was investigated in a basket trial of patients with R/R NHL and demonstrated only an ORR of 40% in FL and 36% in DLBCL.[55] However, pembrolizumab was combined with rituximab and resulted in an ORR rate of 67% and a CR rate of 50% in R/R FL.[56] Optimal combinations need to be identified to improve the modest outcomes with single-agent checkpoint inhibitors.

CD47 is a normal marker of "self" and is involved in the homeostasis of red blood cells, platelets, clearance of apoptotic cells, and, importantly, the ability of tumor cells to evade phagocytosis based on their greater expression of the protein.[57] Thus, CD47 serves as a "Don't eat me" protein. Several drugs in development block the Don't eat me signal, in 1 case by presenting a decoy receptor, delivering an "Eat me" signal to macrophages. Such drugs can activate both the innate and adaptive immune responses. In a recent study by Advani and colleagues,[57] the combination of 5F9 and rituximab resulted in an ORR of 50%, with 71% in FL and 40% in DLBCL. These drugs appear well tolerated, except for anemia with Hu5F9-G4, and warrant further study. For more details regarding this topic, see Alex F. Herrera's article, "Noncellular Immune Therapies for Non-Hodgkin Lymphoma," in this issue.

COMBINATIONS INCORPORATING TARGETED AGENTS

Several obstacles must be surmounted if cure of patients with NHL and CLL with targeted agents is to be realized (**Table 3**).[58] Simply combining targeted agents with standard chemotherapy does not guarantee an improved outcome. Whereas ibrutinib, everolimus, bortezomib, and lenalidomide each demonstrated preferential activity for the nongerminal center subtype of DLBCL, randomized trials evaluating the addition these agents to standard CHOP have, thus far, failed to demonstrate benefit.[59–61]

In several histologies, treatment strategies are moving away from chemoimmunotherapy and focusing on targeted agents alone (**Fig. 2**). A current controversy in CLL/SLL is whether current combinations are preferable to sequencing of agents.[58] Doublets or triplets are more likely to be effective on NHL; however, which agents to mix remains enigmatic and will likely vary by histology and also by patient. Despite the tolerability of individual targeted agents, numerous combinations have either failed to demonstrate improved efficacy, or have led to unanticipated, disastrous

Table 3 Targeted agent in NHL	
Agent	**Target**
Obinutuzumab/ublituximab	CD20
MOR-208	CD19
Polatuzumab vedotin	CD79b
Blinatumomab	CD3/CD19
Ibrutinib, Acalabrutinib	BTK
Idelalisib, Copanlisib, Umbralisib	PI3K
Venetoclax (ABT-199)	Bcl-2
Tazemetostat	EZH2
Selinexor (KPT-330)	XPO-1
Lenalidomide	Multiple
Nivolumab/pembrolizumab	PD-1
Atezolizumab	PD-L1

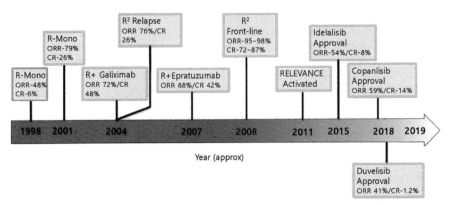

Fig. 2. Timeline for chemo-free world for follicular lymphoma. CR, complete response; Mono, monotherapy; ORR, overall response rate; R, rituximab; R2, rituximab plus lenalidomide.

consequences.[62–64] Carefully conducted clinical trials are essential before exposing patients to untested doublets or triplets.[65] Comparing responders with nonresponders using next-generation sequencing and other technologies may generate enlightening hypotheses.[58] Improved methods of efficiently testing combinations of the large number of agents and next generations of those agents directed at a variety of targets are needed. Novel statistical designs are required for clinical trials, and reliable surrogate markers to facilitate their completion.[66] The latter might include assessment of minimal residual disease by polymerase chain reaction or a more sensitive clonotypic assay. Most important is the need to identify biomarkers, not only for response and toxicity, but also for mechanisms of resistance, as seen in other lymphoid malignancies. These factors will provide the template for assembling the parts together into an effective and tolerable creation eventually leading to a chemo-free world for patients with lymphoma.[58,65]

REFERENCES

1. Ehrlich P. On immunity with special reference to the cell of life. Proc R Soc London 1900;66:424–48.
2. KÖHler G, Milstein C. Continuous cultures of fused cells secreting antibody of predefined specificity. Nature 1975;256:495.
3. Nadler LM, Ritz J, Hardy R, et al. A unique cell surface antigen identifying lymphoid malignancies of B cell origin. J Clin Invest 1981;67(1):134–40.
4. McLaughlin P, Grillo-López AJ, Link BK, et al. Rituximab chimeric anti-CD20 monoclonal antibody therapy for relapsed indolent lymphoma: half of patients respond to a four-dose treatment program. J Clin Oncol 1998;16(8):2825–33.
5. Colombat P, Salles G, Brousse N, et al. Rituximab (anti-CD20 monoclonal antibody) as single first-line therapy for patients with follicular lymphoma with a low tumor burden: clinical and molecular evaluation. Blood 2001;97(1):101.
6. Hiddemann W, Kneba M, Dreyling M, et al. Frontline therapy with rituximab added to the combination of cyclophosphamide, doxorubicin, vincristine, and prednisone (CHOP) significantly improves the outcome for patients with advanced-stage follicular lymphoma compared with therapy with CHOP alone: results of a

prospective randomized study of the German Low-Grade Lymphoma Study Group. Blood 2005;106(12):3725.

7. Coiffier B, Lepage E, Brière J, et al. CHOP chemotherapy plus rituximab compared with CHOP alone in elderly patients with diffuse large-B-cell lymphoma. N Engl J Med 2002;346(4):235–42.

8. Czuczman MS, Leonard JP, Jung S, et al. Phase II trial of galiximab (anti-CD80 monoclonal antibody) plus rituximab (CALGB 50402): Follicular Lymphoma International Prognostic Index (FLIPI) score is predictive of upfront immunotherapy responsiveness. Ann Oncol 2012;23(9):2356–62.

9. Grant BW, Jung SH, Johnson JL, et al. A phase 2 trial of extended induction epratuzumab and rituximab for previously untreated follicular lymphoma: CALGB 50701. Cancer 2013;119:3797–804.

10. Leonard JP, Jung SH, Johnson J, et al. Randomized trial of lenalidomide alone versus lenalidomide plus rituximab in patients with recurrent follicular lymphoma: CALGB 50401 (Alliance). J Clin Oncol 2015;33(31):3635–40.

11. Martin P, Jung SH, Pitcher B, et al. A phase II trial of lenalidomide plus rituximab in previously untreated follicular non-Hodgkin's lymphoma (NHL): CALGB 50803 (Alliance). Ann Oncol 2017;28(11):2806–12.

12. Morschhauser F, Fowler NH, Feugier P, et al. Rituximab plus lenalidomide in advanced untreated follicular lymphoma. N Engl J Med 2018;379(10):934–47.

13. Leonard JP, Trněný M, Izutsu K, et al. AUGMENT: a phase III randomized study of lenalidomide plus rituximab (R2) Vs rituximab/placebo in patients with relapsed/refractory indolent non-Hodgkin lymphoma. Blood 2018;132(Suppl 1):445.

14. Marcus R, Davies A, Ando K, et al. Obinutuzumab for the first-line treatment of follicular lymphoma. N Engl J Med 2017;377(14):1331–44.

15. Goede V, Fischer K, Busch R, et al. Obinutuzumab plus chlorambucil in patients with CLL and coexisting conditions. N Engl J Med 2014;370(12):1101–10.

16. Sehn LH, Chua N, Mayer J, et al. Obinutuzumab plus bendamustine versus bendamustine monotherapy in patients with rituximab-refractory indolent non-Hodgkin lymphoma (GADOLIN): a randomised, controlled, open-label, multicentre, phase 3 trial. Lancet Oncol 2016;17(8):1081–93.

17. Cheson BD, Chua N, Mayer J, et al. Overall survival benefit in patients with rituximab-refractory indolent non-Hodgkin lymphoma who received obinutuzumab plus bendamustine induction and obinutuzumab maintenance in the GADOLIN study. J Clin Oncol 2018;36(22):2259–66.

18. Vitolo U, Trněný M, Belada D, et al. Obinutuzumab or rituximab plus cyclophosphamide, doxorubicin, vincristine, and prednisone in previously untreated diffuse large B-cell lymphoma. J Clin Oncol 2017;35(31):3529–37.

19. Salles GA, Duell J, González-Barca E, et al. Single-arm phase II study of MOR208 combined with lenalidomide in patients with relapsed or refractory diffuse large B-Cell lymphoma: L-mind. Blood 2017;130(Suppl 1):4123.

20. Connors JM, Jurczak W, Straus DJ, et al. Brentuximab vedotin with chemotherapy for stage III or IV Hodgkin's lymphoma. N Engl J Med 2017;378(4):331–44.

21. Younes A, Gopal AK, Smith SE, et al. Results of a pivotal phase II study of brentuximab vedotin for patients with relapsed or refractory Hodgkin's lymphoma. J Clin Oncol 2012;30(18):2183–9.

22. Younes A, Bartlett NL, Leonard JP, et al. Brentuximab vedotin (SGN-35) for relapsed CD30-positive lymphomas. N Engl J Med 2010;363(19):1812–21.

23. Horwitz S, O'Connor OA, Pro B, et al. Brentuximab vedotin with chemotherapy for CD30-positive peripheral T-cell lymphoma (ECHELON-2): a global, double-blind, randomised, phase 3 trial. Lancet 2019;393(10168):229–40.

24. Morschhauser F, Flinn I, Advani RH, et al. Updated results of a phase II randomized study (ROMULUS) of polatuzumab vedotin or pinatuzumab vedotin plus rituximab in patients with relapsed/refractory non-Hodgkin lymphoma. Blood 2014; 124(21):4457.

25. Sehn LH, Kamdar M, Herrera AF, et al. Randomized phase 2 trial of polatuzumab vedotin (pola) with bendamustine and rituximab (BR) in relapsed/refractory (r/r) FL and DLBCL. J Clin Oncol 2018;36(15_suppl):7507.

26. Viardot A, Goebeler M-E, Hess G, et al. Phase 2 study of the bispecific T-cell engager (BiTE) antibody blinatumomab in relapsed/refractory diffuse large B-cell lymphoma. Blood 2016;127(11):1410.

27. Schuster SJ, Bishop MR, Tam CS, et al. Tisagenlecleucel in adult relapsed or refractory diffuse large B-cell lymphoma. N Engl J Med 2019;380(1):45–56.

28. Burger JA, Tedeschi A, Barr PM, et al. Ibrutinib as initial therapy for patients with chronic lymphocytic leukemia. N Engl J Med 2015;373(25):2425–37.

29. Woyach JA, Ruppert AS, Heerema NA, et al. Ibrutinib regimens versus chemoimmunotherapy in older patients with untreated CLL. N Engl J Med 2018;379(26): 2517–28.

30. Itchaki G, Brown JR. Experience with ibrutinib for first-line use in patients with chronic lymphocytic leukemia. Ther Adv Hematol 2018;9(1):3–19.

31. Byrd JC, Owen R, Brien SM, et al. Pooled analysis of safety data from clinical trials evaluating acalabrutinib monotherapy in hematologic malignancies. Blood 2017;130(Suppl 1):4326.

32. Poulain S, Roumier C, Decambron A, et al. MYD88 L265P mutation in Waldenstrom macroglobulinemia. Blood 2013;121(22):4504.

33. Dimopoulos MA, Tedeschi A, Trotman J, et al. Phase 3 trial of ibrutinib plus rituximab in Waldenström's macroglobulinemia. N Engl J Med 2018;378(25): 2399–410.

34. Owen R, McCarthy H, Rule S, et al. Acalabrutinib in patients (pts) with Waldenström macroglobulinemia (WM). J Clin Oncol 2018;36(15 suppl):7501.

35. Wang ML, Rule S, Martin P, et al. Targeting BTK with ibrutinib in relapsed or refractory mantle-cell lymphoma. N Engl J Med 2013;369(6):507–16.

36. Noy A, de Vos S, Thieblemont C, et al. Targeting BTK with ibrutinib in relapsed/ refractory marginal zone lymphoma. Blood 2017. https://doi.org/10.1182/blood-2016-10-747345.

37. Wilson WH, Young RM, Schmitz R, et al. Targeting B cell receptor signaling with ibrutinib in diffuse large B cell lymphoma. Nat Med 2015;21:922.

38. Gopal AK, Schuster SJ, Fowler NH, et al. Ibrutinib as treatment for patients with relapsed/refractory follicular lymphoma: results from the open-label, multicenter, phase II DAWN study. J Clin Oncol 2018;36(23):2405–12.

39. Yahiaoui OI, Nunes JA, Castanier C, et al. Constitutive AKT activation in follicular lymphoma. BMC Cancer 2014;14:565.

40. Psyrri A, Papageorgiou S, Liakata E, et al. Phosphatidylinositol 3'-kinase catalytic subunit alpha gene amplification contributes to the pathogenesis of mantle cell lymphoma. Clin Cancer Res 2009;15(18):5724–32.

41. Go H, Jang JY, Kim PJ, et al. MicroRNA-21 plays an oncogenic role by targeting FOXO1 and activating the PI3K/AKT pathway in diffuse large B-cell lymphoma. Oncotarget 2015;6(17):15035–49.

42. Gopal AK, Kahl BS, de Vos S, et al. PI3Kdelta inhibition by idelalisib in patients with relapsed indolent lymphoma. N Engl J Med 2014;370(11):1008–18.

43. Yazdy MS, Ujjani C. Current challenges in the management of follicular lymphoma. Int J Hematol Oncol 2017;6(1):13–24.

44. Dreyling M, Morschhauser F, Bouabdallah K, et al. Phase II study of copanlisib, a PI3K inhibitor, in relapsed or refractory, indolent or aggressive lymphoma. Ann Oncol 2017;28(9):2169–78.

45. Cheson BD, O'Brien S, Ewer MS, et al. Optimal management of adverse events from copanlisib in the treatment of patients with non-Hodgkin lymphomas. Clin Lymphoma Myeloma Leuk 2019;19(3):135–41.

46. Flinn IW, Hillmen P, Montillo M, et al. The phase 3 DUO trial: duvelisib vs ofatumumab in relapsed and refractory CLL/SLL. Blood 2018;132(23):2446–55.

47. Burris HA 3rd, Flinn IW, Patel MR, et al. Umbralisib, a novel PI3Kdelta and casein kinase-1epsilon inhibitor, in relapsed or refractory chronic lymphocytic leukaemia and lymphoma: an open-label, phase 1, dose-escalation, first-in-human study. Lancet Oncol 2018;19(4):486–96.

48. Stilgenbauer S, Eichhorst B, Schetelig J, et al. Venetoclax in relapsed or refractory chronic lymphocytic leukaemia with 17p deletion: a multicentre, open-label, phase 2 study. Lancet Oncol 2016;17(6):768–78.

49. Seymour JF, Kipps TJ, Eichhorst B, et al. Venetoclax-rituximab in relapsed or refractory chronic lymphocytic leukemia. N Engl J Med 2018;378(12):1107–20.

50. Davids MS, Roberts AW, Seymour JF, et al. Phase I first-in-human study of venetoclax in patients with relapsed or refractory non-Hodgkin lymphoma. J Clin Oncol 2017;35(8):826–33.

51. Liu D, Mamorska-Dyga A. Syk inhibitors in clinical development for hematological malignancies. J Hematol Oncol 2017;10(1):145.

52. Friedberg JW, Sharman J, Sweetenham J, et al. Inhibition of Syk with fostamatinib disodium has significant clinical activity in non-Hodgkin lymphoma and chronic lymphocytic leukemia. Blood 2010;115(13):2578–85.

53. Pagel J, Morschhauser F, Herve T, et al. Interim update from a phase 2 multicenter study of tazemetostat, an EZH2 inhibitor, in patients with relapsed or refractory (R/R) follicular lymphoma (FL). Clin Lymphoma Myeloma Leuk 2018;18: S278–9.

54. Kuruvilla J, Savona M, Baz R, et al. Selective inhibition of nuclear export with selinexor in patients with non-Hodgkin lymphoma. Blood 2017;129(24):3175–83.

55. Lesokhin AM, Ansell SM, Armand P, et al. Nivolumab in patients with relapsed or refractory hematologic malignancy: preliminary results of a phase Ib study. J Clin Oncol 2016;34(23):2698–704.

56. Nastoupil L, Westin J, Fowler N, et al. High complete response rates with pembrolizumab in combination with rituximab in patients with relapsed follicular lymphoma: results of an open-label, phase II Study. Blood 2017;130:414.

57. Advani R, Flinn I, Popplewell L, et al. CD47 blockade by Hu5F9-G4 and rituximab in non-Hodgkin's lymphoma. N Engl J Med 2018;379(18):1711–21.

58. Sarraf Yazdy M, Mato AR, Cheson BD. Combinations or sequences of targeted agents in CLL: is the whole greater than the sum of its parts (Aristotle, 360 BC)? Blood 2019;133(2):121–9.

59. Younes A, Thieblemont C, Morschhauser F, et al. Combination of ibrutinib with rituximab, cyclophosphamide, doxorubicin, vincristine, and prednisone (R-CHOP) for treatment-naive patients with CD20-positive B-cell non-Hodgkin lymphoma: a non-randomised, phase 1b study. Lancet Oncol 2014;15(9):1019–26.

60. Nowakowski GS, Chiappella A, Witzig TE, et al. ROBUST: lenalidomide-R-CHOP versus placebo-R-CHOP in previously untreated ABC-type diffuse large B-cell lymphoma. Future Oncol 2016;12(13):1553–63.

61. Leonard JP, Kolibaba KS, Reeves JA, et al. Randomized phase II study of R-CHOP with or without bortezomib in previously untreated patients with

non-germinal center B-cell-like diffuse large B-cell lymphoma. J Clin Oncol 2017;35(31):3538–46.

62. Ujjani CS, Jung SH, Pitcher B, et al. Phase 1 trial of rituximab, lenalidomide, and ibrutinib in previously untreated follicular lymphoma: Alliance A051103. Blood 2016;128(21):2510–6.

63. Barr PM, Saylors GB, Spurgeon SE, et al. Phase 2 study of idelalisib and entospletinib: pneumonitis limits combination therapy in relapsed refractory CLL and NHL. Blood 2016;127(20):2411–5.

64. Smith SM, Pitcher B, Jung S-H, et al. Unexpected and serious toxicity observed with combined idelalisib, lenalidomide and rituximab in relapsed/refractory B cell lymphomas: alliance A051201 and A051202. Blood 2014;124(21):3091.

65. Cheson BD. Releasing follicular lymphoma from the curse of Frankenstein. The ASCO Post 2018. February 25.

66. Narkhede MS, Cheson BD. Surrogate endpoints and risk adaptive strategies in previously untreated follicular lymphoma. Clin Lymphoma Myeloma Leuk 2018; 18(7):447–51.

Printed and bound by CPI Group (UK) Ltd, Croydon, CR0 4YY

03/10/2024

01040405-0017